The Respiratory System

SYSTEMS OF THE BODY

The Respiratory System

BASIC SCIENCE AND CLINICAL CONDITIONS

THIRD EDITION

Caroline Thomas BSc, MBChB, FRCA
Consultant in Anaesthesia, Leeds Teaching Hospitals NHS Trust
Honorary Senior Clinical Lecturer, University of Leeds
Leeds, UK

Gunchu Randhawa BSc, MBChB, FRCA, FFICM
Consultant in Intensive Care Medicine and Anaesthesia
Faculty Tutor in Intensive Care Medicine
Leeds Teaching Hospitals NHS Trust
Honorary Senior Lecturer, University of Leeds
Leeds, UK

Series Editor
Stephen Hughes BSc, MSc, MBBS, FRCSEd, FRCEM, FHEA
Consultant in Emergency Medicine, Broomfield Hospital
Senior Lecturer in Medicine, School of Medicine, Anglia Ruskin University
Chelmsford, UK

For additional online content visit ExpertConsult.com

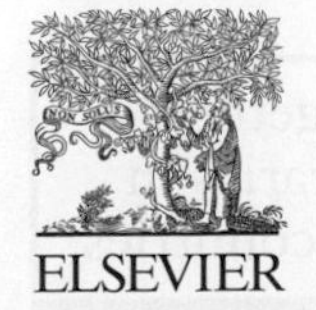

First edition 2003
Second edition 2010

Notices

Practitioners and researchers must always rely on their own experience and knowledge in evaluating and using any information, methods, compounds or experiments described herein. Because of rapid advances in the medical sciences, in particular, independent verification of diagnoses and drug dosages should be made. To the fullest extent of the law, no responsibility is assumed by Elsevier, authors, editors or contributors for any injury and/or damage to persons or property as a matter of products liability, negligence or otherwise, or from any use or operation of any methods, products, instructions, or ideas contained in the material herein.

ISBN: 978-0-7020-8284-9

Publisher: Jeremy Bowes
Content Project Manager: Fariha Nadeem
Design: Margaret Reid
Illustration Manager: Anitha Rajarathnam
Marketing Manager: Deborah Watkins

Copyedited by Editage, a unit of Cactus Communications Services Pte. Ltd.
Typeset by TNQ Technologies Pvt. Ltd.

Printed in Scotland

Last digit is the print number: 9 8 7 6 5 4 3 2 1

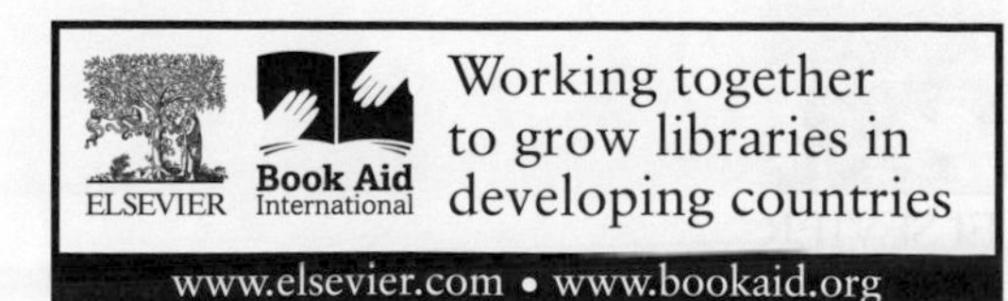

For my parents, Dilbag and Gurbans (G.R.)

For my parents, Andrew and Shirley (C.T.)

SERIES EDITOR FOREWORD

Most students now study medicine through a form of integrated curriculum. These courses blend basic science with exposure to clinical medicine from an early stage. These students have the good fortune to be left in no doubt, from the outset, why they are studying medicine. I teach in a medical school that delivers a fully integrated curriculum and I can compare it with the traditional model according to which I received my early medical education. That comparison is very favourable.

Unlike many other texts, the *Systems of the Body* series has been designed very specifically to support an integrated approach to learning medicine. Our carefully selected panel of authors drawn from across the English-speaking world have combined basic science with clinical application. Links to clinical skills, clinical investigation and therapeutics are made clear throughout.

The aim is to offer highly accessible guidance for all student types and stages. It will be invaluable to those who are approaching the subject for the first time or who may have found a topic challenging when using other more traditionally configured resources – as well as greatly assist all students wishing to excel as their course progresses. The clear layout and writing style, together with detail that informs without overwhelming, go a long way to supporting students. It may also provide welcome reminders to postgraduates facing their own examinations.

Whatever curriculum you follow, wherever you are in the world, and whichever stage you are at, we know that the *Systems of the Body* volumes will serve as great places to start when learning something new and enable you to effectively piece together the essential components of each major body system, in a modern clinical context.

Good luck!

Stephen Hughes, MSc MBBS FRCSEd FRCEM FHEA
Senior Lecturer in Medicine
Anglia Ruskin University
Chelmsford, UK
and
Consultant, Emergency Medicine
Broomfield Hospital
Chelmsford, UK

PREFACE

In the digital era, one may wonder whether there remains a need for the traditional textbook. Undergraduate medical and health science students are confronted with a mass of information on the basic science of the respiratory system. This text distils and contextualises this information, approaching complex concepts in an understandable way to enable the development of a solid knowledge base. Each chapter begins with clearly defined objectives and addresses a discrete aspect of respiratory physiology. Summaries of each subsection include a recap of the key points. Normal structure and function are explained to allow the understanding of the disruptive effects of respiratory system diseases.

An integrated approach is adopted throughout the *Systems of the Body* series. This third edition of The Respiratory System has been updated to reflect the integrated nature of modern science courses. Pathology and pharmacology are woven into the information on basic science to illustrate their relevance and to aid understanding. Updated clinical cases are included throughout the book to illustrate important concepts and new clinical skills sections have been added, in relevant chapters, to ease the transition from theory to practice. Efforts have been made to ensure this edition is written in accessible language and updated references have been included to reflect current knowledge and practice. Suggestions for further reading include recent review and educational journal articles to enhance understanding of respiratory physiology. New self-assessment materials have been produced to accompany the print information in the eBook.

The authors wrote this book while working clinically in critical care and anaesthesia during the COVID-19 pandemic. The medical management of patients with a new disease entity, such as SARS-COV-2, clearly illustrates the value of a sound understanding of normal respiratory physiology and the processes which may disrupt it. This appreciation of basic principles is the foundation upon which patient and population management strategies are based.

ACKNOWLEDGEMENTS

The authors would like to thank Drs. Andrew Davies and Carl Moores for their work on the previous edition, and Dr Andrew Lumb (Department of Anaesthesia, St James University Hospital and Honorary Clinical Associate Professor at the University of Leeds) for helpful comments during the preparation of this manuscript.

INTRODUCTION 1

Introduction 2
What is respiration? 2
The need for respiration 2
Diffusion and gas transport 3
Timing in circulation and respiration 3
Basic science of respiration 3
Respiratory symbols—the language of the respiratory system 4
Centimetre, gram, second and système international units 4
Drugs 5
Symptoms of respiratory disease 5

STRUCTURE AND FUNCTION OF THE RESPIRATORY SYSTEM 9

Introduction 10
Embryology 10
Airways 10
Mouth and nose 11
Larynx 12
Trachea 13
Intrathoracic airways 13
Histological structure of the airways 14
Supporting tissues 16
Pulmonary vasculature 18
Lymphatics 19
Nerves 19
Mechanics of breathing 20
Defences against the environment 21
Conditioning air 21
Inhaled particles 21
Smoking and air pollution 23
Metabolic activity 23
Metabolism and production of biologically active substances 24
Non-respiratory functions of the lung 24

ELASTIC PROPERTIES OF THE RESPIRATORY SYSTEM 29

Introduction 30
Compliance and elastance 30

AIRFLOW AND RESISTANCE IN THE RESPIRATORY SYSTEM 43

Introduction 44
Bringing about airflow 44
Laminar and turbulent flow 45
Factors affecting flow 45
Respiratory system resistance 46
Work of breathing 50
Assessing and measuring resistance in the respiratory system 52
Asthma 54
Chronic obstructive pulmonary disease 57

PULMONARY VENTILATION 61

Introduction 62
Lung volumes, capacities and spirometry 62
Spirometric abnormalities in disease 63

DIFFUSION OF GASES BETWEEN AIR AND BLOOD 77

Introduction 78
Diffusion and the significance of partial pressure 78
Factors affecting the rate of diffusion 78
Factors affecting diffusing capacity 79
Measuring diffusing capacity 81
The management of inadequate diffusion 82
Carbon dioxide and other gases 83

THE PULMONARY CIRCULATION 85

The bronchial circulation 86
The pulmonary circulation 86
The pulmonary circulation – structure and function 86
Matching ventilation and perfusion 89
Regional differences in ventilation in the lungs 92
Ventilation/perfusion matching and its effect on blood oxygen and carbon dioxide content 93

CARRIAGE OF GASES BY THE BLOOD AND ACID/BASE BALANCE 101

Introduction – why do we need to transport gases in the blood? 102
Oxygen transport 102
Haemoglobin 103
Why is haemoglobin kept in red cells? 107
Haemoglobin variants 107
Carbon dioxide transport 109
Acid–base balance 111
Calculation and illustration of acid–base status 115
Clinical measurements 115

NERVOUS CONTROL OF BREATHING 121

Introduction 122
Central control of breathing 123
Medullary respiratory centres 124
Conscious control of breathing 125
Pattern of breathing in chronic obstructive pulmonary disease 126
Respiratory muscle innervation 127
Neuromuscular disorders 128
Afferent inputs to the respiratory centre 130
Pulmonary afferents 130
Upper airway afferents – the nose, pharynx, and larynx 132
Musculoskeletal afferents 133

CHEMICAL CONTROL OF BREATHING 137

Introduction 138
Hypercapnia 138
Central chemoreceptors 139
Hypoxia 140
Peripheral chemoreceptors 140
Cheyne–Stokes breathing 142
Long-term hypoxic stimulation 142
Effects of anaesthesia on chemical control of breathing 143
Asphyxia 143

LUNG FUNCTION TESTS 147

Introduction 148
Measuring lung volumes and capacities 148
Measuring lung mechanics 150
Measuring diffusing capacity 150
Blood gas analysis 152
Measuring oxygen levels 152
Measuring the uniformity of ventilation and perfusion 152
Multiple-breath washout curves 153
Functional testing 154

Appendix: basic science 159

Glossary 165

Index 171

1

INTRODUCTION

Chapter objectives

After studying this chapter, you should be able to:

1. Define respiration.
2. Explain the role of respiration in human homeostasis.
3. Describe the pivotal roles of diffusion and gas transport, via the circulation, in respiration.
4. Give examples of the importance of named physical phenomena in specific clinical conditions.
5. Explain the rationale of respiratory symbols.
6. Give examples of classes of drugs that affect the respiratory system.
7. Describe some common symptoms in respiratory diseases.
8. Have an approach to the examination of the respiratory system, and to the interpretation of chest X-rays.

Introduction

The aim of this book is to provide an understanding of the respiratory system, including its structure, function, and some of the diseases and conditions that affect it. The anatomy, histology, and physiology of the respiratory system are illustrated by relevant clinical conditions which are designed to deepen the appreciation of normal physiology and illustrate why a sound knowledge of basic science is so important in understanding disease processes. Illustrative clinical cases and clinical skills are highlighted in blue boxes, and there are directions for further reading at the end of each chapter to expand upon the content. To promote understanding, the material is broken down into manageable portions with a coherent theme. Each chapter of the book is based on a particular aspect of the respiratory system and is preceded by a list of objectives—things you should be able to do when you have mastered the material in that chapter. Each chapter also links to questions related to the material covered. Key terms are highlighted in bold (explained in the glossary) or bold italics. At the end of the book, there is an appendix which discusses the basic science relevant to respiration.

This initial chapter introduces some basic terminologies and concepts relevant to the respiratory system. We will consider the symptoms of respiratory disease that patients complain of, discuss how the respiratory system is examined, and look at the features of normal chest X-rays.

What is respiration?

Biochemists use the term ***respiration*** to describe the energy-producing chemical processes that take place in tissues, cells, or even parts of cells. In this book, we will use the physiologist's definition, which is 'an interchange of gases between an organism and its environment'. For all intents and purposes, for human beings this means 'breathing' (Latin, *spiro*, 'I breathe'). The movement of air into and out of the lungs, which most people call breathing, is referred to as **ventilation** in physiological terms. Breathing is brought about by specific structures of the body, including (but not exclusively) the lungs. A description of these structures at the macroscopic (anatomical) and microscopic (histological) levels helps us understand the processes of the respiratory system and the disruption of these processes and structures (pathology) in disease.

The part of our environment involved in this 'interchange of gases' mentioned in the previous paragraph is, of course, the air around us. Our need for air was obvious to even our most distant ancestors; for example, Anaximenes of Miletus (c.570 BCE) observed that air (Greek, *pneuma*, 'breath') was essential to life. What was not clear to the ancients was what the air was used for. Aristotle, drawing on theories dating from the 5th century BCE, which noted the rapid and repeated movements of the heart, relegated the function of the lungs to that of a sort of radiator, and stated with his usual authority:

> ***...as the heart might easily be raised to too high a temperature by hurtful irritation (by its rapid movements) the genii placed the lungs in its neighbourhood, which adhere to it and fill the cavity of the thorax, in order that air vessels might moderate the great heat.***

Galen (CE 130–199), probably more by an accident of metaphor rather than based on any scientific evidence, came close to describing the true nature of respiration when he compared it to a lamp burning in a gourd:

> ***When an animal inspires it is, I think, similar to a perforated gourd, but when respiration is prevented at the appropriate place on the trachea, you may compare it to a gourd unperforated and everywhere closed.***

If Galen had the benefit of modern gas analysis facilities, he would have found even closer parallels between breathing and burning, with oxygen being consumed and carbon dioxide (CO_2) being produced in both cases. Indeed, the basic premise underlying the complicated process of respiration is that it starts with an inflow of oxygen and ends with an outflow of CO_2. These two flows are the first and final results of the complex metabolism of the body, and this book describes the respiratory system that facilitates these flows and why they are needed.

The need for respiration

One definition of the success of a species, in evolutionary terms, is how well it can maintain a constant composition of the fluid surrounding its individual cells (its internal environment), despite changes in its external environment (surroundings getting dryer, colder, warmer, etc.). This process is called **homeostasis** and requires energy. Most of the energy generated by our tissues is the result of the oxidation of food substrates, and this is the reason we need an inflow of oxygen. A continuous supply of oxygen is important for maintaining essential energy stores in the tissues of the body. The word 'oxygen' means 'acid producer' (Greek, *oxy*, 'acid'; *gen*, 'to produce'), and the major product of our oxidative metabolism is the acid gas CO_2. CO_2 reacts with water to form carbonic acid (Chapter 8); thus, the accumulation of CO_2 would result in acidification of the body fluids, which would lead to failure of essential systems (e.g. enzyme action within the body) and ultimately death. This highlights the importance of the respiratory system in eliminating CO_2 from the body. The mechanisms to ensure this occurs can be demonstrated by rebreathing from a plastic bag for a few minutes. The unpleasant sensation that forces you to stop this rather dangerous experiment is due to overstimulation of the reflex that controls breathing to remove CO_2.

Ventilation allows the flow of oxygen into, and CO_2 out of, the human body. However, to fulfil the needs of our cells, oxygen must enter the bloodstream and be carried to the cells, where it can be utilised, and the CO_2 produced by the cells must enter the bloodstream and be transported to the lungs, where it can be eliminated. Hence, a discussion of respiratory physiology must consider all processes involved in gas transport.

Diffusion and gas transport

The flows of oxygen and CO_2 into and out of the body take place as a result of one very basic physical phenomenon: **diffusion**, which results in the movement of molecules in liquids and gases from regions of high concentration to regions of lower concentration. Microscopic organisms, such as the humble amoeba, can rely solely on this phenomenon to carry oxygen to and remove CO_2 from a single cell. Multicellular creatures are too large to rely on diffusion alone; the distances gases would have to diffuse to reach each cell are too great, and the movement of gas is therefore too slow to maintain life.

In human beings, the same passive process of diffusion alone supplies and removes O_2 and CO_2 from our bodies (there is no active chemical transport), but we rely on the circulation to transport these gases to distant cells. The lungs promote diffusion by having an enormous, very thin surface area through which diffusion can easily take place. A surface of over 90 m^2 is enclosed in a lung volume of less than 10 L. This functional 90 m^2 is often reduced by disease, thickening of the membrane, excess fluid in the lungs, or reduced supply of air or blood. The circulation of blood forms the transport link between the diffusion site of the lungs and the diffusion site of the capillaries within the tissues. The distances involved in this link are enormous, in molecular terms, and diffusion would be totally useless for transporting gas over the metre or so between the lungs and distal tissues of our bodies (Fig. 1.1). This transport is accomplished within seconds by circulation.

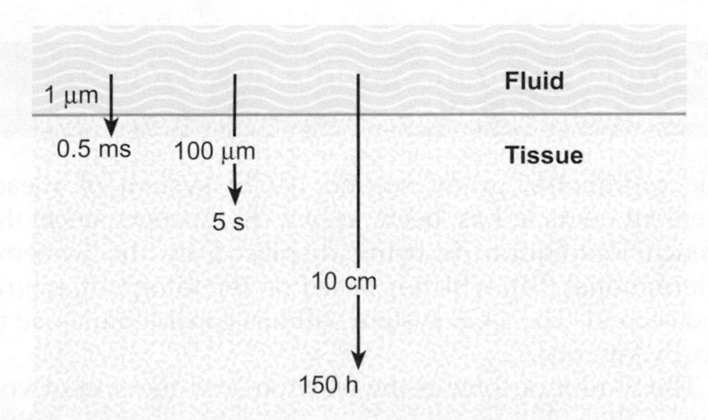

Fig. 1.1 Time course of diffusion over increasing distances. This figure illustrates how the time needed for diffusion to take place increases as the distance involved increases. The absolute times shown in this example would be for a fairly large molecule, such as a neurotransmitter.

Timing in circulation and respiration

The processes of breathing and beating of the heart are both cyclic events. One involves the inhalation and exhalation of air, and the other involves filling of the heart with blood and its ejection into the circulation. The time courses of these two cycles are very different: at rest, you may take 12 breaths within a minute while the heart beats 60 times, ejecting 5 L of blood through the lungs (Fig. 1.2).

The composition of air in the lungs changes as a result of two effects. During inspiration, it is altered by the addition of fresh air to that already in the lungs and the effects of exchange with the blood passing through the lungs. Expiration, in this context, is equivalent to breath-holding because no new air is added; the only effect is due to the exchange of gases in the lungs with those in the blood. These changes in the composition of the air in the lungs are picked up by the blood flowing in the pulmonary circulation, which therefore shows cyclic changes in its composition that coincide with the breathing cycle (see Fig. 1.2).

Basic science of respiration

Basic science is integral to understanding respiration in normal and diseased states. Examples of these phenomena and their clinical relevance are illustrated in Figure 1.3.

Taking examples from this list of phenomena, we see that solids, such as lung tissue and the chest wall, are elastic; this elasticity of our respiratory system determines part of our work of breathing. Liquids exert vapour pressure, a property important in humidifying the air we breathe and in the administration of volatile anaesthetics. Gases exert partial pressure, the understanding of which is essential to the monitoring, through arterial blood gas sampling, of how well the lungs work. The volume of a mass of gas is described by laws relating it to temperature and pressure, and the resistance to the flow of gases is related to the dimensions of the tube in which it is flowing.

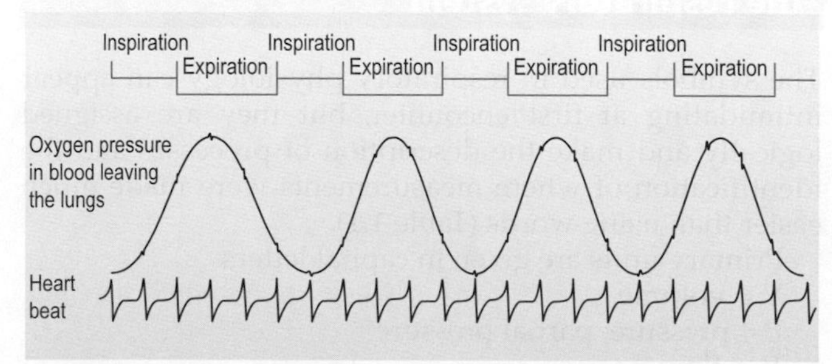

Fig. 1.2 Timing. Because the heart beats so much faster than the respiratory cycle, there is effectively a continuous flow of blood through the lungs during inspiration and expiration. Expiration is like breath-holding—no fresh air is added, and the composition of blood leaving the lungs changes accordingly.

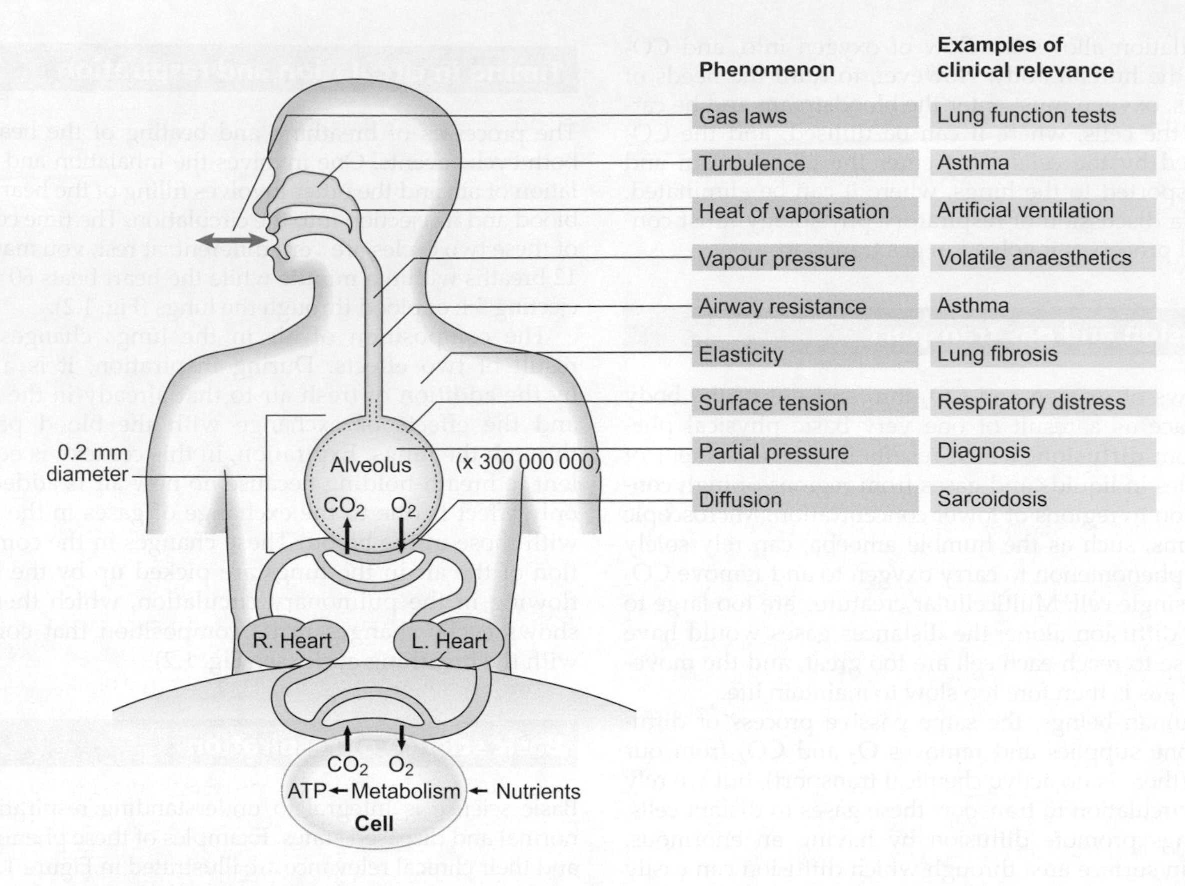

Fig. 1.3 An overview of respiration, showing the physical phenomena that make it up and the clinical situations where understanding these phenomena are important.

These examples of the importance of the basic sciences in understanding the respiratory system do not mean that a great deal, or a great depth, of knowledge is required. The Appendix contains all that is required to understand the contents of this book. However, there is a vocabulary specific to the respiratory system which is important to understand.

Respiratory symbols—the language of the respiratory system

The symbols used in respiratory physiology can appear intimidating at first encounter, but they are assigned logically and make the description of processes and the identification of where measurements were made much easier than using words (Table 1.1).

Primary units are given in capital letters:

V = volume
P = pressure, partial pressure
$\dot{V}$ = flow

Locations in the gas phase are also given capital letters, but smaller than the primary units:

A = alveolar
B = barometric
E = expired

Locations in blood are identified by lower-case letters:

a = arterial
v = venous
c = capillary

The primary symbol is written first, followed by the qualifying symbol at a lower level, for example, PAO_2 = alveolar partial pressure of oxygen.

Centimetre, gram, second and système international units

The centimetre, gram, second (CGS) system of measurement, which has been in use in Europe since the French Revolution, is being displaced by the Système International (SI), which is based on the kilogram, metre, and second. The CGS system still has considerable use in North America.

The SI unit of force is the Newton, and the unit of volume is the cubic metre (m^3); as the cubic metre is rather large, the cubic decimetre (dm^3), which is equivalent to a litre, is frequently used. The unit of pressure, in the SI system, is the Newton per square meter or Pascal (Pa). The Pa

Table 1.1 The major respiratory symbols

Variable					
P	Pressure, tension, or partial pressure				
V	Volume of gas				
$\dot{V}$	Volume of gas per unit time (flow)				
Q	Volume of blood				
$\dot{Q}$,	Volume of blood per unit time (flow)				
C	Content				
F	Fractional concentration in dry gas				
R	Resistance				
G	Conductance				
Location in blood		**location in gas**		**other suffixes**	
A	Arterial	A	Alveolar	pl	Pleural space
C	Capillary	I	Inspired	aw	Airway
V	Venous	E	Expired	W	Chest wall
$\dot{V}$,	Mixed venous	T	Tidal	el	Elastic
		L	Lung	res	Resistive
		B	Barometric	tot	Total
		D	Dead space		
				Prefix	
				S	Specific
Examples					
VT				Tidal volume	
PaO_2				Oxygen tension in arterial blood	
$\dot{V}E$				Expired minute volume	
sRaw				Specific airway resistance	

is too small for practical use, and thus, the kilopascal (kPa) is used; 1 kPa = 7.5 mmHg or 10 cm of water. Usefully, the barometric pressure at sea level is close to 100 kPa, which makes the arithmetic of calculating partial pressures easier. In the SI system, concentration is represented in moles per litre, where a mole is 6.02×10^{23} molecules of the substance in solution. Measurement of blood pressure is still widely expressed in mmHg, probably because it is usually measured using a mercury manometer.

Drugs

There are a vast number of drugs used to target conditions affecting the respiratory system, and an equally long list of drugs that may have side effects affecting the respiratory system: bronchodilators, steroids, neuromuscular blockers, analgesics, immunosuppressants, and antimicrobials, to name just a few classes. A detailed account of these drugs and their actions is beyond the scope of this book, but relevant drugs are mentioned in context. In addition, there are multiple therapies used to treat respiratory conditions, including physiotherapy, oxygen therapy, and non-invasive and invasive ventilation.

Symptoms of respiratory disease

Patients with respiratory disease complain of symptoms, which fall into a few broad groups.

1. *Cough.* Cough is probably the most common symptom of respiratory disease and is usually a response to irritation of the respiratory tract. Cough is one of the most important features of chronic bronchitis; it also occurs in patients with chest infections as well as in asthmatics, where it may be particularly common at night.
2. *Sputum.* Sputum is the substance coughed up from the respiratory tract. The colour of sputum may give a clue as to its cause; for example, respiratory tract infection usually results in thick, yellow or green sputum, whereas pink, frothy sputum may indicate pulmonary oedema.
3. *Haemoptysis.* Haemoptysis means coughing up blood. Haemoptysis may indicate a chest infection or may be a symptom of more serious respiratory diseases, such as tuberculosis or bronchial carcinoma.
4. *Breathlessness.* Breathlessness is a symptom of a range of respiratory diseases as well as being a symptom of cardiac failure. *Dyspnoea* is a particular type of breathlessness, described as 'air hunger'.
5. *Wheezing.* Wheezes are characteristic musical sounds caused by gas flow through narrowed airways. Patients may complain of wheezing, and it may be audible on auscultation of the chest. It is characteristic of pulmonary diseases, such as asthma, chronic bronchitis, and chest infection, all of which can result in airway narrowing.
6. *Stridor.* Stridor is an abnormal, high-pitched sound produced by a partially obstructed upper airway. It is usually heard on inspiration.
7. *Chest pain.* In certain respiratory conditions, patients may complain of chest pain. Such conditions include infection, pleuritis, pulmonary infarction, and pneumothorax.

Clinical skill - examination of the respiratory system

A clinical examination of the respiratory system includes examination of the hands, tongue, neck, and chest wall, as well as percussion (tapping) and auscultation (listening with a stethoscope) of the chest. A detailed description is not necessary to understand this book. However, these are some key features to note.

1. *Finger clubbing.* Inspecting a patient's hands is an important part of examining the respiratory system. In addition to looking for peripheral cyanosis (see the next description), it is important to look for finger clubbing. Clubbing is present when the normal angle at the nail bed is lost, the curvature of the nail is increased, and there is increased mobility of the nail on the nail bed (the nail fluctuates) (Fig. 1.4). It is not known, for certain, why finger clubbing occurs, but it is present in a number of respiratory diseases, including bronchial carcinoma, bronchiectasis, and pulmonary fibrosis. Clubbing is also present in some non-respiratory diseases.

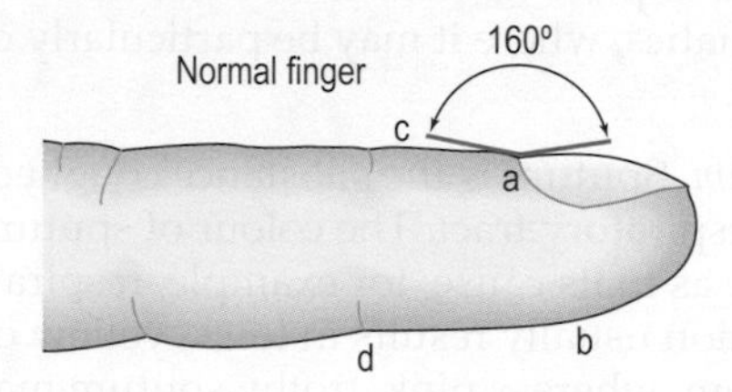

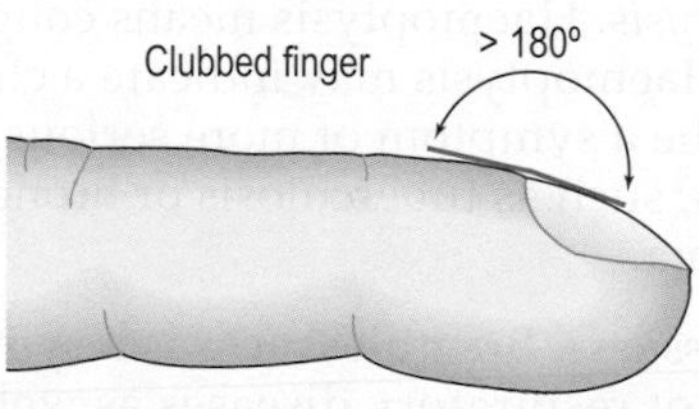

Fig. 1.4 Finger clubbing. In clubbed fingers the angle of the nailbed is lost and there is increased mobility of the nail on the nailbed.

2. *Cyanosis.* Cyanosis refers to a blue tinge to the skin or mucus membranes and indicates the presence of deoxygenated haemoglobin (Chapter 8). Cyanosis may be either central or peripheral. Central cyanosis refers to the blueness of the lips and the tongue. Because these organs are covered by the mucosa rather than the skin, cyanosis is more evident there than in the face, for example. Blood does not travel far from the heart to reach the tongue and lips; therefore, if they are cyanosed, it suggests that blood leaving the left ventricle is deoxygenated, either because of lung disease or certain forms of heart abnormality. Peripheral cyanosis refers to the blueness of the extremities and is usually most evident in the fingernails and toenails. In the absence of central cyanosis, inadequate circulation to the periphery is usually suggested by peripheral cyanosis.
3. *Trachea.* The trachea can be felt in the neck above the sternal notch and is examined to assess whether it is lying in the midline or is deviated to one side. Tracheal deviation can occur in a number of lung diseases, where the trachea is pulled toward (e.g., in patients with pneumonia) or away from (e.g., in patients with pneumothorax) the pathology.
4. *Inspection of the chest.* The examination of the chest itself starts with an inspection. The shape of the chest may be abnormal; for example, in chronic obstructive pulmonary disease, the chest is often unusually expanded and rounded (the so-called barrel chest). Surgical scars or other abnormalities of the skin on the chest wall may be present. The patient may also be asked to take a deep breath, and the movements of the chest wall are noted. Movements of the chest wall may be limited by abnormalities of the spine or the chest wall itself, or by abnormalities of the underlying lung(s).
5. *Percussion.* Percussion essentially means tapping the patient's chest and listening to the sound that is produced. Normally, the chest sounds hollow or resonant if the underlying lung is filled with air; a dull sound is heard if there is fluid in the intrapleural space (pleural effusion) or if the alveoli of the underlying lung are filled with fluid. If there is a pneumothorax, with air between the chest wall and the lung, percussion may be hyperresonant; in other words, the chest sounds are more hollow than normal.
6. *Auscultation.* Auscultation refers to listening to the lungs using a stethoscope. Normally, it is possible to hear air quietly entering and leaving the lungs without there being any added sounds. Additional breath sounds are called vesicular sounds. Breath sounds may be absent or very quiet if pleural effusion or pneumothorax is present. There may also be sounds present in addition to the breath sounds. Where gas passes through narrowed airways, a sound like a musical note may be produced. These sounds are called wheeze or rhonchi, and are usually heard during expiration, and are most likely to be heard in patients with asthma or chronic bronchitis; however, if the airway narrowing is very severe, no gas flow takes place and there is no wheeze. Crackles or crepitations may also be heard during auscultation. Crackles probably represent the opening of closed airways and are most commonly heard in patients with chronic bronchitis, pulmonary fibrosis, or pulmonary oedema.

Clinical skill - interpreting a chest X-ray

This section will introduce you to the appearance of a normal chest X-ray so that you can appreciate the abnormal chest X-ray appearances that are associated with some respiratory conditions.

Usually, a chest X-ray is taken with the front of the patient's chest against a photographic plate. The patient's elbows are bent forward so that the shoulder blades move around to the side of the ribcage and X-rays pass through the patient. This type of X-ray is called a posteroanterior view because the X-rays travel from behind the patient (posterior) to the front (anterior). X-ray shadows of structures within the chest are cast onto the photographic plate; structures which are nearer to the plate (i.e., those in the front of the chest) appear clearer than those further away from the plate, which may appear distorted or blurred.

If a patient is too unwell to stand in front of the photographic plate (e.g., if they are too ill to leave bed), the X-ray may be taken with the photographic plate behind the patient and with the X-rays administered from in front of the patient (an anteroposterior chest X-ray (Fig. 1.5)); a lateral chest X-ray may also be taken from the side (Fig. 1.6).

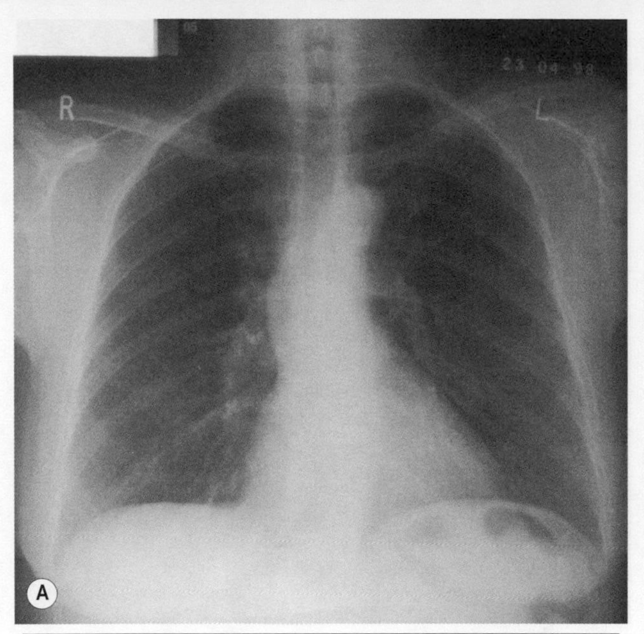

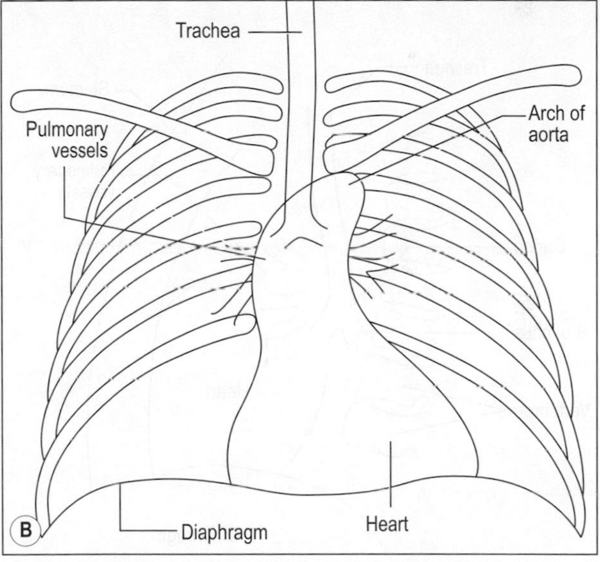

Fig. 1.5 Normal anteroposterior chest X-ray.

Continued

Clinical skill - interpreting a chest X-ray—cont'd

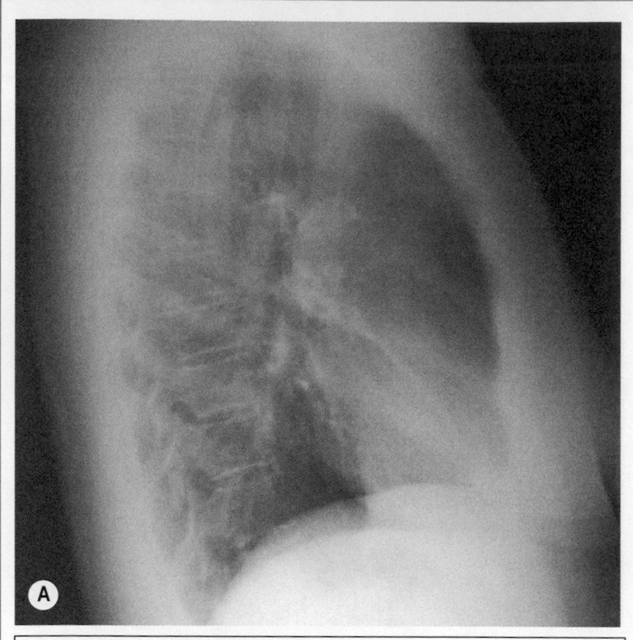

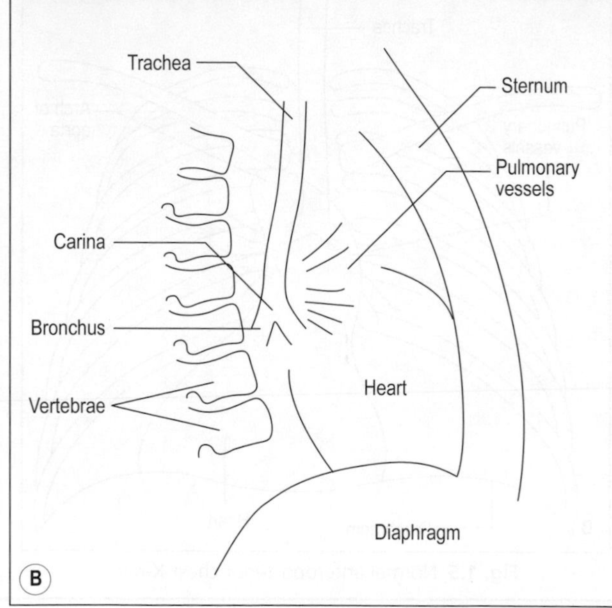

Fig. 1.6 Normal lateral chest X-ray.

It is important to remember the way an X-ray film is developed when you look at one for the first time. Structures such as bones, which block X-rays, appear white on the X-ray film. Structures such as the lungs and blood vessels, which partially block the passage of X-rays, appear grey. Gas-filled structures, like the lungs, which absorb little X-ray energy, appear black.

On the chest X-ray of a healthy person in Fig. 1.5, the following structures are visible:

1. *Bones.* The ribs, sternum, and thoracic vertebrae can usually be seen on a chest X-ray.
2. *Heart.* The outline of the heart is clearly visible. If the heart is enlarged (e.g., due to heart disease), this will be evident. The border of the heart may not appear sharp and distinct if the lung tissue around it is diseased.
3. *Aorta.* The outline of the aorta is usually visible as it arises from the heart and arches around in the thorax.
4. *Trachea.* Because the trachea is filled with air, through which X-rays can easily pass, it appears as a dark structure in the midline. It is usually possible to see the carina, where the trachea divides into the two main bronchi.
5. *Pulmonary vessels.* The pulmonary vessels are visible as they pass from the heart into the lungs.
6. *Diaphragm.* . The outline of the diaphragm is usually clearly visible. The right-hand side of the diaphragm is usually higher than the left side. A collapsed lung or damage to the phrenic nerve may cause the diaphragm to shift upwards, whereas emphysema and other diseases that increase lung volume may cause the diaphragm to be shifted downwards. If the outline of the diaphragm is not sharp, particularly where the shadows of the diaphragm and the ribs intersect (the costophrenic angle), fluid in the intrapleural space adjacent to the diaphragm is suggested.
7. *Lungs.* As the lungs are filled mainly with air, X-rays pass through them easily and they appear relatively dark on a chest X-ray. However, it is generally possible to make out the shadows of large blood vessels as they pass through the lung tissue. If there is fluid in the alveoli (e.g., as a result of oedema or infection), the lung fields will appear lighter as fewer X-rays will pass through them. If an area within the lungs appears darker than normal, this suggests that there is more air present than usual. This might be a result of emphysema or pneumothorax.

References and further reading

MacMillan Rodney, W., MacMillan Rodney, J.R., Arnold, K.M.R., 2020. Principles of X-ray interpretation. In: Fowler, G.C. (Ed.), Pfenninger and Fowler's Procedures for Primary Care, fourth ed. Elsevier.

Swartz, M.H., 2021. The chest. Textbook of Physical Diagnosis: History and Examination, eighth ed. Elsevier.

Waldmann, C., Rhodes, A., Soni, N., Handy, J., 2019. Respiratory drugs. Oxford Desk Reference: Critical Care, second ed. Oxford University Press.

STRUCTURE AND FUNCTION OF THE RESPIRATORY SYSTEM

2

Chapter objectives

After studying this chapter, you should be able to:

1. Explain the embryological origins of the respiratory system.
2. Describe the structures of the upper airway.
3. Distinguish between the structures of conducting and respiratory airways and relate these to their functions.
4. Outline the structure of the bronchial tree and how this is disrupted in disease.
5. Describe the histology of the regions of the lung and relate it to function and pathology.
6. Explain the special features of the pulmonary circulation and pulmonary hypertension.
7. Outline the afferent and efferent innervation of the lungs.
8. Describe the gross structure of the chest and thoracic viscera and the way they bring about breathing.
9. Understand the role of airway structure and function regarding air conditioning and the effects of pollution on the respiratory system.
10. List the metabolic and non-respiratory functions of the respiratory system.

Introduction

Just as each part of the respiratory system has a particular function, each part also has its particular pathologies. The structure of the respiratory system is intimately related to function in both health and disease, and understanding the structure helps to understand both respiratory system function and pathology. We will first describe the development of the human lung, and then the structure of the airways and the tissues that surround them.

Embryology

An appreciation of the way in which human lungs develop aids in understanding certain disease states.

The lungs undergo five overlapping phases of development, as shown in Table 2.1.

Developmental stage	*Approximate gestation*	*Key features*
Embryonic	0–6 weeks	Laryngotracheal bud forms and elongates
Pseudoglandular	5–16 weeks	Formation of conducting airways
Canalicular	16–26 weeks	Formation of bronchioles and vascularisation
Saccular	26–40 weeks	Formation of alveolar ducts and sacs, capillary network develops, epithelial cells differentiate into types I and II pneumocytes
Alveolar	Week 28 of gestation to 8 years of age	Increase in number of alveoli and capillaries

The respiratory system starts as an outpouching (the ***laryngotracheal bud***) on the ventral surface of the digestive tract endoderm (Fig. 2.1) at 4 weeks of gestation. As the bud elongates, the proximal portion forms the trachea, and the distal end bifurcates to form the two main bronchi. During the pseudoglandular phase, the bronchi successively branch to form the conducting airways of the bronchial tree, with around 17 generations of subdivisions present by 6 months of gestation and a further 6 divisions occurring after birth, to eventually yield the 23 generations of the airway seen in the adult lung. During the canalicular phase, the respiratory bronchioles and alveolar ducts develop and vascularise. Unlike the respiratory epithelium (derived from the endoderm), the cartilage, muscle, and connective tissue, which make up the rest of the lung structure, develop from the embryonic mesoderm. During the saccular phase, ongoing development of the capillary networks in the lungs occurs, and the terminal sacs or primitive alveoli develop. The epithelium differentiates from simple cuboidal cells to type I (responsible for gas exchange) and type II (responsible for surfactant production) pneumocytes.

The number of alveoli continues to increase throughout the alveolar phase and into childhood, accounting for the increase in lung volume throughout early childhood. Development of the lung is therefore incomplete at birth, and any degree of prematurity risks respiratory compromise. Although the respiratory system is capable of gas exchange in the saccular phase of embryonic development, type II pneumocytes are still immature, and surfactant production may be inadequate and promote airway collapse. For this reason, premature babies may develop ***respiratory distress of the newborn,*** which is discussed further in Chapter 3.

Airways

The airways are anatomically divided into the upper (extrathoracic) airway, comprising the mouth, nose, larynx, and upper trachea, and the lower (intrathoracic) airway, comprising the lower trachea, left and right main bronchi, and multiple bronchial generations. Functionally, the respiratory system can be divided into the conducting zone (nose to bronchioles), which carries gases, and the respiratory zone (alveolar ducts and alveoli) where gas exchange occurs.

Table 2.1 Dimensions of some of the airways of the human tracheobronchial tree. Note the enormous increase in cross-sectional area and the percentage of the total volume occurring in the last few generations.

Generation	*Name*	*Diameter (cm)*	*Total cross-sectional area (cm²)*	*Cumulative volume (%)*	*Number*
0	Trachea	1.80	2.5	1.7	1
10	Small bronchi	0.13	13.0	4.0	10^3
14	Bronchioles	0.08	45.0	7.0	10^4
18	Respiratory bronchioles	0.05	540.0	31.0	3×10^5
24	Alveoli	0.04	8×10^5	100.0	3×10^8

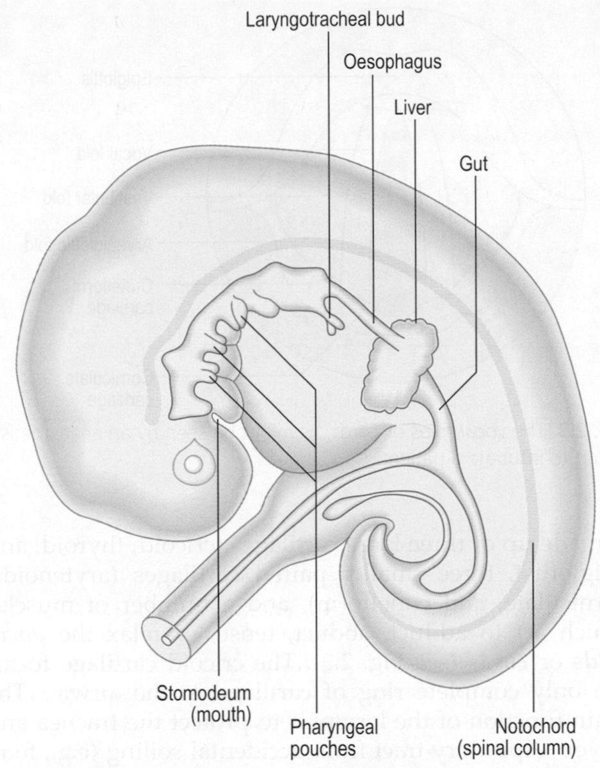

Fig. 2.1 Lateral view of a 4-week human embryo. The *laryngotracheal bud* is beginning to divide to form the two lungs.

Mouth and nose

The structures of the upper airways can be seen in sagittal sections of the head and neck (Figure 2.2). The nose extends from the nostrils (external nares) to the *choanae* (internal nares), which empty into the nasopharynx. Humans normally breathe through the nose during quiet breathing, via the mouth during exertion or when the nasal air passages are blocked. In Figure 2.2, the subject is breathing through the nose, as evidenced by the lips being closed and the tongue laying against the palate. When breathing through the mouth (e.g., when blowing out a candle or sucking through a straw), the soft palate arches upward to form a seal against the top of the pharynx. Newborn babies are predominantly nose breathers, which may contribute to their ability to suckle and breathe at the same time. Other animal species, such as rabbits, manage to eat and breathe at the same time by having lateral food channels, on either side of the larynx, that bypass the airway, whereas marine mammals, such as whales, have completely separate air and food channels.

The major function of the upper airway is to 'condition' the inspired air (see Air Conditioning section, in this chapter). Most of this air conditioning occurs in the vascular mucosa covering the nasal *turbinates*, three projections of bone arising from the lateral walls of the nasal cavity. The large surface area of this mucosa (150 cm^2) makes the nose efficient at filtering, warming, and humidifying inspired air, but the resistance to breathing through the nose is almost twice that of breathing through the mouth. Most of this resistance comes from the nasal valves at the proximal end of each nostril. This point represents the narrowest total cross-sectional area of the respiratory system.

Passage of air through the nose can be further impeded by mucosal inflammation (rhinitis) during the common cold. A small, inflammation-induced reduction in the diameter

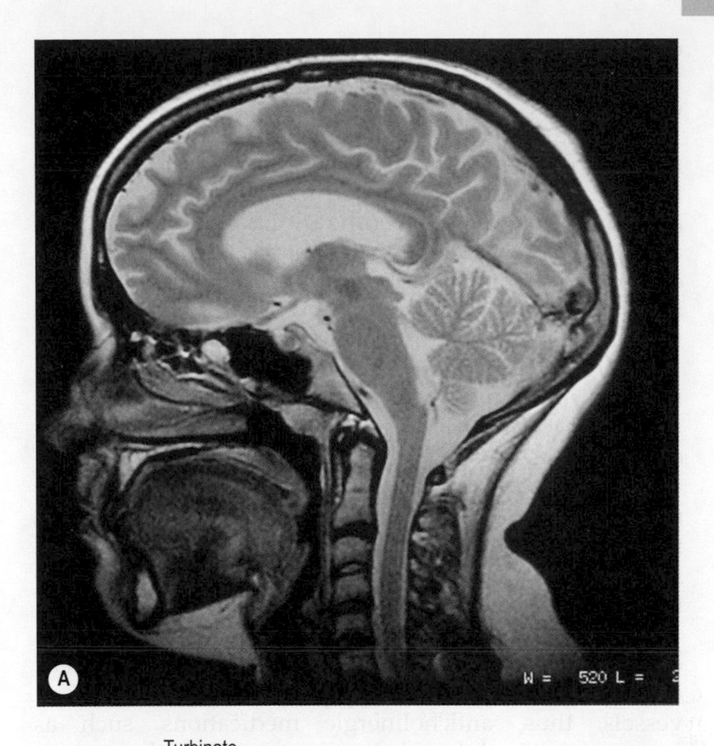

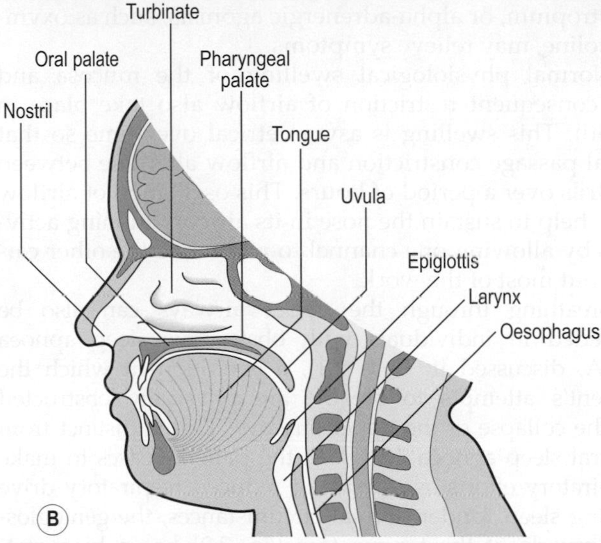

Fig. 2.2 Paramedial magnetic resonance imaging scan of the head and neck. The mouth is closed, and the subject is breathing through his nose.

of the airways produces a relatively large reduction in air flow. Rhinitis can have an infective, allergic, or vasomotor origin.

Infective rhinitis is most frequently caused by rhinoviruses or coronaviruses. Transient vasoconstriction of the mucous membrane is followed by vasodilation, oedema, and mucus production. Secondary bacterial infection can also occur and make the secretions viscid with pus, cells, and bacteria, which contribute to the obstruction of breathing. The inflammation may spread to the sinuses, causing the congestion symptoms that are typical of sinusitis.

Allergic rhinitis may be triggered by pollen, animal fur, or house dust mites. The house dust mite, *Dermatophagoides pteronyssinus*, is invisible to the unaided eye and lives on shed skin scales. Its allergens can provoke asthma and rhinitis. In this case, symptoms may be relieved by topical antihistamines, corticosteroids (e.g., a fluticasone nasal spray), or by environmental measures, such as regular hot washing of bedding, regular cleaning, and minimising the use of soft furnishings.

Vasomotor rhinitis is thought to be the result of an excess of parasympathetic activity over sympathetic activity in the nerves supplying the mucosal blood vessels; thus, anticholinergic medications, such as ipratropium, or alpha-adrenergic agonists, such as oxymetazoline, may relieve symptoms.

Normal physiological swelling of the mucosa and the consequent restriction of airflow also take place in health. This swelling is asymmetrical over time so that nasal passage constriction and airflow alternate between nostrils over a period of hours. This oscillation of airflow may help to sustain the nose in its air-conditioning activities by allowing one channel to rest while the other carries out most of the work.

Breathing through the upper airways can also be impeded in individuals with obstructive sleep apnoea (OSA, discussed in Case 2.1), a condition in which the patient's attempts to breathe are physically obstructed by the collapse of the upper airways. This is distinct from central sleep apnoea, in which the patient ceases to make respiratory efforts as a result of reduced respiratory drive during sleep. Under normal circumstances, the genioglossus muscle of the tongue (see Fig. 2.2) has a high resting tone in the conscious person and holds the tongue forward, preventing it from obstructing the airway. During sleep, particularly in individuals with OSA, the tongue falls against the back wall of the pharynx and can obstruct breathing. This is also seen after induction of general anaesthesia, where it can be resolved by a jaw thrust or the insertion of an endotracheal tube or laryngeal mask to bypass the obstruction. The muscle tone of the pharynx itself also reduces during sleep; in patients with OSA, the pharynx collapses under the negative pressure of inspiration.

Larynx

The larynx is a box-like, funnel-shaped structure at the top of the trachea, located at vertebral levels C3–C6/7. It is made up of three large cartilages (cricoid, thyroid, and epiglottis), three smaller paired cartilages (arytenoids, corniculate, and cuneiform), and a number of muscles which act to adduct, abduct, tense, or relax the ***vocal folds*** or ***cords*** (see Fig. 2.3). The cricoid cartilage forms the only complete ring of cartilage in the airway. The main function of the larynx is to protect the trachea and lower respiratory tract from accidental soiling (e.g., food inhalation). Other functions include phonation, coughing, and contributing to control of ventilation.

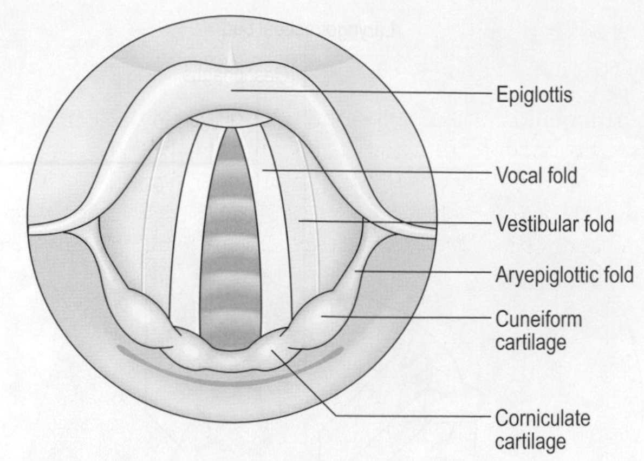

Fig. 2.3 The *vocal folds* or cords, as might be seen by an anaesthetist about to intubate a patient.

The epiglottis is attached only to the wall of the larynx along one edge, meaning it can move to cover or reveal the opening to the larynx, like a trapdoor. During swallowing, the larynx elevates, which helps to open up the oesophagus. At the same time, the tongue moves backwards, forcing the epiglottis to move backwards and effectively seal over the laryngeal inlet, which stops food entering the trachea, known as 'aspiration'. If this system of preventing solids from entering the airways fails, powerful cough reflexes can be provoked by nerves in the lining of the larynx and trachea. The innervation of the larynx is described in Chapter 9.

The vocal cords are like two curtains of muscle which can adduct (come together) to close off the lumen of the larynx or abduct (move apart) to open the lumen. The cords are abducted during respiration to allow for airflow. They can be further abducted during forced inspiration to increase the diameter of the airway, thereby reducing resistance to air flow. Phonation during speech (production of sound) occurs through the vibration of air through adducted vocal cords. The vocal cords must also adduct and then rapidly abduct to produce an effective cough. Vocal cord closure is not always normal; in some circumstances, particularly around instrumentation of the airway, ***laryngospasm*** may develop, where the vocal cords become so tightly adducted that they remain airtight against the greatest breathing efforts a subject can make. A laryngospasm may occur during induction of or emergence from anaesthesia and can be relieved by applying continuous positive airway pressure through a tight-fitting facemask, or by sedation and paralysis.

Trachea

The trachea is a tube-shaped structure which extends from the larynx (at about the C6 vertebral level, in adults) to the carina (at approximately the T4 vertebral level, in adults), where it divides into the left and right main bronchi. The trachea is composed of multiple horseshoe-shaped, incomplete rings of cartilage, which help it to hold its shape and structure. Posteriorly, the rings are incomplete, and the posterior wall is made up of the linear ***trachealis muscle***. Tracheal stenosis can occur as a result of scar tissue formation after tracheostomy or as a result of trauma, neoplasm, or connective tissue disorders.

The trachea can be inspected using a bronchoscope. These instruments may be rigid or, more commonly, flexible (Figure 2.4). Flexible bronchoscopes are able to pass further down into the bronchial tree. Bronchoscopes have channels to allow suction (e.g., to clear mucous plugs) and to pass instruments (e.g., biopsy forceps) to sample lesions.

Intrathoracic airways

The conducting airways carry air to the respiratory airways where gas exchange occurs.

In bronchitic patients, secretions can fill small airways, solidify, and may even be coughed up as small casts which resemble parts of a tree. The intrathoracic airways are often referred to as bronchial trees due to the branching nature of the airways. The trachea (which resembles the trunk) is the first and largest of approximately 23 generations of airways (represented in Figure 2.5). Each airway divides into two smaller airways (known as ***dichotomous branching***), although the two divisions are not always equal in size. Despite the reduction in the diameters of the individual airways at each generation (Table 2.1), the serial branching means that the total cross-sectional area of the airways increases vastly with each successive generation (Figure 2.6). Note that the figure uses a logarithmic scale; the cross-sectional area increases even more than may be first appreciated. The increase in area means that the velocity of the air falls

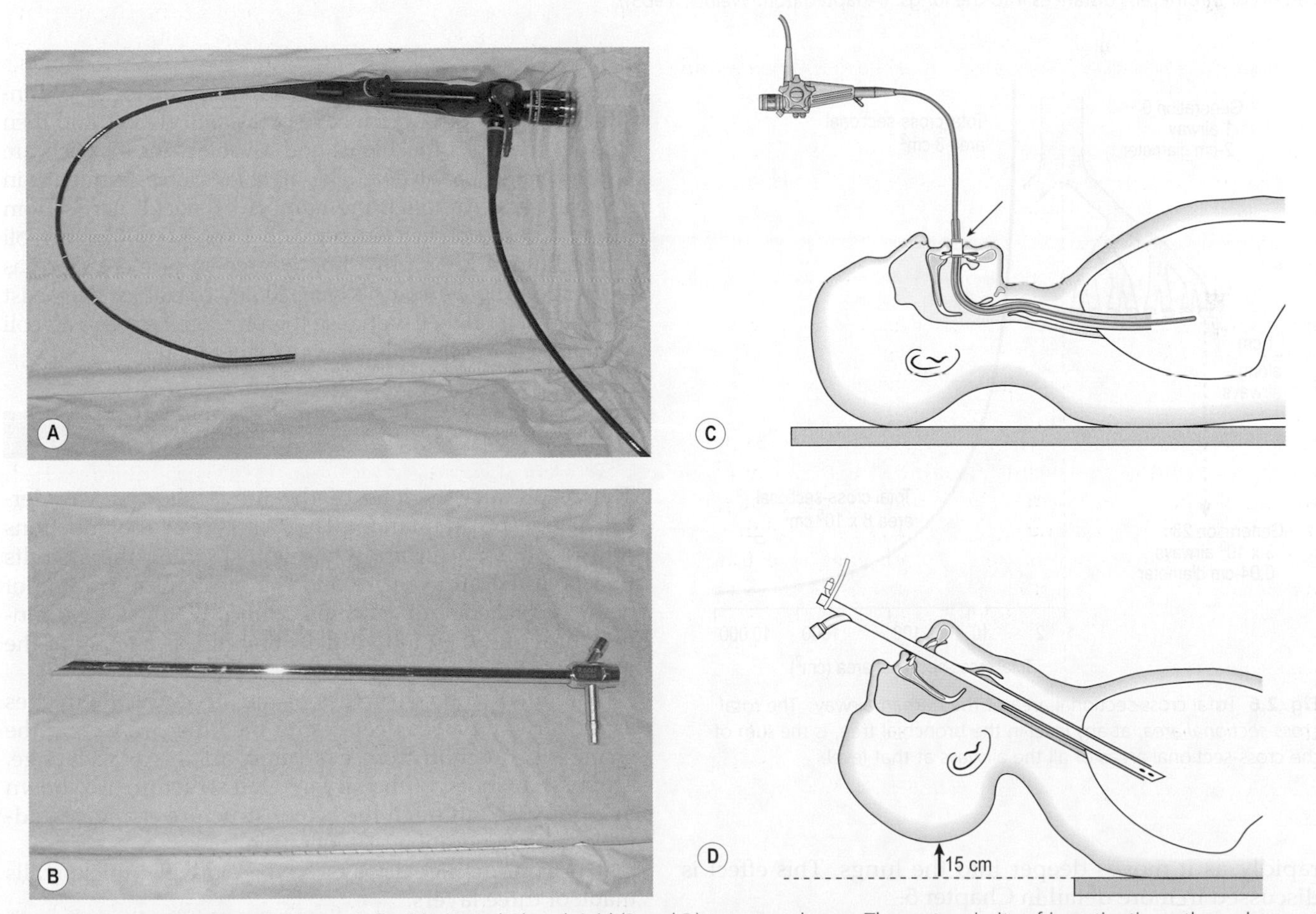

Fig. 2.4 Bronchoscopes. Both fibreoptic flexible (A and C) and rigid (B and D) types are shown. The vast majority of investigations, these days, are carried out using the flexible type. To insert a rigid bronchoscope, the patient's head has to be raised and rotated as shown.

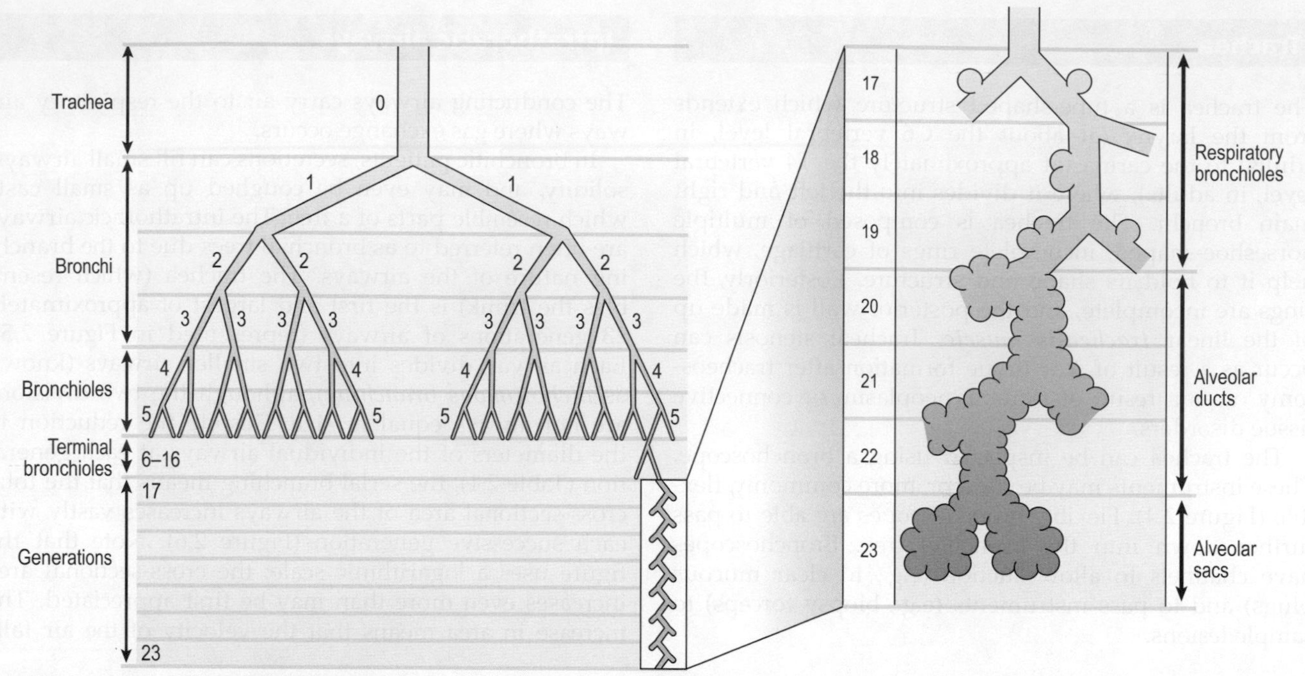

Fig. 2.5 The naming of airways. There is, of course, a gradual change in structure from one type of airway to another. A particular type of airway can occur at different distances into the lungs. (Adapted from Weibel, 1963.)

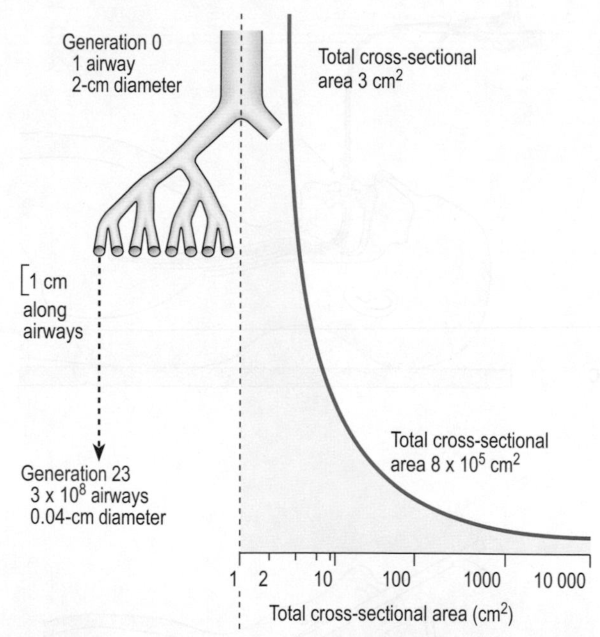

Fig. 2.6 Total cross-sectional area of the human airway. The *total cross-sectional area*, at any level in the bronchial tree, is the sum of the cross-sectional areas of all the airways at that level.

rapidly as it moves deeper into the lungs. This effect is discussed in more detail in Chapter 5.

The first 15 generations of airways are purely conducting pipes. As no gas exchange occurs here, the volume of these airways is called **dead space** (approximately 150 mL).

The terminal bronchioles of generation 16 divide into transitional bronchioles which have occasional alveoli, and then into respiratory bronchioles and alveolar ducts which are entirely lined by alveoli. The alveolar ducts terminate in alveolar sacs. Although the number of alveoli varies from person to person, there are typically over 300 million alveoli in the human lung, providing a huge surface area for gas exchange. The ***pores of Kohn***, 10-μm openings that exist between alveoli, help equalise the pressure between alveoli and provide a collateral pathway for aeration.

Histological structure of the airways

The respiratory regions of the lungs show a wonderful degree of adaptation. They carry out the functions of a respiratory surface while withstanding the assaults of a polluted atmosphere and the mechanical trauma of being stretched and relaxed around 12 times per minute, throughout an individual's lifetime, as a result of the movements of breathing.

The microscopic structure of the airway wall changes as the airway passes deeper into the lungs, reflecting the change in function from gas transport to gas exchange. Three 'snapshots' of the airway wall structure are shown in Figure 2.7, although the actual structure changes gradually from generation to generation.

The conducting airways have relatively thick walls made of three layers:

1. The outermost layer is ***connective tissue***, with supporting cartilage to keep the large airways open.

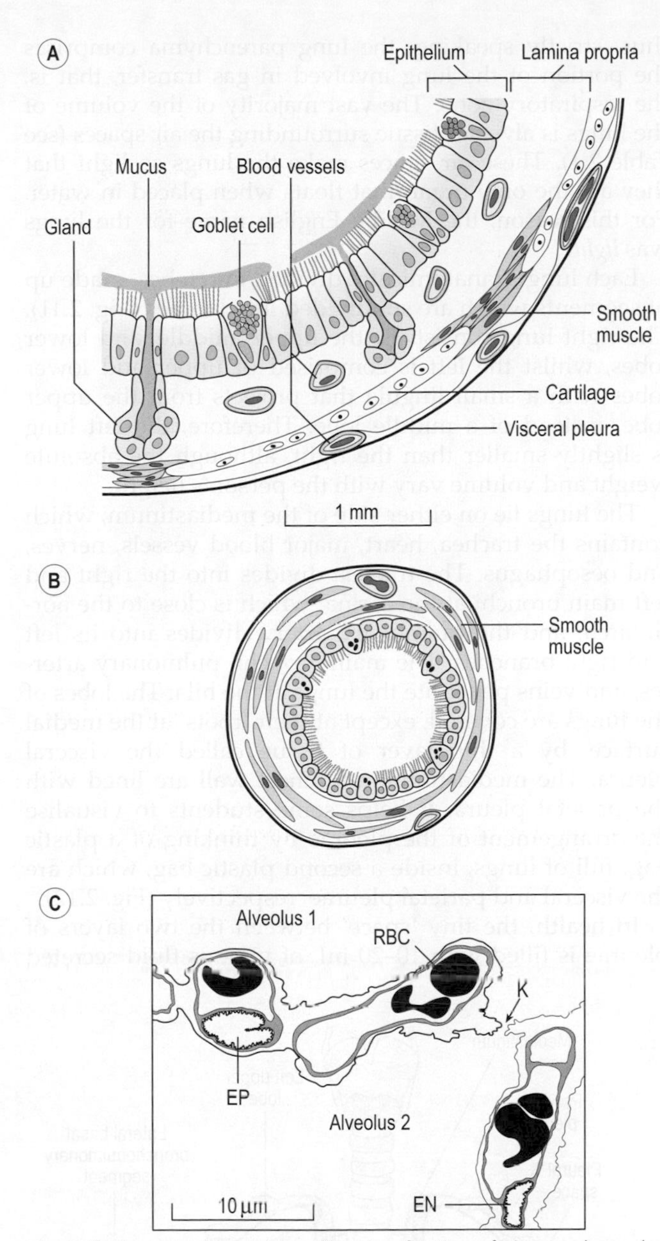

Fig. 2.7 Airway wall structure. The classification of airways depends on the structural characteristics illustrated here. (A) Bronchus, (B) bronchiole, (C) alveolus. EN, endothelial nucleus; EP, epithelial nucleus; K, pores of Kohn; RBC, red blood cell.

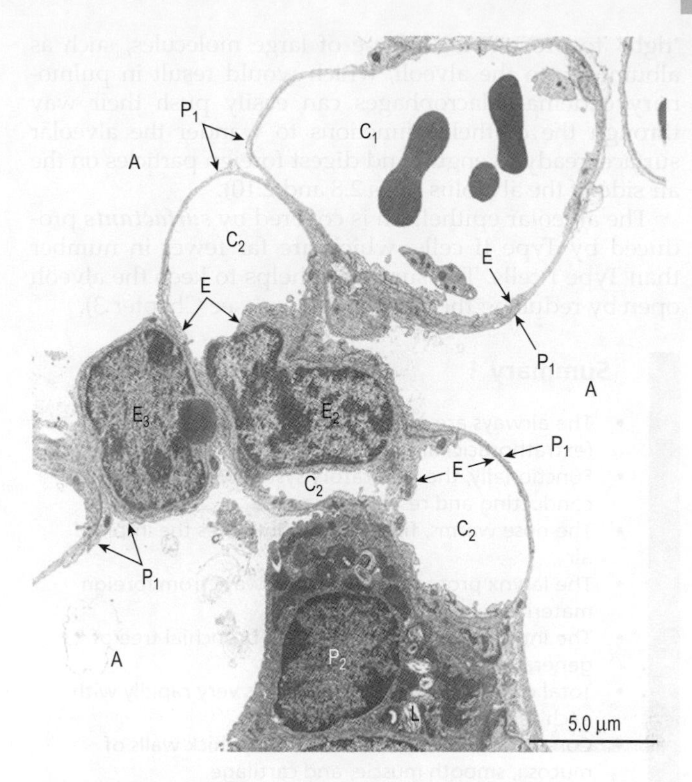

Fig. 2.8 Scanning electron micrograph of an alveolus. A, alveolus; C1, C2, C3, capillaries; E, endothelial cell; L, lamellar bodies; P1, Type I pneumocytes; P2, type II pneumocyte. (From B. Young, J.W. Heath 2000. Wheater's Functional Histology: A Text and Colour Atlas. Edinburgh: Churchill Livingstone.)

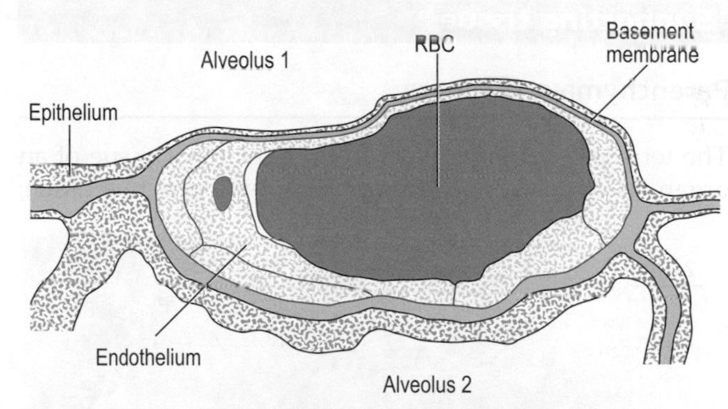

Fig. 2.9 The alveolar–capillary membrane. This diagram of an electron micrograph shows the way the alveolar and capillary cells on one side of the alveolar septum fuse to form an ultrathin layer which offers little barrier to diffusion. The other side of the septum is thicker and provides physical support. RBC, red blood cell.

2. The middle layer is ***smooth muscle***, which reduces in thickness from the large airways down to the entrances to the alveoli.
3. The inner mucosal surface is ***a ciliated epithelium*** with mucus-secreting goblet cells. This makes up the *mucociliary escalator*, which is important for removing inhaled particles from the lungs.

In contrast to the conducting airways, the alveolar wall is very thin (25 nm) to permit gas exchange. The wall is formed by squamous epithelial cells. Type I epithelial cells make up about 95% of the lining of the respiratory zone (Fig. 2.8). These are fused with the pulmonary capillary endothelium, making an ultrathin layer that is ideal for gas diffusion. The pulmonary capillaries are only fused/thinned on one side, leaving the cells on the other side more robust to support the capillary in its place (Fig. 2.9). The junctions between the endothelial cells of the capillaries are 'leaky' and allow an easy flux of water and solutes between the plasma and the interstitial space. The junctions between the epithelial cells, however, are sufficiently 'tight' to prevent the escape of large molecules, such as albumin, into the alveoli, which would result in pulmonary oedema. Macrophages can easily push their way through the epithelial junctions to wander the alveolar surface, ready to engulf and digest foreign particles on the air side of the alveolus (Figs 2.8 and 2.10).

The alveolar epithelium is covered by ***surfactants*** produced by Type II cells, which are far fewer in number than Type I cells. The surfactant helps to keep the alveoli open by reducing the surface tension (see Chapter 3).

Summary 1

- The airways are anatomically divided into upper (extrathoracic) and lower (intrathoracic) airways.
- Functionally, the respiratory system is divided into conducting and respiratory zones.
- The nose warms, filters, and humidifies the inspired air
- The larynx protects the lower airways from foreign materials.
- The intrathoracic airways form a bronchial tree of 23 generations.
- Total cross-sectional area increases very rapidly with each successive airway generation.
- Conducting airways have relatively thick walls of mucosa, smooth muscle, and cartilage.
- The mucosa is ciliated and forms an 'escalator', carrying dust out of the lungs to the mouth.
- Alveoli have very thin walls with squamous epithelium consisting of Type I and II pneumocytes.

Supporting tissues

Parenchyma and pleura

The term ***parenchyma*** refers to the functional tissue of an organ, as opposed to the supporting or connective tissue; thus, strictly speaking, the lung parenchyma comprises the portion of the lung involved in gas transfer, that is, the respiratory zone. The vast majority of the volume of the lungs is alveolar tissue surrounding the air spaces (see Table 2.1). These air spaces make the lungs so light that they are the only organ that floats when placed in water. For this reason, the Middle English name for the lungs was *light*.

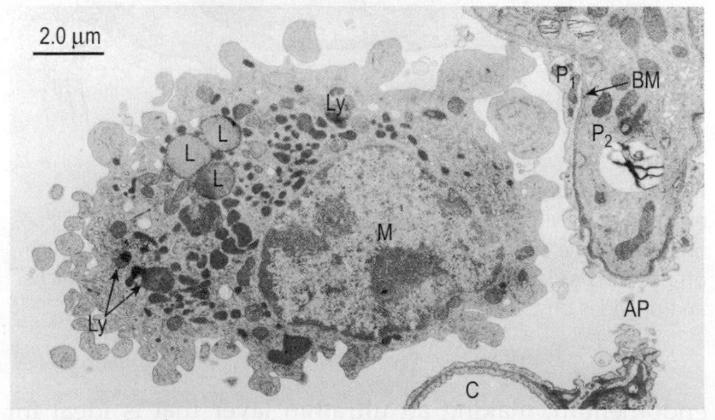

Fig. 2.10 Alveolar macrophage. Formed from monocytes produced in the bone marrow, these phagocytic cells contain enzymes destructive to microorganisms. These enzymes can produce emphysema in patients deficient in the protective protein α1-antitrypsin. AP, alveolar pore; BM, basement membrane; C, septal capillary; L, lipid droplets; Ly, lysosomes; M, macrophage; P_1, Type 1 pneumocyte;. (From B. Young and J.W. Heath 2000. Wheater's Functional Histology: A Text and Colour Atlas. Edinburgh: Churchill Livingstone.)

Each lung is anatomically divided into lobes, made up of segments which are subdivided into lobules (Fig. 2.11). The right lung consists of the upper, middle, and lower lobes, whilst the left is comprised of upper and lower lobes with a small lingula that projects from the upper lobe, instead of a middle lobe. Therefore, the left lung is slightly smaller than the right, although the absolute weight and volume vary with the person's height.

The lungs lie on either side of the mediastinum, which contains the trachea, heart, major blood vessels, nerves, and oesophagus. The trachea divides into the right and left main bronchi at the carina, which is close to the aortic arch, and the pulmonary artery divides into its left and right branches. The main bronchi, pulmonary arteries, and veins penetrate the lungs at the hila. The lobes of the lungs are covered, except at their 'roots' at the medial surface, by a thin layer of tissue called the visceral pleura. The mediastinum and chest wall are lined with the parietal pleura. It helps some students to visualise the arrangement of the pleurae by thinking of a plastic bag, full of lungs, inside a second plastic bag, which are the visceral and parietal pleurae, respectively (Fig. 2.12).

In health, the tiny 'space' between the two layers of pleurae is filled with 10–20 mL of viscous fluid secreted

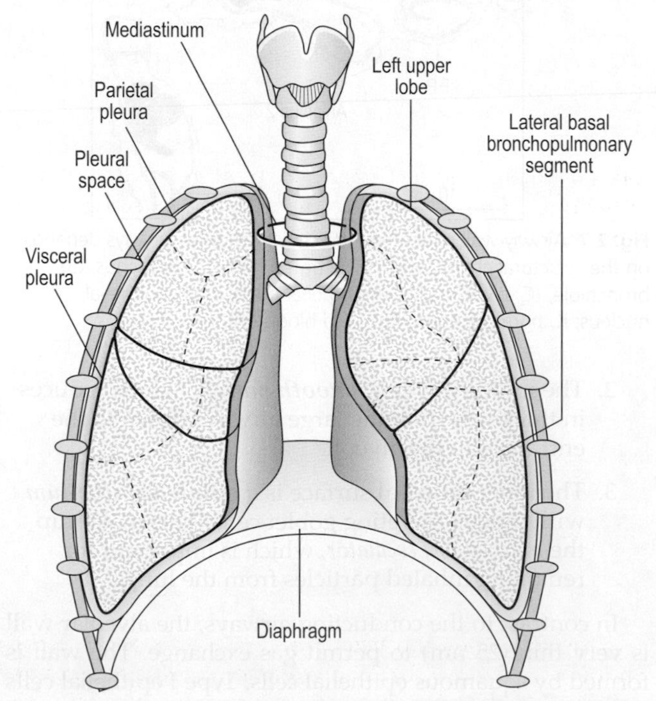

Fig. 2.11 Gross anatomy of the lungs. Each lung is divided into lobes made up of segments subdivided into lobules by fibrous tissue.

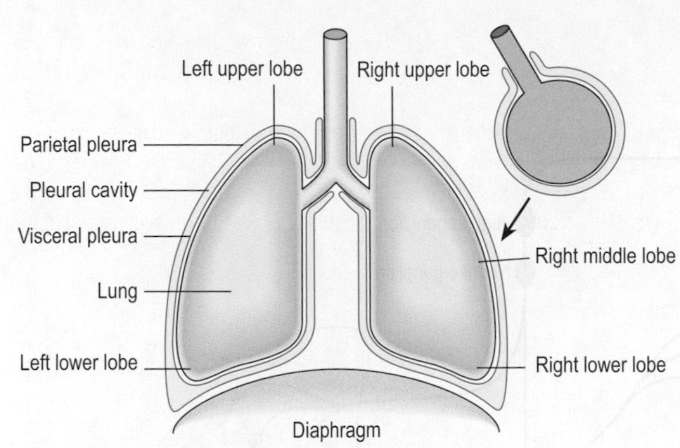

Fig. 2.12 Schematic diagram of the pleurae. It is important to remember that there is no real 'space' between the pleurae, just a few millilitres of slippery fluid.

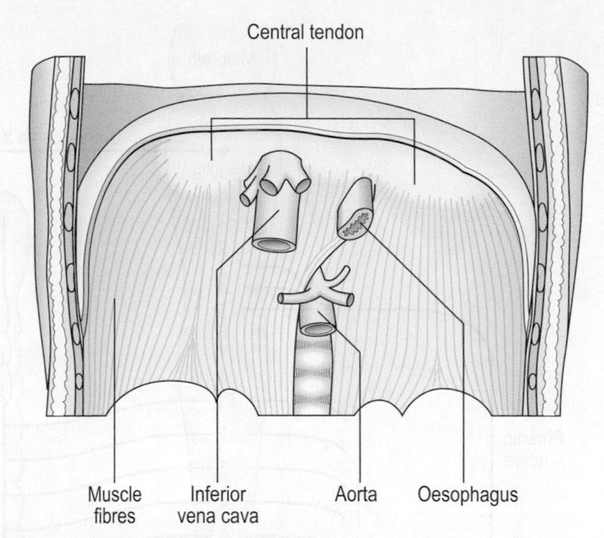

Fig. 2.13 The diaphragm in coronal section. This figure illustrates how far into the chest the diaphragm bulges. This enables it to act like the piston in a syringe as its muscle fibres shorten when stimulated by the bilateral phrenic nerves.

by the pleurae. This lubricates them as they rub against each other during breathing. In conditions such as cancer or pneumonia, the pleura can become inflamed (*pleurisy*), meaning the two layers swell and rub against each other with every breath, causing 'pleuritic chest pain', a sharp, localised pain associated with inspiration or coughing.

Pathologically, blood (**haemothorax**), air (**pneumothorax**), excess fluid (**pleural effusion**), or pus (**empyema**) can accumulate in the pleural space, restricting normal movement of the lungs during respiration and/or causing lung collapse. Pleural effusions result from a variety of conditions, such as cancer, pneumonia, and congestive heart failure. The pleural fluid can be aspirated through a needle and examined to help elucidate its cause. Effusions containing little protein are called ***transudates*** (found in conditions such as congestive heart failure and liver cirrhosis), whereas high protein effusions are called ***exudates*** (found in patients with malignancies, infections, and trauma). As the pleural space is not essential for life (indeed, elephants do not have one at all), surgeons can artificially obliterate the pleural space to treat recurrent pleural effusions. This procedure is called ***pleurodesis*** and involves fixing the lungs to the chest wall.

Diaphragm and chest wall

The diaphragm is a sheet of muscle surrounding a large central tendon (Fig 2.13). It has two main functions:

1. to separate the thoracic cavity from the abdominal cavity, and
2. to contribute to the change in volume of the thoracic cavity required to produce inspiration and expiration (see 'Mechanics of Breathing', later in this chapter).

The central tendon lies around the level of the eighth thoracic vertebra (T8). The edges of the diaphragm are attached to the xiphisternum, the lower margins of the ribcage, and the upper lumbar vertebrae. There are three openings through the diaphragm, which convey the inferior vena cava, oesophagus, and aorta through the structure (Fig. 2.13).

The diaphragm is innervated by the left and right phrenic nerves which originate from cervical cord segments C3, C4, and C5. Both nerves run from the neck through the mediastinum, piercing the diaphragm and innervating it from its inferior surface (Fig 2.14). Therefore, if a patient suffers a high cervical spinal cord injury, they lose diaphragmatic function entirely if the injury is above C3. The phrenic nerves can be injured anywhere along their paths.

The chest wall is comprised of skin, fat, muscles, and the ribcage (Fig. 2.15). The ribcage consists of 12 ribs, the sternum anteriorly, and the spinal column posteriorly. Ribs 1–7 are referred to as true ribs because they directly connect to the sternum and manubrium via costal cartilages. Ribs 8–10 are referred to as false ribs because their costal cartilages conjoin to form a single indirect connection to the sternum via the costal arch. Ribs 11 and 12 are referred to as floating ribs because their anterior extremities are not attached to the sternum. At the spinal column, the ribs articulate with vertebrae T1–T12 by costovertebral joints, which may involve more than one vertebra.

Between the ribs are the three layers of the intercostal muscles:

1. external intercostals, running forward and downward,
2. internal intercostals, at right angles to the externals, therefore running downward and posteriorly, and
3. innermost intercostals, whose fibres run in the same direction as those of the internals.

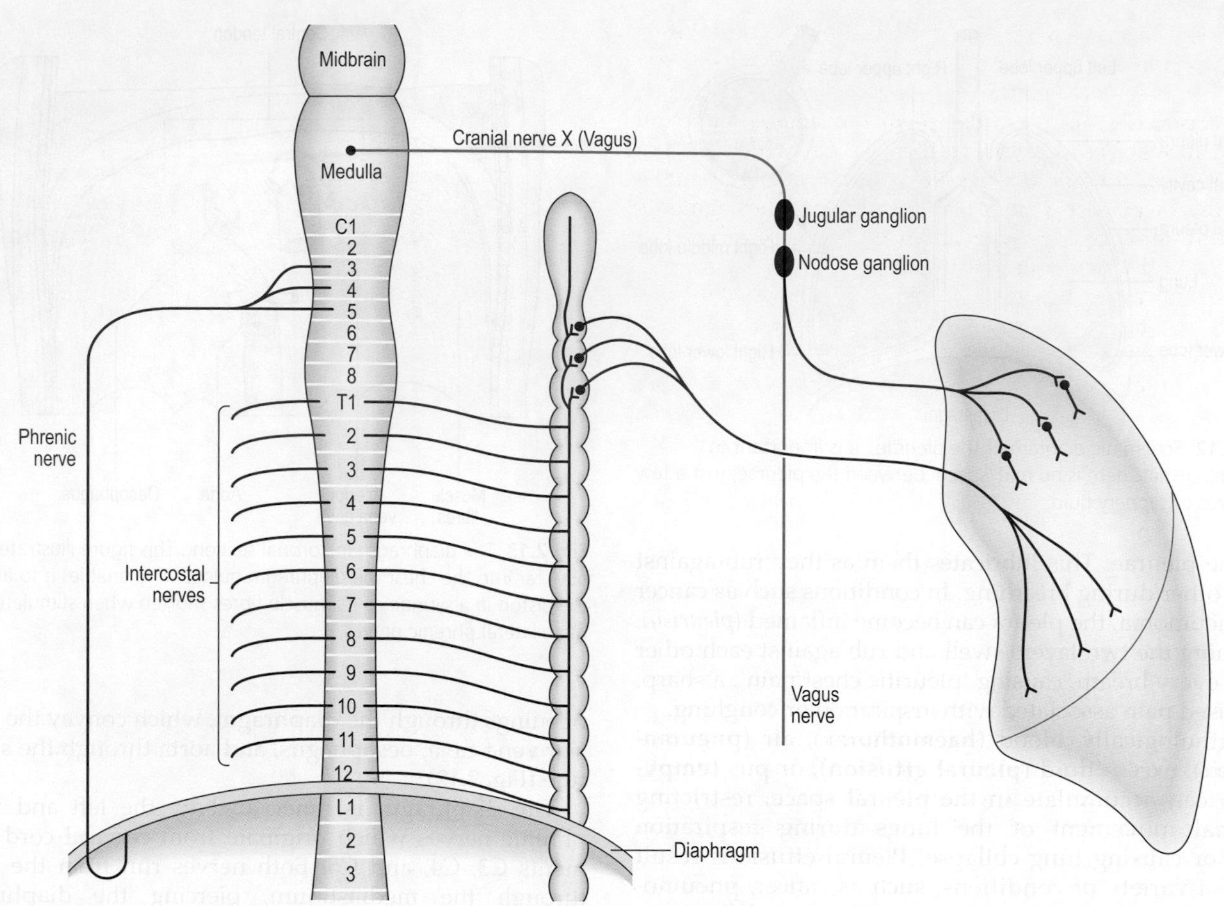

Fig. 2.14 Innervation of the diaphragm, intercostal muscles, and lungs. The efferent (motor) systems are shown. The afferent (sensory) system is mainly in the *vagus nerves*.

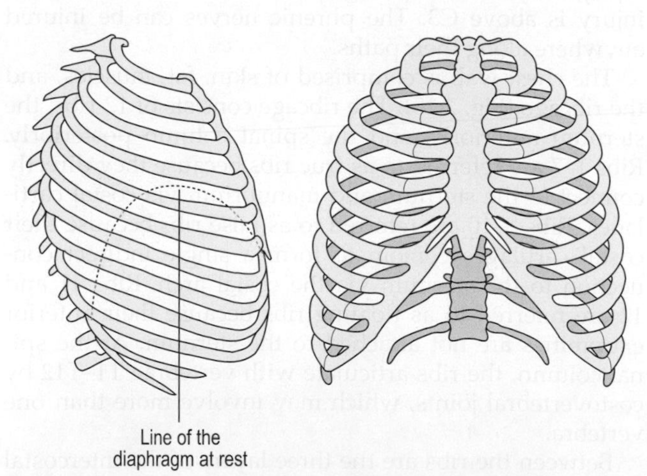

Fig. 2.15 The ribcage. This 'cage' is much more flexible than prepared specimens or models sometimes suggest. The intercostal muscles stretch between the ribs.

These muscles are innervated by the intercostal nerves from the anterior primary rami of spinal cord segments T1–T11 (Fig. 2.14).

The diaphragm and intercostal muscles are the primary muscles of respiration. During exertion, or in disease states where the primary muscles are not functioning adequately, accessory muscles of respiration may also be used. These include neck muscles, such as the sternocleidomastoid and scalenes, which aid inspiration, and the spinal flexors and abdominal muscles, such as the quadratus lumborum, rectus abdominis, internal and external obliques, and tranversus abdominis, which aid expiration.

Pulmonary vasculature

The pulmonary circulation has evolved to facilitate the high-volume gas exchange required to meet the oxygen demands of the body. The lungs receive the entire volume of the cardiac output during each cardiac cycle but maintain low pressure to prevent damage to the delicate gas exchange barrier; therefore the pulmonary circulation is a high-flow, low-pressure system, with only one-sixth of the resistance to blood flow found in the systemic circulation. This is reflected in the thin walls of arteries. There are two pulmonary arteries which branch and follow the airways through the lungs in connective tissue sheaths.

Unlike systemic arterioles, the pulmonary arterioles have very little smooth muscle in their walls. The arterioles carry deoxygenated blood to the capillaries which snake along several alveolar walls, one after the other, before reaching the venules. Together, the arterioles, capillaries, and venules form the ***microcirculation*** of the lungs. Venules join to form veins, which, unlike the arteries, do not travel with the airways but make their own way along the septa that separate the segments of the lung, carrying oxygenated blood back to the left atrium via the four pulmonary veins.

The airways and pulmonary blood vessels down as far as the terminal bronchioles receive their nutrition from the bronchial circulation, which is part of the systemic circulation rather than the pulmonary circulation. Part of the bronchial circulation returns to the systemic venous system in the normal way, but part drains into the pulmonary veins, 'contaminating' their oxygenated blood with deoxygenated blood. This situation constitutes a 'shunt' (see Chapter 7).

The pulmonary mean arterial pressure is normally about 15 mmHg. Hypertension (high blood pressure) can occur in both the pulmonary and systemic circulation. ***Pulmonary hypertension*** may arise as the result of extrapulmonary reasons, such as mitral stenosis or left ventricular failure, which prevent the heart from pumping away the blood returning from the lungs. Congenital defects which allow blood to pass from the left (high-pressure, systemic) side of the heart to the right (low pressure, pulmonary) side of the heart also produce pulmonary hypertension. However, the most common cause of pulmonary hypertension is changes in the pulmonary vessels. They may be blocked by emboli, circulating fat, amniotic fluid, or cancer cells. They may be obliterated by the destruction of the architecture of the capillary beds by emphysema, or the smooth muscle in their walls may be provoked to contract by low oxygen tension that results from high altitude or diseases such as bronchitis and emphysema.

The clinical features of pulmonary hypertension are mainly the result of the increased pressure, producing oedema in the lung and imposing a load on the relatively thin-walled right heart. A patient with pulmonary hypertension complains of chest pain, dyspnoea, and fatigue. Heart sounds are modified, and an electrocardiogram often demonstrates right ventricular hypertrophy.

Lymphatics

The perivascular spaces of the alveolar wall are drained by the lymph vessels. The lymph system of the lungs begins as tiny, blind-ended vessels just above the alveoli. These join to form lymphatics in close proximity to the blood vessels and airways. They are an important feature in the control of fluid balance in the lung and can contain considerable amounts of lymph, particularly during pulmonary oedema when they produce characteristic 'butterfly shadows' on chest X-rays (Fig. 2.16).

As in other tissues, the lymphatic system plays a key role in the immune defence of the lungs. This is achieved through immediate hypersensitivity, antibody-dependent cytotoxicity, immune complex reactions, and cell-mediated immune reactions.

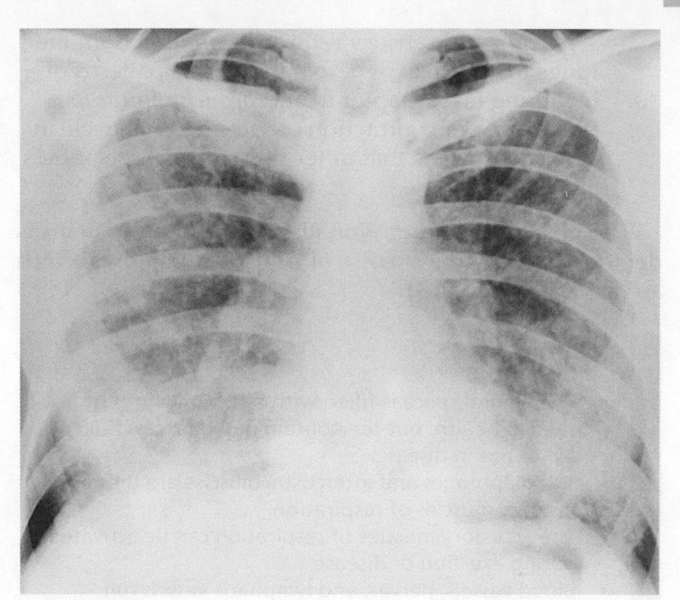

Fig. 2.16 X-ray showing a 'butterfly shadow' in a patient with pulmonary oedema.

Nerves

The nerves supplying the airways and vasculature of the lungs are separate from those supplying the respiratory muscles. Innervation of the respiratory system is discussed in greater detail in Chapter 9.

The nerves of the lungs are derived from the pulmonary plexuses. There are three main types:

1. *Parasympathetic nerves.* These originate from the vagus nerve. Long preganglionic fibres synapse in ganglia on the bronchi. The short postganglionic fibres release acetylcholine at the bronchial smooth muscle, causing it to contract and resulting in bronchoconstriction (Fig. 2.14). Parasympathetic efferents also cause vasodilation of the pulmonary vessels and stimulate the secretion of mucus from the bronchial glands.

2. *Sympathetic nerves.* These arise from the sympathetic trunks and cause ***vasoconstriction*** of the pulmonary vessels and ***relaxation*** of the bronchial smooth muscle. This bronchodilatory action makes drugs, which are sympathetic agonists (such as adrenaline and salbutamol) useful in the treatment of asthma.

3. *Visceral afferents.* Afferent nerves from receptors near the alveoli (J receptors), in the smooth muscle of airways (stretch receptors), and free nerve endings between the epithelial cells of the airways (rapidly adapting irritant receptors) conduct

sensation and sensory reflex information from the lungs to the brain, where it influences patterns of breathing (see Chapter 9) and ***bronchomotor** tone* (the degree of contraction of the smooth muscle in the airway walls that determines the calibre of the airways).

The limited importance of all these nervous systems is demonstrated by the success of transplanted lungs which are, in fact, denervated!

Summary 2

- The pleural space is filled with a few millilitres of fluid in health, but can contain blood, excess fluid, air, or pus in disease.
- The diaphragm and intercostal muscles are the primary muscles of respiration.
- The accessory muscles of respiration can be activated during exertion or disease.
- Blood vessels, nerves, and lymphatic vessels run parallel to the airways
- The bronchial circulation supplies the lung tissues.
- The pulmonary circulation is involved in gas exchange and is a high-flow, low-pressure system.
- Parasympathetic efferents cause bronchoconstriction, while sympathetic efferents cause bronchodilation.

Mechanics of breathing

Lung movements are passive and are brought about by external forces on the respiratory muscles. The lungs are held to the walls of the thoracic cavity by the visceral and parietal plurae, as described earlier in this chapter. To understand the mechanics of breathing, it is important to appreciate that the lungs themselves do not have muscles that contribute to this process. Smooth muscle is present in the airways, but it controls the airway diameter. Second, air will only flow from a region of high pressure to a region of low pressure. During inspiration, the pressure in the elastic alveoli is lowered relative to the atmospheric pressure by expanding the thorax. Therefore air is sucked into the lungs. During expiration, pressure in the lungs is increased by decreasing the size of the thorax which leads to exhalation.

The reduction in pressure around the lungs which brings about inspiration is mainly the result of the activity of the phrenic nerves. They cause the diaphragm to flatten and descend like a plunger in a syringe. This draws air into the chest. During quiet breathing, inspiration is the only *active* part of breathing; expiration is largely passive and is the result of the *elastic recoil* of the lungs pulling them and the diaphragm back into their resting positions.

The central tendon of the diaphragm moves 1-2 cm during quiet breathing, but can move up to around 10 cm during vigorous breathing. The movement of the diaphragm normally accounts for about 75% of the volume of breathing but is not essential for life; if the diaphragm is paralysed, other respiratory muscles can take over, to a large degree. During quiet breathing, only some (and not always the same) diaphragmatic muscle fibres contract with each inspiration. This may explain why we rarely suffer from fatigue of the diaphragm.

If we liken the diaphragm to the plunger of a syringe, the ribs can be likened to the syringe walls. However, the action of the intercostal muscles on the ribs (mainly the second to tenth ribs) can alter the diameter of the chest and actively draw air into and expel it from the lungs. This is largely because the ribs are set at an angle, sloping down from the horizontal, and are capable of being raised and lowered (see Fig. 2.13).

The external intercostal muscles cause two types of movement during inspiration:

1. 'Pump-handle' movements, in which the anterior end of each rib is elevated like the action of an old-fashioned water pump.
2. 'Bucket-handle' movements, in which the diameter of the chest increases, each rib on either side acting like the raising of the handle of a bucket from the horizontal position.

Both types of action increase the diameter of the chest and, thus, draw air into the lungs by reducing the pressure in the chest. Not only do the external intercostal muscles help bring about this reduction in pressure, but by stiffening the chest wall during inspiration, they prevent a 'sucking-in' of the chest (just as you can suck in your cheeks) that would take place if they did not contract. The actions of the intercostal muscles account for approximately 25% of the maximum voluntary ventilation. Patients with more than one rib broken in more than one place have a 'flail segment,' where that part of the chest wall moves in during inspiration and out during expiration.

Although expiration is largely passive during quiet breathing, expiratory muscles contract actively during vigorous breathing or if the airways are obstructed by disease. Under these conditions, the abdominal muscles are the most important muscles during expiration. By squeezing the contents of the abdomen up against the diaphragm, they force it up into the chest, thereby expelling air from the lungs. These abdominal muscles are especially active during coughing or sneezing, as will be apparent if you press your fingers into the abdomen and cough. The internal and innermost intercostal muscles, like the external intercostal muscles, occupy the spaces between the ribs and are innervated by segmental nerves. They pull the ribs down, reduce the diameter of the chest, and contribute to expiration. They also reinforce the spaces between the ribs and prevent the chest from bulging during expiration, as do the external intercostals.

The changes in the size and shape of the chest brought about by the activity of the diaphragm, intercostals, and accessory muscles are transmitted to the outer surface of the lungs. Any change in pressure on the surface of the lung is rapidly transmitted to the air within the alveoli. It is important to understand that the actual pressure in the fluid between the layers of the pleura, that form the covering of the lungs, and the lining of the chest is not the same as the pressure within the alveoli, a concept explored in more detail in Chapter 5.

Summary 3

- There are no muscles in the lungs that bring about breathing.
- Inspiration is brought about mainly by the descending diaphragm, like the plunger in a syringe.
- Expiration is largely passive due to the elasticity of the lungs, as in balloon deflation.
- Active expiration, as in exercise, involves accessory muscles, including the muscles of the abdomen.

Defences against the environment

To enable efficient gas exchange, the interface between air and blood is thin, moist, and vascular. Unfortunately, as a result, it is not especially physically robust. Therefore, as an evolutionary advantage, this interface between the respiratory surfaces of the lungs and the environment is protected from damage by the air and airborne hazards. As part of the protection, the larger, conducting airways are lined with a mucous layer, which is propelled out of the airways by the movements of cilia on the epithelial cells lining the airways.

Conditioning air

Air is cold and dry compared with the respiratory surface of the lungs. If the mucosal surfaces of the airway were to become similarly cold and dry, processes such as ciliary function and gas exchange would be impaired. Therefore conditioning (warming and humidification) of the inspired air is necessary. The temperature and humidity gradients are greatest between inspired air and the mucosa of the nose and upper airways; therefore most of the conditioning takes place in these regions. During quiet breathing, air is fully conditioned by the time it reaches the trachea. Air transit through the nose takes < 0.1 s under these conditions, but the temperature can be raised from 20°C to 31°C by the time the air leaves the internal nares and to 35°C by the time it reaches the mid-trachea. Humidification takes place equally rapidly, and inspired air is close to saturation by the time it reaches the pharynx. The humidification of inspired air places a thermal demand on the body because of the high latent heat of vaporisation of water. Five times as much heat is used to vaporise water to saturate the inspired air than is used to warm the air. Thus, this-air conditioning process is a metabolic 'expense', but up to 40% of this expense is recovered from the expired air which warms and moistens the nasal mucosa as we breathe out. Desert animals, such as camels and gerbils, have highly developed turbinate systems in their noses which recover far more heat and water than do ours.

This countercurrent exchange of heat and water in the nose is well demonstrated under cold conditions when the mucosa of the nose is much colder than the exhaled air from deep in the lungs. Under these conditions, sufficient water may condense to form a drop at the end of the nose. This is a purely natural physical phenomenon, not 'a cold' or other pathological condition.

At rest, most people breathe through their nose, although 15% of the population are habitual mouth breathers. We resort to mouth breathing during heavy exercise. The mouth is surprisingly good at air conditioning, and by the time air reaches the glottis, its conditions are similar whether a person is breathing through the nose or mouth. The disadvantage of mouth breathing arises during expiration, when much less heat and water are recovered. We have all experienced the discomfort of a dry mouth, which often accompanies the nasal obstruction during a cold.

Inhaled particles

The respiratory system is presented with around 10,000 L of inhaled air within a 24-hour period, and with it, many chemical and biological particles. As the conducting airways are much more robust than respiratory surfaces, they play an important role in protecting the lower airways.

Factors such as the size and velocity of a particle affect how far it can travel into the respiratory tract, where it is deposited, and by which process it is deposited (Fig. 2.17). Particles which reach the wall of the airways are trapped by a mucus layer and travel, via the mucociliary escalator (see Histological Structure of the Airways, earlier in this chapter), at a rate of about 2 mm s^{-1}, to the pharynx to be swallowed. The mucous blanket which traps the particles is 5–10 μm thick and consists of two layers: the outer gel layer that rests on a less viscous layer in which the cilia beat toward the mouth at a frequency of about 20 Hz.

Large drops fall faster than smaller ones; Stoke's law states that the terminal velocity of a falling sphere is proportional to the square of its radius. Particles that are inhaled more quickly can penetrate further into the respiratory tract. Particles are displaced from the airstream, towards the surfaces of the respiratory tract, by ***impaction***, ***sedimentation***, and ***diffusion***. Large particles (> 8 μm in diameter) do not tend to get further than the pharynx. Those with diameters of 3–8 μm fall out of the airstream owing to the effect of inertia in the turbulent airflow of the upper airways. They reach the walls of the airways and are deposited by impaction. Smaller particles (1–3 μm) survive the turbulence of the upper airways but are removed by sedimentation in the small airways and alveoli. Sedimentation is the process by which small particles moving at a lower velocity in the small

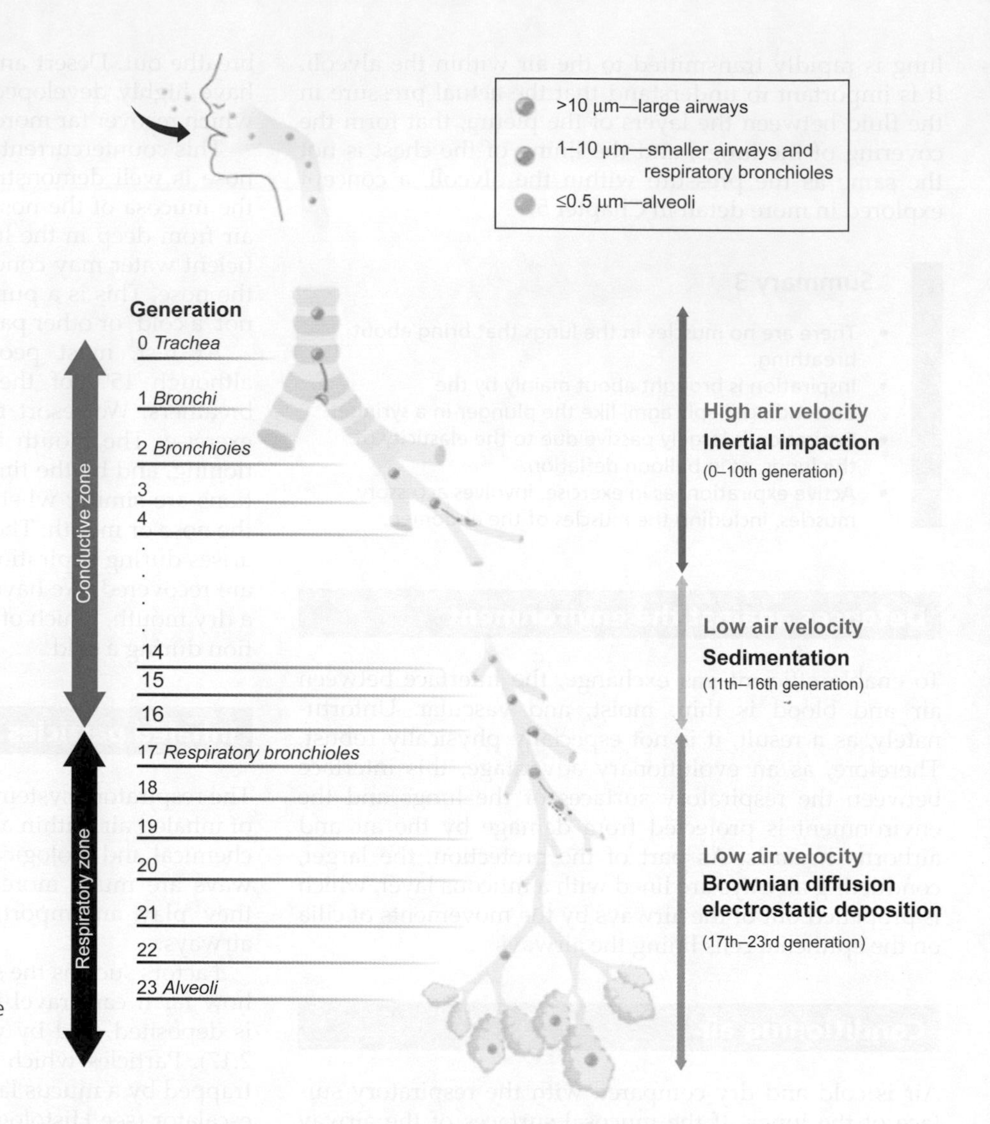

Fig. 2.17 The size and velocity of a particle affect the process and site of deposition. (From Garcia-Mouton C et al. Eur J Pharm Biopharm. 2019).

airways fall out of suspension because of gravity and settle. The smallest particles (< 1 µm) are subject to 'jostling' by gas molecules until they bump into the walls of a small airway or alveolus. This diffusion is caused by the Brownian motion of the smallest particles and gas molecules. Particles of this size may be inhaled and promptly exhaled again, although some may bump into the wall of a small airway or alveolus. In this region, particles are stuck to the walls by surface tension because there is no secretion of mucus, and as such, they are also beyond the end of the ciliary escalator.

In the alveolar region, amoeboid macrophages (Fig. 2.10) engulf particles and carry them to the escalator or take them into the blood or lymph. When the particle load is large, the macrophages deposit this around the respiratory bronchioles; pathologists in a coal-mining area will have seen the black 'halos' so formed. Bacteria are particularly susceptible to the attention of macrophages, which kill them with enzymes and oxygen-based free radicals (see the Metabolic Activity section later in this chapter) or transport them out of the lungs. The activities of these phagocytic cells ensure that the alveolar region of the lung remains sterile. The free radicals and proteases produced by macrophages to deal with foreign materials also have the potential to damage the lung itself. Figure 2.18 illustrates the effect of particle size on the location of deposition in the respiratory tract.

There is a practical application for understanding the behaviour of particles of varying sizes. Drugs can be delivered topically via the respiratory tract to relieve the symptoms of diseases (e.g., asthma), or the respiratory route can be used as a method of delivering a drug that is absorbed systemically. These drugs are delivered as aerosols via nebulisers or inhalers. An aerosol is a cloud of particles or droplets that remains stable and suspended in the air for some time. The size of the particle and the patient's breathing pattern are factors which can be altered to ensure that the drug reaches the intended part of the respiratory tract. The use of inhalers requires

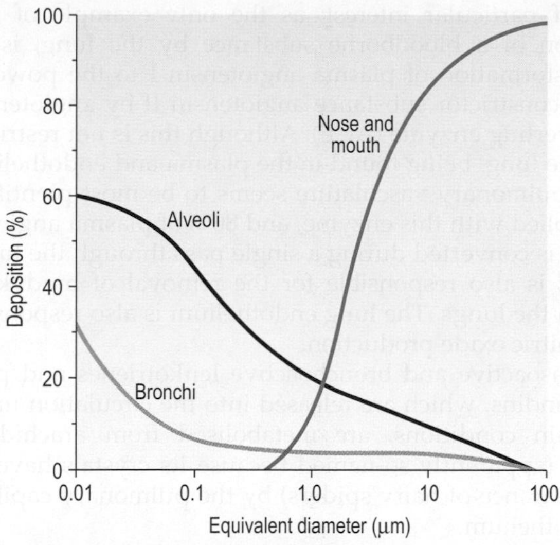

Fig. 2.18 Deposition of particles in the lung. Notice that the aerodynamic diameter is represented using a log scale and that there is a point, at about a bronchial diameter of 0.5 mm, where deposition is minimal.

slow, deep breathing to ensure adequate penetration. The use of a spacer device can be helpful, as it reduces the need for a breath to be coordinated with the activation of the inhaler. It also allows the largest particles to fall out of the aerosol prior to inhalation, which can reduce systemic side effects. This can be a problem if large quantities of larger particles that impact the pharynx are absorbed. Nebulisers turn a liquid drug into a fine mist, which is then supplied as a constant flow to the patient, removing the need for a coordinated effort to inhale. However, large doses can lead to problematic side effects, and the equipment required to nebulise a drug is far more complex and expensive than that required by an inhaler.

Smoking and air pollution

Particulate matter accounts for only a small fraction, by weight, of the pollutants we breathe; gases and vapours also pose a serious threat. Fig. 2.19 indicates the contribution of suspended particulate matter, as well as the sources of the pollution we encounter. Despite decreases in some parts of the world, air pollution remains a major global issue and is associated with diseases such as cardiac disease and lung cancer. The World Health Organisation sets standards for the maximum acceptable levels of pollutants. In his 1604 '*Counterblaste to Tobacco*', King James I of England described smoking, then becoming increasingly fashionable, as '*a custom loathsome to the eye, hateful to the nose, harmful to the brain, and dangerous to the lungs*'. However, 350 years would lapse before firm evidence was gathered to support his assertions. Smoking is now recognised as the leading cause of preventable illness and premature death in the UK, accounting for almost 100,000 deaths annually; worldwide, this number is six million. Although, in the UK, the number of people smoking regularly is decreasing, in some parts of the world, the rate continues to rise, with an associated burden on global health. More than 4500 chemicals are inhaled in tobacco smoke, the majority of which have harmful effects. Smoking causes 90% of lung cancers, and approximately 20% of smokers develop chronic obstructive pulmonary disease. An excessive level of carbon monoxide is a feature of both those suffering the effects of air pollution and of smoking. This has a particularly deleterious effect on the carriage of oxygen by the blood (see Chapter 8).

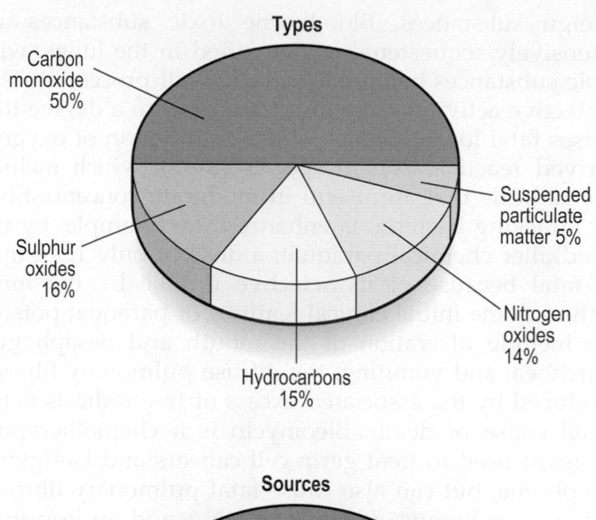

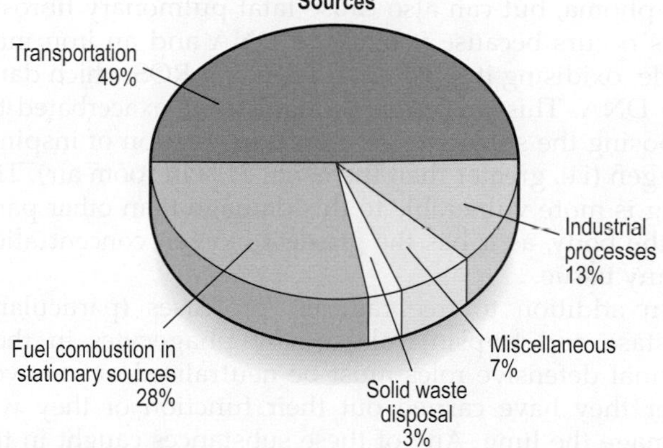

Fig. 2.19 Air pollutants and their sources. Note the contribution made by automobiles.

Metabolic activity

Lung tissue metabolism is unremarkable, having a metabolic rate only slightly higher than the average for the whole body. Although it is the major extrahepatic site for mixed-function oxidation by the cytochrome P450 system, lung tissue is, gram for gram, much less active than the liver. The major role of the P450 system in the lungs may therefore be in the detoxification of inhaled foreign substances. Bloodborne toxic substances are extensively sequestered or detoxified in the lungs, with basic substances being particularly well processed. This protective activity of the lung can occur to a degree that causes fatal local damage. The accumulation of oxygen-derived reactive oxygen species (ROS), which include free radicals that are useful in moderate concentrations for attacking bacteria, is enhanced, for example, by the weedkiller chemical paraquat; a dose of only 1.5 g may be fatal because of its selective uptake by the lung. Although the initial clinical features of paraquat poisoning include ulceration of the mouth and oesophagus, diarrhoea, and vomiting, the diffuse pulmonary fibrosis produced by the associated excess of free radicals is the usual cause of death. Bleomycin is a chemotherapeutic agent used to treat germ cell cancers and Hodgkin's lymphoma, but can also cause fatal pulmonary fibrosis. This occurs because it binds to DNA and an iron molecule, oxidising it to Fe^{3+} and releasing ROS which damage DNA. This process is thought to be exacerbated by exposing the subject to an increased fraction of inspired oxygen (i.e. greater than the usual 21% in room air). The lung is more vulnerable to this damage than other parts of the body, as it has the greatest oxygen concentration of any tissue.

In addition to free radicals, proteases (particularly elastase and trypsin) released by phagocytes in their normal defensive roles must be neutralised or removed after they have carried out their function or they will damage the lung. Any of these substances caught in the mucociliary escalator will be carried out in the lungs. In addition, their activity is terminated by conjugation with α_1-antitrypsin in the plasma. The importance of this mechanism is demonstrated by the high incidence and severity of pulmonary emphysema in people who lack antitrypsin because of a genetic deficiency.

Metabolism and production of biologically active substances

The lungs are in series with the systemic circulation and receive the whole cardiac output; thus they are ideally situated to metabolise and control levels of substances circulating in the blood. They utilise the enormous surface area of the endothelium (100 m^2) to remove or degrade substances that have effects that need to be rapidly terminated once they have carried out their function. These include noradrenaline (norepinephrine), adenosine triphosphate, adenosine diphosphate, adenosine monophosphate, bradykinin, 5-hydroxytryptamine, leukotrienes, prostaglandin-$E_{1 \text{ and } 2}$, and prostaglandin-$F_{2\alpha}$. Substances which are more generally active and sustained in their actions pass through the pulmonary circulation unchanged and include adrenaline (epinephrine), angiotensin II, dopamine, histamine, salbutamol, prostaglandin I_2, and prostaglandin A_2.

Of particular interest, as the only example of activation of a bloodborne substance by the lung, is the transformation of plasma angiotensin I to the powerful vasoconstrictor substance angiotensin II by angiotensin-converting enzyme (ACE). Although this is not restricted to the lung, being found in the plasma and endothelium, the pulmonary vasculature seems to be most plentifully supplied with this enzyme, and 80% of plasma angiotensin I is converted during a single pass through the lungs. ACE is also responsible for the removal of bradykinin from the lungs. The lung endothelium is also responsible for nitric oxide production.

Vasoactive and bronchoactive leukotrienes and prostaglandins, which are released into the circulation under certain conditions, are metabolised from arachidonic acid (apparently so-named because its crystals have the appearance of hairy spiders) by the pulmonary capillary endothelium.

In addition to modifying the blood, the lungs also produce mucopolysaccharides as part of the production of bronchial mucus and secrete immunoglobulins (Ig) into the airways to defend against infection. The production of surfactant by Type II pneumocytes is discussed in Chapter 3.

Non-respiratory functions of the lung

Blood filtration

The lung receives the entire outflow of right-ventricle blood and is perfectly placed to filter particulate matter, protecting the vulnerable cerebral and coronary circulations. Emboli returning to the right heart via the vena cava from the systemic circulation comprise the major filtered load. The lungs filter clumps of fibrin, platelets, agglutinated white and red blood cells, fat droplets, and droplets of amniotic fluid during pregnancy. It is interesting to note that the 7-μm capillary diameter of the pulmonary circulation is not regarded as the overall pore size of the 'filter'; It is well recognised that gas and fat emboli exceeding this size can pass through the pulmonary circulation to access the systemic circulation. Precapillary and intrapulmonary arteriovenous anastomoses exist, which allow the passage of particulate matter, and abnormal intracardiac communications also exist (e.g., the 'probe-patent' foramen ovale found in over 25% of postmortem examinations). Due to the relative pressures of the right and left atria, these normally remain closed but can open if the pressure of the right atrium is increased by a pulmonary embolus.

Blood fluidity

In addition to trapping blood clots, the lung contributes to blood fluidity by being the richest source of factors that promote (thromboplastin) or inhibit (heparin) clotting. The balance between their effects maintains the fluidity of the blood. Thrombi are cleared more rapidly from the lungs than from other organs because the lungs have well-developed proteolytic systems; any blood clots already formed are broken down by the proteolytic enzyme plasmin, activated from its inactive precursor in the plasma by factors found in large quantities in the pulmonary endothelium.

Blood capacity

The pulmonary blood volume is about 500 mL in a recumbent man of around 70 kg. This volume can be halved by increases in pressure within the chest, such as forced expiration against a closed larynx. On the other hand, the volume of blood in the chest can be doubled by forced inspiration. This phenomenon allows the pulmonary circulation to act as a reservoir, for example, at the start of exercise, when the output of the left ventricle rapidly increases. The activity of the sympathetic nervous system may influence the capacity of the system by triggering the contraction of smooth muscle in the blood vessel walls.

Cooling

In animals, the high latent heat of vaporisation of water makes its evaporation from the respiratory surface a useful mechanism for cooling. This mechanism is less evident in humans, perhaps because we use evaporation from our hairless skin. However, a residue of this mechanism can be seen if you stay too long in a very hot bath or if you have a fever; in such circumstances, you will notice that you begin to breathe through your mouth.

Voluntary control of breathing

Breathing is unique among the major functions of the body, in that it is both voluntarily and involuntarily controlled. For example, our hearts and kidneys pump and filter blood without our awareness. However, we cannot control the rate at which they work. Breathing goes on unconsciously for most of the time (except for individuals suffering from 'Ondine's Curse', a syndrome of congenital central hypoventilation, see Chapter 9), but we can take control of our breathing, for example, to allow us to speak.

Our respiratory muscles help other systems of the body in many non-respiratory ways. When lifting a heavy weight, our breathing stops and the muscles of the chest contract to form a rigid cage against which the muscles of the arms can act.

The diaphragm and abdominal muscles contract simultaneously to raise intra-abdominal pressure during vomiting, defecation, and labour. Conversely, inspiration is switched off while swallowing food or drinks to prevent their inhalation. Changes in patterns of breathing can signal emotion, amicable or otherwise, and above all, we use our respiratory system to power speech and vocalisation.

Summary 4

- Relatively large particles are deposited in the nose and pharynx by impaction.
- Smaller particles are deposited in the small airways by sedimentation.
- Sedimented particles are removed to the mouth by the mucociliary escalator.
- Macrophages deal with particles that reach the alveoli
- The pulmonary circulation forms an important filter of the blood, particularly blood clots.

Case 2.1 Structure of the respiratory system

Obstructive sleep apnoea

Mr Sinclair is 50 years old. He is overweight for his height: he is 168 cm tall but weighs 102 kg, with a body mass index of 36 kg m^{-2} He also drinks rather heavily and is a smoker.

For the past two years, Mrs Sinclair has slept in a different room from Mr Sinclair because of his very loud snoring and restlessness at night. Recently, Mr Sinclair has been feeling increasingly tired during the day, and he has been regularly falling asleep when he arrives home from work. Over the past month or so, he has found it difficult to concentrate at work and, on one recent occasion, he was caught sleeping at his desk by his manager, and he is facing disciplinary action. Mrs Sinclair eventually persuaded her husband to visit his doctor.

Mr Sinclair's doctor referred him to a specialist in sleep medicine. The doctor suggested that he may be suffering from obstructive sleep apnoea (OSA). He explained that during periods of deep sleep, Mr Sinclair's airway was becoming obstructed. During an episode of obstruction, Mr Sinclair's sleep becomes lighter until the obstruction is overcome. These episodes of obstruction and sleep interruption are responsible for Mr Sinclair's daytime sleepiness. The doctor went on to suggest that Mr Sinclair be treated with a nasal continuous positive airway pressure device.

In this section we will consider:

1. What causes obstructive sleep apnoea?
2. What are the signs, symptoms, and treatments of obstructive sleep apnoea?

Case 2.1 Structure of the respiratory system

Causes of OSA

For efficient gas flow to take place from the mouth to the alveoli, the airways that make up the respiratory system need to be open and patent. The trachea and larger airways are held open by partial rings of cartilage within their walls. The smaller airways and alveoli are held open by the tension in the lung tissue surrounding them.

Case 2.1 Structure of the respiratory system

Above the larynx, the airway is held open by the actions of airway-dilating muscles, including the genioglossus and palatopharyngeus. Were it not for the actions of these muscles, the upper airway would collapse, particularly when an individual is in the supine position. During sleep, the skeletal muscle tone, throughout the body, is reduced; this applies equally to the muscles which keep the upper airway patent. Therefore the upper airway normally narrows during sleep.

In patients with OSA, airway narrowing is more pronounced than normal, leading to periods of airway obstruction. There are a number of reasons why this happens, but obesity is the most important. It is thought that, in obese patients, the pressure exerted by the fat in the neck tends to cause the airway to collapse. When the tone of the genioglossus and palatopharyngeus is reduced, as during sleep, airway obstruction may result.

The airway may remain obstructed for only a few seconds, or it may be well over a minute before the patient takes his next breath. During this time, the patient may become hypoxic and will begin to make vigorous efforts to try and breathe against the obstructed airway. Furthermore, he will become increasingly aroused from his sleep. Eventually, he regains the tone in his airway-dilating muscles, and the airway obstruction is relieved (patients do not usually waken). After the obstruction has been relieved, ventilation resumes and the patient's sleep deepens. This leads to reduced tone in the airway-dilating muscles and the cycle starts to repeat itself.

Although obesity is probably the most important factor leading to OSA, there are other predisposing factors. These include anatomical variations predisposing to airway narrowing, such as enlarged tonsils, airway tumours, and abnormalities of the mandible. Sedative drugs, including alcohol, may also predispose patients to OSA, probably by affecting sleep patterns and reducing muscle tone. A small number of OSA cases may be explained by abnormalities in neuromuscular function.

Case 2.1 Structure of the respiratory system

Signs and symptoms of OSA

Often, the first person to complain about a patient's OSA is his or her partner. OSA is invariably associated with loud snoring as the airway becomes narrowed; this, combined with the cycles of obstruction and arousal, can lead to a very poor night's sleep for anyone in the same room. By the time a patient presents for treatment, their partner has often resorted to sleeping alone.

The main symptom that the patient complains of is daytime somnolence. Because their sleep patterns are disrupted by cycles of apnoea and arousal, these patients are very tired and sleepy during the day. This may begin to impinge upon the patient's work and home life as their ability to concentrate for long periods of time begins to diminish. At worst, the patient may have a tendency to lose concentration or even fall asleep at the wheel of their car—motor accidents are more common in patients with OSA.

Other symptoms that the patient may complain of include morning headaches and night sweating, and relatives may notice personality changes. For reasons that are not fully understood, patients often complain of having to get up to urinate during the night, sometimes on a few occasions.

Treatment is aimed at reducing the incidence of airway obstruction. The patient is advised to lose weight and limit alcohol consumption, particularly before retiring to bed.

The most effective form of treatment, and the one tried by Mr Sinclair, is continuous positive airway pressure, often delivered via a nasal mask. At night, the patient wears a small mask strapped over the nose to form an airtight seal. A continuous positive pressure, generated by a small machine, is applied to the mask. This pressure is transmitted to the upper airways to prevent their collapse.

Surgical treatment of the condition was once popular but is now rarely performed. Uvulopalatopharyngoplasty involves removing the uvula and part of the soft palate. It has only a limited success rate and is associated with complications, including fluid refluxing into the nose during drinking, and is, therefore, infrequently performed, today.

References and further reading

Doll, H., 1950. Smoking and carcinoma of the lung. Br. Med. J. 2, 739–748.

Garcia-Mouton C, Hidalgo A, Cruz A, Pérez-Gi J. The Lord of the lungs: the essential role of pulmonary surfactant upon inhalation of nanoparticles. Eur J Pharm Biopharm 2019;144:230–43.

Lumb, T., 2020. Functional anatomy of the respiratory tract. In: Lumb, A.B., Thomas, C.R. (Eds.), Nunn's Applied Respiratory Physiology. Elsevier, London, pp. 2–13.

Ochs, et al., 2004. The number of alveoli in the human lung. Am. J. Respir. Crit. Care Med. 169, 120–124.

Silverman, G., Collins, 1997. Metabolic function of the pulmonary endothelium. In: Crystal, R.G., West, J.B., Barnes, P.J., Weibel, E.R. (Eds.), The Lung: Scientific Foundations. Raven Press, New York.
Weibel, 1963. Morphometry of the Human Lung. Academic Press, New York.
Weibel, 1997. Design and morphometry of the pulmonary gas exchanger. In: Crystal, R.G., West, J.B., Barnes, P.J., Weibel, E.R. (Eds.), The Lung: Scientific Foundations. Raven Press, New York.
Young, H., 2000. Wheater's Functional Histology: A Text and Colour Atlas. Churchill Livingstone, Edinburgh.

3 ELASTIC PROPERTIES OF THE RESPIRATORY SYSTEM

Chapter objectives

After studying this chapter, you should be able to:

1. Define compliance and elastance.
2. Describe why compliance changes in disease states.
3. Explain why lung compliance is increased by filling an isolated healthy lung with water.
4. Understand that the interaction between the lungs and chest wall produces negative intrapleural pressure.
5. Explain hysteresis in the context of the relationship between pressure and volume in the lung.
6. Understand the relationship between radius and pressure in bubbles.
7. Explain the significance of the properties of the liquid lining of the lungs and their disturbance in prematurity.
8. Describe how static and dynamic compliance are measured.

Introduction

One of the properties of the respiratory system most often changed by disease is the ease with which it can be expanded and contracted during breathing. The lungs and thoracic cage (the ribcage and diaphragm) are elastic structures, which can be distorted and then return to their original shape when the distorting force is removed. As we learned in Chapter 2, the lungs have no muscles capable of changing their shape to bring about breathing. During spontaneous breathing, the sources of the distorting force are the internal and external intercostal muscles of the thoracic cage, along with the most important inspiratory muscle, the diaphragm. These muscles alter the intrapleural pressure to allow the lungs to change in volume as they fill with air.

In artificial ventilation, distortion is usually produced by a pressure gradient between the airway and the atmosphere. The lungs are not attached to the chest wall, but rather pressed closely to it; the small space between the visceral and parietal pleura is the **intrapleural space** and contains 10–20 mL of viscous fluid (see Chapter 2). Because of this separation, we can consider the properties of the lungs and chest wall separately, whilst bearing in mind that, in life, they work together. The response of the lung to the effects of either the respiratory muscles or a ventilator is determined by the impedance of the respiratory system. This impedance has several sources, including the ***elastic resistance*** of the lungs and the chest wall, and resistance from ***surface forces*** at the very large interface between gas and liquid at the alveolar surface; these are measured when no air or gas is flowing in the airways. Additional factors contributing to impedance are those related to resistance; these occur when air or gas is flowing in the airways and are considered in Chapter 4.

Simple models may be used to describe how changes in the volume of the elastic lungs are brought about by the changes in the pressure around them. The most commonly used model of lung inflation is a balloon. If a balloon is inflated and the air is prevented from escaping by blocking the neck (Fig. 3.1A), the elastic recoil produces a recoil pressure. The pressure inside the balloon will be the same if no flow is taking place into or out of the balloon. A more physiological model of the respiratory system can be made by suspending a balloon in a jar with a piston, such as a large syringe, at its base (Fig. 3.1B). In this case, the balloon represents the lungs, the jar represents the chest wall, and the piston represents the diaphragm. Lowering the piston reduces the pressure around the balloon (intrapleural pressure) and causes it to fill, representing inhalation.

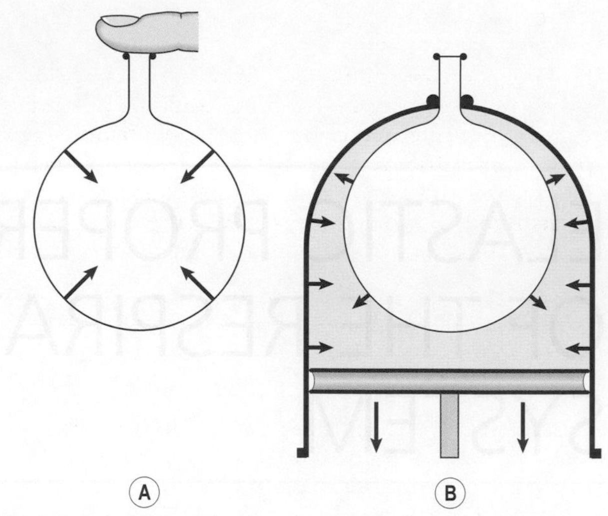

Fig. 3.1 A simple model of breathing. (A) Balloon demonstrating elastic recoil. (B) Physiological model of the respiratory system.

Compliance and elastance

Lung compliance and elastance

Before we consider the elastic properties of the respiratory system further, the concepts of compliance and elastance (see 'Compliance, Elastance, and Elasticity in the Appendix) should be understood. Elasticity is a measure of how easily the lungs can be stretched, conventionally expressed as compliance, and is the change in volume per unit change in pressure. The compliance of the lung is abbreviated as C_L. The **elastance** of the respiratory system reflects its capacity to return to its resting position. Elastance (also known as recoil) is the reciprocal of compliance; thus stiff lungs, which occur in disease states such as acute respiratory distress syndrome (ARDS), have low compliance but high elastance. The potential energy stored as a result of the elastic deformation of the lungs leads to quiet expiration. The compliance of the lungs, lungs and chest wall together, or (rarely) the chest wall alone may be measured. Lung compliance can be measured as either **static compliance**, where pressure and volume are measured when no breathing movements are taking place, or as dynamic compliance, which is measured during the end-inspiratory and end-expiratory points of cyclical breathing when no flow is taking place.

The following overview is useful when considering compliance:

Compliance = the change in volume/unit change in pressure, usually expressed as litres (L) or millilitres (mL) per kilopascal (kPa) (or per centimetres of water). The lung compliance of an average, healthy, young male is approximately 1.5 L kPa^{-1}, or 150 mL cm^{-1} H_2O.

Elastance = 1/compliance

Elastance is the reciprocal of compliance and is expressed in kPa (or centimetres of water) per L (or mL).

Factors affecting lung compliance

The elastic properties of the lungs, and hence their compliance, depend almost equally on two major factors: the elasticity of the lung tissue and the liquid lining of the alveoli.

Effects of disease on lung compliance

Healthy lungs are at optimal compliance, but compliance is affected by most lung diseases. It should be noted that decreased compliance increases the work of breathing (see Chapter 4). In restrictive lung diseases, the compliance of the lung is reduced because a pressure greater than normal is required to achieve the same increase in volume. Obstructive lung disease can also affect lung compliance.

- ***Pulmonary fibrosis*** is an example of a restrictive lung disease in which the lungs are stiffened by the laying down of collagen and fibrin bundles.
- ***Acute respiratory distress syndrome*** is characterised by greatly reduced lung compliance. There is widespread inflammation and increased alveolar capillary membrane permeability, leading to fluid-filled or collapsed alveoli.
- ***Pneumonia*** causes decreased compliance due to inflammation of the lung parenchyma, which results in an accumulation of exudate and collapse of the alveoli and airways. The decrease in volume implies that higher pressures are required to inflate the lungs.
- In ***respiratory distress syndrome of the new-born***, the small alveoli and the immature nature of the liquid lining of the lungs lead to poorly compliant lungs, which are difficult to inflate and are prone to collapse.
- ***Asthma*** is an obstructive lung disease (see Chapter 4) that causes episodes of inflammation and contraction of the bronchial (i.e. small airway) smooth muscle. During normal breathing, the pressure–volume relationship is unaltered; however, when the respiratory rate increases, greater pressure is needed to overcome the airway resistance to airflow and the volume of each breath decreases, leading to a decrease in compliance. During asthma attacks, air can also become trapped in the lungs because of the difficulty in exhaling through constricted small airways; thus each breath is taken from a volume greater than the functional residual capacity (FRC), which also adversely affects compliance.
- ***Emphysema*** leads to an increase in ***static*** compliance because the parenchyma of the lungs is destroyed, resulting in poor elastic recoil. Even in emphysema, however, ***dynamic*** compliance is decreased because of the disordered distribution of ventilation, resulting in variations in the volume of different areas of the lungs.

Other factors affecting lung compliance

- ***Lung volume.*** Compliance is related to lung volume. As above, the lung compliance of an average, healthy, young male is about 1.5 L kPa^{-1}, or 150 mL cm^{-1} H_2O. A man has greater compliance than a mouse due to the difference in the amount of lung being inflated. This can be taken into account by measuring *specific lung compliance* (sC_L) (see later in this chapter). Comparing sC_L values, there is little difference in the values between men and women or between adults and children. The lung volume at which compliance is measured also exerts an effect and is greatest at the FRC.
- ***Pulmonary blood volume.*** Increased pulmonary blood volume or congestion of the pulmonary veins leads to reduced C_L.
- ***Airway resistance.*** An increase in airway resistance leads to a decrease in dynamic compliance. Static compliance is unaffected by the means by which it is measured.
- ***Age.*** Structural changes in lung elastin fibres may cause small increases in compliance with increasing age, but the effect of healthy ageing on compliance tends to be minimal. This is because around half of contributors to C_L are related to surface forces, which do not alter with age.
- ***Posture.*** FRC is reduced when a person is supine, and even smaller if the individual is tilted head-down; it is highest when in the standing position. Compliance is also altered by changes in posture.

Compliance of the thoracic cage

The term chest wall compliance (C_W) is frequently used to describe what should be called thoracic cage compliance. This is because the diaphragm and the abdominal contents pressing on it represent an important element of this component of respiratory mechanics which, unlike the lungs, contains no element of surface tension. At the end of expiration, the lungs do not collapse completely because of the opposing outward force of the thorax holding them out in a slightly expanded condition; the lung volume at the end of a normal expiration is the FRC. At FRC, the outward recoil of the chest wall is exactly matched by the inward recoil of the lungs. The elasticity of the thorax initially helps inspiration; a neutral position is reached at about two-thirds of the **vital capacity**, after that the direction of the elastic forces favours expiration (Fig. 3.2). Perhaps surprisingly, considering their very different structures, the compliance of the thoracic cage is about the same as that of the lungs (1.5 L kPa^{-1}). The compliance of the thoracic cage is very difficult to measure in a spontaneously breathing subject as it can only be properly assessed when the respiratory muscles are totally relaxed. For this reason, it is best determined in anaesthetised patients.

As in the lungs, thoracic cage compliance is influenced by disease, and perhaps even more so than the lungs, by posture and position. Ossification of the costal cartilages and scars resulting from burns to the chest reduce compliance. The diaphragm passively transmits intra-abdominal pressure due to factors such as obesity, venous congestion, or pregnancy; for this reason, changes in posture can reduce the static compliance of the total respiratory system by up to 60% (e.g. when moving from the supine to the prone position).

Total compliance

Total compliance is the compliance of the lungs and chest wall, together, and is abbreviated as C_{tot}. Because the lungs fit inside the thorax rather like an inner tube inside a tyre, they must be treated as elements in *parallel* rather than in ***series*** when their properties are considered together (Fig. 3.3).

We can see that the pressure gradient for both the lungs and chest wall is the gradient from the intrapleural space to the atmosphere. Therefore they are parallel to each other in terms of the pressure gradients. When adding the C_L and C_W values to determine C_{tot}, we must use the relationship appropriate for parallel structures and add reciprocals:

$$1/C_{tot} = 1/C_L + 1/C_W$$

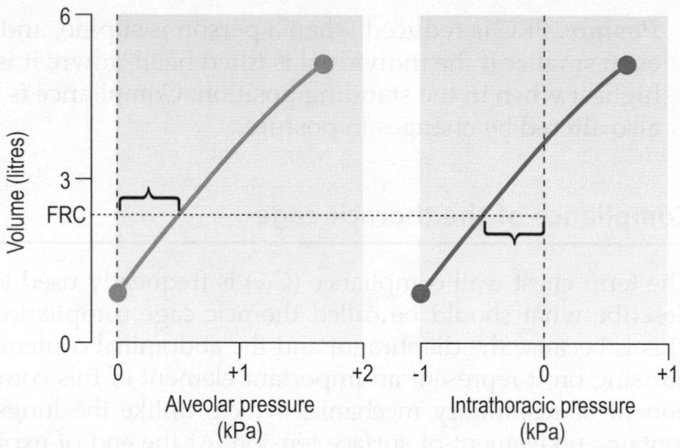

Fig. 3.2 The pressure–volume relationship for (A) excised lungs and (B) an empty thorax. At the functional residual capacity, the recoil pressures of both structures have the same magnitude but opposite signs. Also, the slopes of these lines are similar, showing that the lungs and chest wall have about the same compliance.

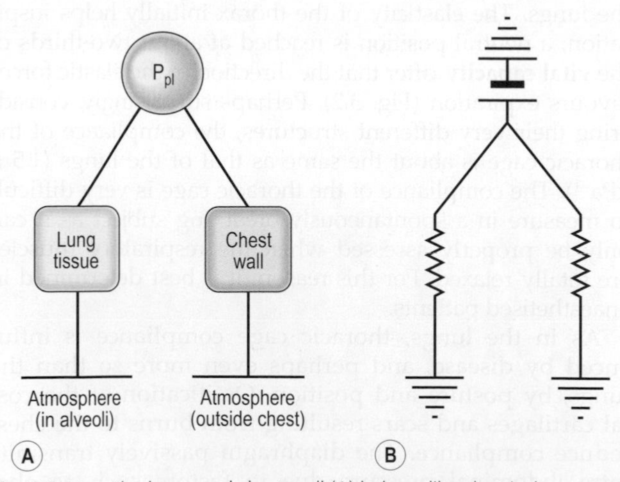

Fig. 3.3 How the lungs and chest wall (A) behave like electrical components (B) in parallel when summed together. P_{pl}, intrapleural pressure.

Because the compliance of the lungs and that of the chest wall are approximately the same (1.5 L kPa^{-1}), a ventilator needs to apply twice the normal change in intrapleural pressure to the air in the lungs of a paralysed patient, compared with a normal patient, to produce a normal volume change.

Intrapleural pressure (P_{pl})

For an object to be stretched or in some other way distorted, it must be subjected to a force. In the case of a three-dimensional object, this force may be pressure. In our simple model of breathing (Fig. 3.1A), inspiration is represented by inflation of a balloon and expiration by deflation. The pressure that brings about inflation in Figure 3.1A is applied to the inside, and a pressure gradient exists from the inside of the balloon to the outside. The other, more complicated way for us to inflate the balloon would be to reduce the pressure outside it using the jar and plunger (Fig. 3.1B). Again, there is a pressure gradient from the inside to the outside of the balloon, and this represents the way we inflate our lungs.

At the end of an expiration, when there is no contraction of the respiratory muscles, there is tension in the thorax between the lungs, the elasticity of which causes them to collapse, and the chest wall, the elasticity of which causes it to spring outward. These two structures are 'locked together' by the intrapleural fluid in the intrapleural space. Because it is a fluid and therefore minimally compressible or expandable, and the intrapleural space is airtight, the lungs are firmly pressed to the chest wall in a manner similar to a suction cup applied to a window. The tension between the lungs attempting to collapse and the chest wall attempting to spring outwards is most clearly seen during surgery. For example, during a cardiac procedure when the sternum is split (a sternotomy) to allow surgical access to the heart or during a thoracotomy that allows access to the lung, the lungs are observed to collapse and the ribs to spring out. Another way of visualising what is happening in the space between the lungs and chest wall is to imagine a syringe with two plungers being pulled in opposite directions (Fig. 3.4).

You can see from such a model that intrapleural pressure is negative with respect to atmospheric pressure. Although not immediately obvious, the P_{pl} is also negative with respect to the air pressure within the alveoli

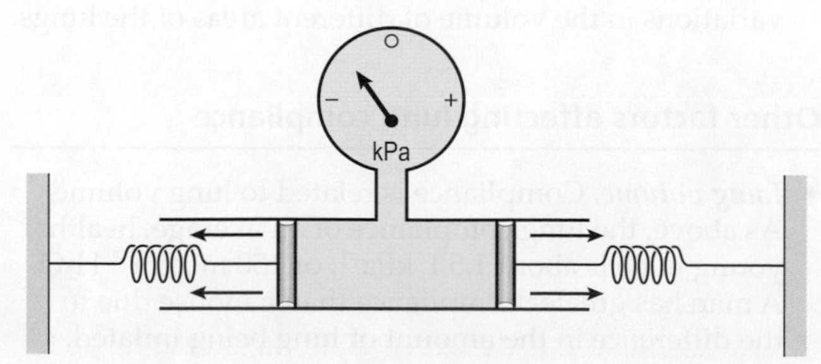

Fig. 3.4 How negative intrapleural pressure is generated.

because the alveoli are connected to the atmosphere by a system of open tubes, the bronchial tree (Fig. 3.5). This means that any communication made between the intrapleural space and either the atmosphere or the alveoli will allow the pressure surrounding the lung to rise and the lung to collapse; this dangerous condition is called a 'pneumothorax' (see Chapter 5).

Because the lungs are suspended from the trachea and rest on the diaphragm, they behave like a very soft spring held at one end and supported from underneath. Gravity causes the lungs to 'slump' under their own weight (Fig. 3.6), causing the chest to behave as if it is filled with a liquid having the average density of the lungs. The pressure increases with descent below the surface of the liquid at a rate dependent on the density of the liquid. Therefore the P_{pl} increases (in fact, becomes less negative) when moving from the apex to the base of the lung. At the end of expiration, the pressure is about –0.8 kPa at the top of the lungs and –0.2 kPa at the base. That this pressure gradient depends on the effect of gravity on the contents of the thorax is clearly demonstrated by the fact that it reverses if the subject in which it is being measured stands on their head.

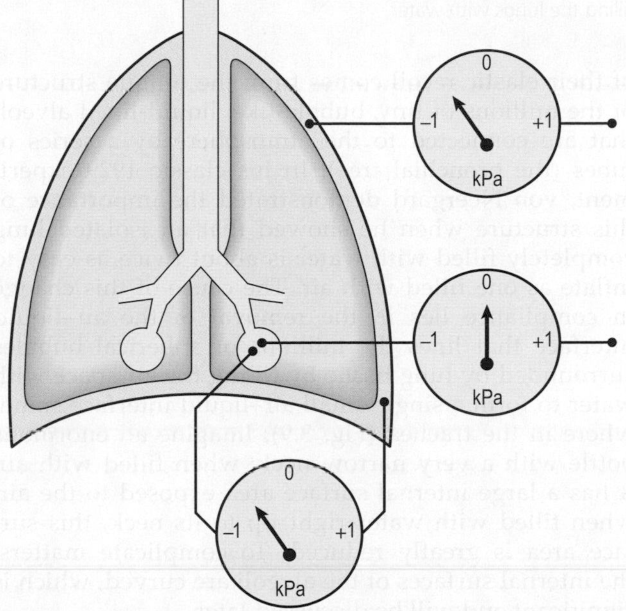

Fig. 3.5 Alveolar and intrapleural pressure compared to atmospheric pressure (100 kPa absolute) at the end of expiration. These lung pressures become more negative during inspiration and are more negative at the apex than at the base of the lung.

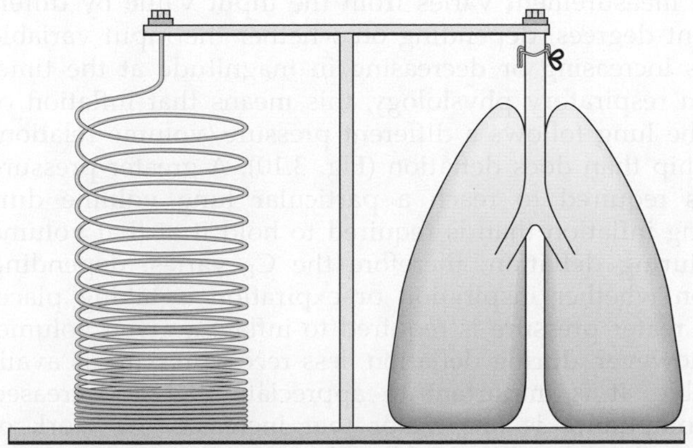

Fig. 3.6 How the lung behaves like a soft spring.

The negative pressure that surrounds the lung expand it to a given volume. If these pressures did not change, the lung volume would not change, and we could not breathe. We cause our lungs to breathe by changing the negative pressure around them by making the diaphragm contract and, like the plunger of a syringe, drawing air into the chest. It should be appreciated that the P_{pl} becomes more negative to bring about inspiration and then becomes less negative during expiration.

The P_{pl} can be measured by inserting a hollow needle between the ribs and into the intrapleural space. Because of the technical challenges of this procedure, and as we are usually more interested in ***changes*** in intrapleural pressure than their absolute values, we frequently measure pressure changes in the oesophagus. The oesophagus is a flexible tube running through the thorax. Because of this property and trajectory, the pressure changes within the oesophagus closely follow the P_{pl} changes and may be used as a surrogate for P_{pl} changes.

It should be noted that mechanical ventilation, used during the support of patients in the operating theatres, intensive care units, or during the transfer of critically ill patients, employs the delivery of ventilation under positive pressure (positive pressure ventilation); therefore physiological negative pressures no longer exist. Intrathoracic pressure becomes positive in this situation, and the ventilator delivers the cyclical inspiratory/expiratory phases.

Summary 1

- Elastic structures return to their original shape when the forces distorting them are removed. Compliance is a measure of how easily a structure can be distended.
- The major components of C_L are the elastic nature of the tissues and the surface forces at air/fluid interfaces in the lining of the lungs.
- The thoracic cage does not have surface tension effects. Its elastic recoil (outwards) is due solely to its elastic tissues.
- Many factors affect C_L and C_W, including disease.
- The lungs are separated from the chest wall by a thin layer of intrapleural fluid.
- The intrapleural fluid is under negative pressure, compared with the atmosphere, due to the recoils of the lungs and chest wall being in opposite directions.

Physical basis of lung compliance

Two major factors affect C_L almost equally: the ***elasticity of the lung tissue*** and the ***liquid lining of the alveoli.***

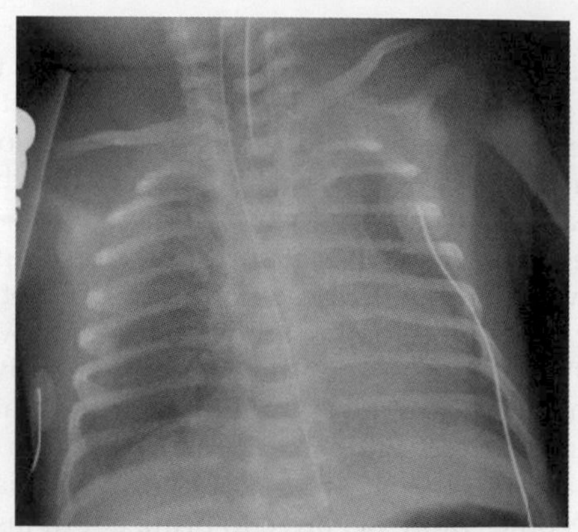

Fig. 3.7 X-ray of the lungs of a child with respiratory distress syndrome. The 'ground glass' appearance of the lungs is clearly visible as is an air bronchogram. (Source: Chan et al., 2019.)

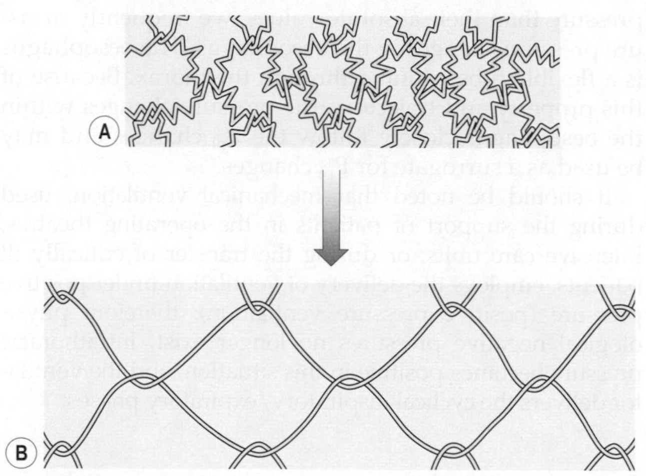

Fig. 3.8 How a nylon stocking stretches when put on (A and B).

Lung tissue elasticity

It might be reasonably assumed that the elastic properties of the lungs are due to the yellow elastin fibres within the lung parenchyma, the same fibre type that gives most other organs their elasticity. In fact, only about half of the elastic recoil of the lungs comes from the elastin fibres in the alveolar walls, bronchioles, and capillaries. Also present in the lungs are collagen fibres, which are less easily stretched and limit overexpansion of the lung. The elastin fibres act in a rather complicated way to provide elasticity. The fibres are kinked and bent around each other and, during inspiration, unfold and rearrange in a manner that has been likened to the straightening of the fibres of a nylon stocking when it is put on (Fig. 3.8).

Liquid lining of the lungs

Around half the elastic recoil of the lungs comes from the elastic properties of their tissues, just as there is recoil in an inflated rubber balloon. The remaining half

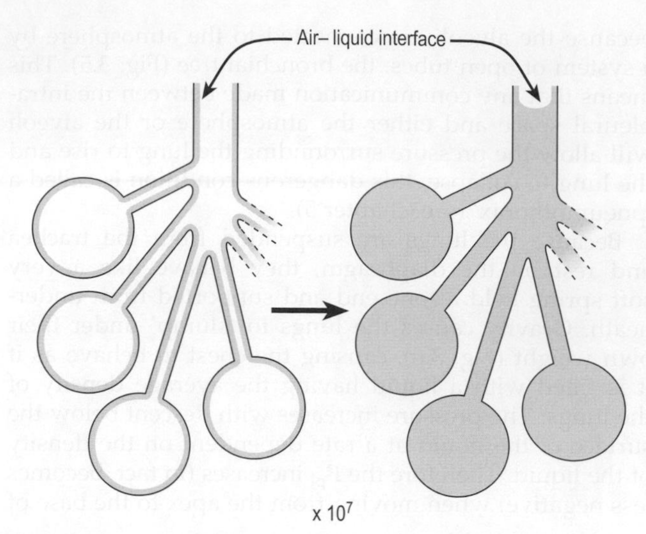

Fig. 3.9 Change in the area of the air–lung interface produced by filling the lungs with water.

of their elastic recoil comes from the unique structure of the millions of tiny, bubble-like, liquid-lined alveoli that are connected to the atmosphere by a series of tubes (the bronchial tree). In his classic 1929 experiment, von Neergard demonstrated the importance of this structure when he showed that an isolated lung completely filled with water is about twice as easy to inflate as one filled with air. The cause of this change in compliance lies in the removal of the air–liquid interface that lines the millions of spherical bubbles surrounded by lung tissue by filling the air space with water to form a single small air–liquid interface somewhere in the trachea (Fig. 3.9). Imagine an enormous bottle with a very narrow neck; when filled with air, it has a large internal surface area exposed to the air; when filled with water right up to its neck, this surface area is greatly reduced. To complicate matters, the internal surfaces of the alveoli are curved, which is significant and will be discussed later.

Not only does filling a lung with fluid make it easier to inflate, it also abolishes the hysteresis seen in the normal lung. Hysteresis (from the Greek *'hysterion'*, meaning 'to lag behind') is the phenomenon whereby a measurement varies from the input value by different degrees, depending on whether the input variable is increasing or decreasing in magnitude at the time. In respiratory physiology, this means that inflation of the lung follows a different pressure/volume relationship than does deflation (Fig. 3.10). A greater pressure is required to reach a particular lung volume during inflation than is required to hold it at that volume during deflation; therefore the C_L varies, depending on whether inspiration or expiration is taking place. Greater pressure is required to inflate a given volume; however, during deflation, less recoil pressure is available. It is important to appreciate that a decreased compliance is one factor that increases the work of breathing (see 'Work of Breathing' in Chapter 4).

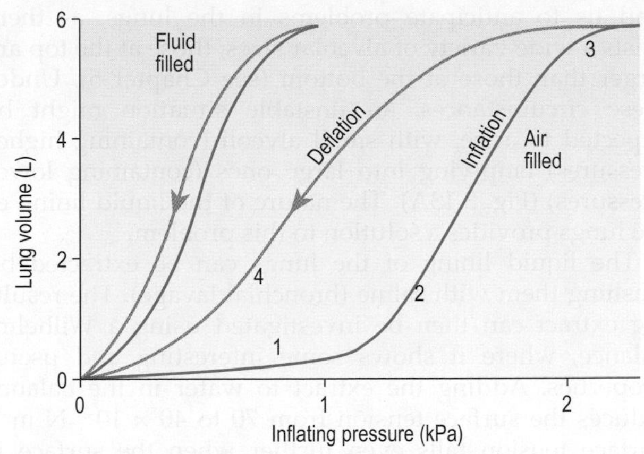

Fig. 3.10 The effect of filling a lung with water, destroying the air–liquid interface; pressure and volume were measured under static conditions. The air-filled lung requires different pressures to hold it at a given volume, depending on whether it is being inflated or deflated (hysteresis). This effect is almost abolished by filling the lung with fluid. Inflating the fluid-filled lung is also much easier than inflating the air-filled lung. The air-filled lung does not begin to inflate until a 'critical opening pressure' of about 1 kPa is reached. At this pressure, alveoli begin to pop open.

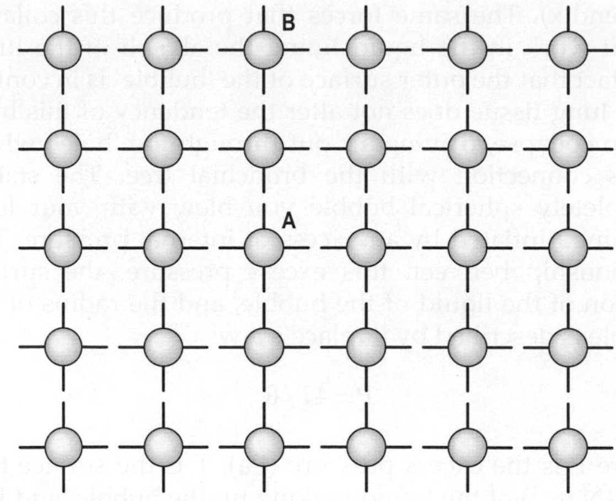

Fig. 3.11 How a surface arises in a liquid. Molecules of a liquid attract each other. The molecule at position *A* is attracted on all sides and so is in a balanced situation. Molecule *B*, at the surface, has no molecules above it and is in tension with those on either side.

These peculiar findings are due to the nature of the bubbles (alveoli) and the properties of the liquid that make up the liquid lining of the lung. We need to consider the nature of the surface of liquids, the nature of bubbles, and the special properties of the liquid lining of the alveoli to understand the static and dynamic compliance of the lungs.

The surface of liquids

Liquids form a clear boundary between themselves and the air. That this boundary is under tension or stress is clearly seen in the liquids we come across in everyday life (e.g. the surface of a cup of coffee, if touched lightly with a spoon, seems to leap up to the spoon). This is the effect of surface tension (Fig. 3.11). The 'skin' or surface of a liquid exists because there is an imbalance of the forces acting on the molecules at the surface (see 'States of Matter', Appendix).

Just as mechanical and chemical systems move to states of minimal energy (maximum entropy), surfaces seek minimal energy and hence minimal area (this is why water droplets are spheres; that shape has the minimum surface area for a given mass). The tendency to reduce the surface area produces tension at the liquid surface, which can be measured using a surface balance (Fig. 3.12). In this process, a bar of metal dips into the liquid and is exposed to the same forces that act on molecules at the surface of liquids. These forces can be measured using a sensitive transducer. The total force depends on the surface tension and the length of the bar; the units of surface tension are therefore N m^{-1}. A surface balance was modified to produce the *Wilhelmi balance* by the ingenious addition of a movable barrier

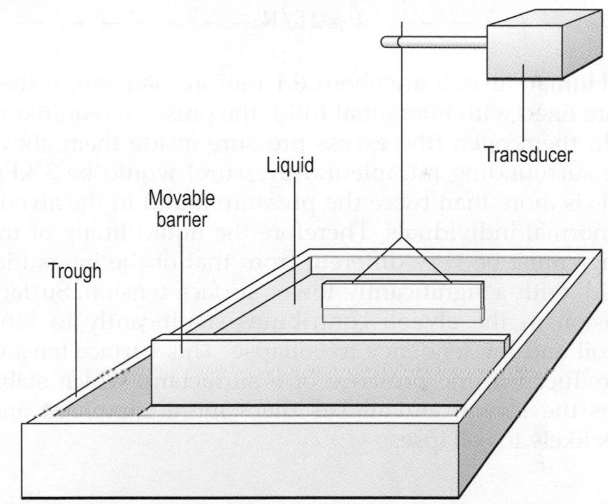

Fig. 3.12 The Wilhelmi balance for measuring surface tension in a liquid while changing its surface area. The movable barrier compresses or expands the surface film. The tension in the surface is measured by the pull on the vertical plate suspended in the liquid.

that can compress the surface of the liquid in the balance trough. Under these circumstances, the depth of the liquid changes as the barrier is moved, but this does not matter because it is the air–liquid interface that is important.

The nature of bubbles

Anyone who has used a pipe or loop to create soap bubbles has demonstrated most of the basic physical principles underlying the elastic recoil of the lung due to its liquid lining. Once a complete sphere has formed, the bubble is stable. However, if you stop blowing while there is a hole in the bubble, the bubble immediately collapses and returns to a flat layer of soap stretched across the pipe or loop (see 'Surface Tension and Bubbles' in the

Appendix). The same forces that produce this collapse are at work in the liquid lining the alveoli of the lung. The fact that the outer surface of the 'bubble' is in contact with lung tissue does not alter the tendency of this bubble to collapse, driving air out through the 'hole', which is its connection with the bronchial tree. The stable, completely spherical bubble you blew with your loop remained inflated by an excess of internal pressure. The relationship between this excess pressure, the surface tension of the liquid of the bubble, and the radius of the bubble is described by Laplace's law:

$$P = 4T/R$$

where P is the excess pressure (Pa), T is the surface tension ($N\ m^{-1}$) of the liquid making up the bubble, and R is the radius (m) of the bubble. Constant 4 appears in this equation because a bubble has two surfaces exposed to air. For alveoli with outer surfaces in contact with the lung tissue, it becomes

$$P = 2T/R$$

Human alveoli are about 0.1 mm in diameter; if they were lined with interstitial fluid, the pressure required to hold them open (the excess pressure inside them above the surrounding intrapleural pressure) would be 3 kPa. This is more than twice the pressure found in the alveoli of normal individuals. Therefore the liquid lining of the lungs must be very different from that of the interstitial fluid, with a significantly lower surface tension. Surface tension in the alveoli contributes significantly to lung recoil and the tendency to collapse. This surface tension is reduced in the presence of a surfactant, which stabilises the alveoli and makes them more compliant and less likely to collapse.

Surfactant in the liquid lining of alveoli

If pure water is placed in the Wilhelmi balance, moving the barrier to and fro (and therefore expanding and contracting the surface) has no effect on the measured surface tension. However, if a phospholipid of the type found lining the alveoli of the lungs is placed on the surface of the liquid, it spreads out to form a layer between the water and the air. Now, the surface tension changes as the barrier advances, forcing the phospholipid molecules closer together, or as it retreats, allowing them to separate. The tension reaches a minimum when all the phospholipid molecules are neatly packed as a single layer on the surface. When the surface area is further reduced, the molecules pile up on each other, and the tension begins to rise again. It is possible to measure the size of the phospholipid molecules using the area of the surface at which the surface tension is minimal.

From Laplace's law, we can see, perhaps counterintuitively, that the pressure in a small bubble is expected to be greater than the pressure in a large bubble. This might lead us to anticipate problems in the lungs, as there exists a wide variety of alveolar sizes; those at the top are larger than those at the bottom (see Chapter 5). Under these circumstances, an unstable situation might be expected to arise, with small alveoli (containing higher pressures) emptying into large ones (containing lower pressures) (Fig. 3.13A). The nature of the liquid lining of the lungs provides a solution to this problem.

The liquid lining of the lungs can be extracted by washing them with saline (bronchial lavage). The resulting extract can then be investigated using a Wilhelmi balance, where it shows some interesting and useful properties. Adding the extract to water in the balance reduces the surface tension from 70 to 40 × 10^{-3} $N\ m^{-1}$. Surface tension falls even further when the surface is compressed, reaching a minimum below 10 × 10^{-2} $N\ m^{-1}$, which is due to surfactant secreted by the Type II pneumocyte cells (see Chapter 2) of the alveolar epithelium (Fig. 3.14).

The surfactant spreads over the inner surface of the alveoli and into the bronchioles; it is made up of dipalmitoyl phosphatidylcholine, and its structure and arrangement at the air–liquid interface are shown in Figure 3.15. The straight structure of these molecules enables them to

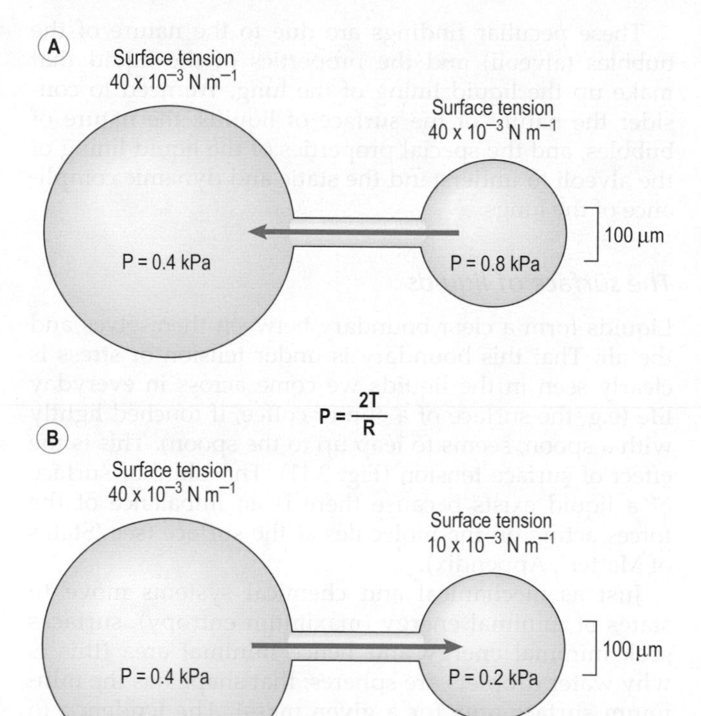

Fig. 3.13 How the special properties of lung surfactant cope with the potential problem of differences in pressure arising in alveoli of different diameters. (A) Two bubbles (alveoli) of different sizes, but having the same surface tension, are connected and the smaller empties into the larger. (B) The sort of change produced by lung inflation and deflation on the surface tension of its liquid lining. The change in tension compensates for the differences in radii and may even overcompensate and cause large alveoli to empty into small ones.

pack more closely during expiration than would other shapes. This packing and unpacking during inspiration and expiration causes the surface tension to decrease and increase in a manner that produces the characteristic hysteresis of the lungs. The change in surface tension also provides a solution to the problem posed earlier regarding alveoli of different sizes having different pressures, and the tendency for the small to empty into the large (Fig. 3.13A). If the surface tension in a large alveolus is sufficiently greater than the tension in a small one, the effect of the larger radius (R) in Laplace's law will be matched or even overpowered by changes in tension (T).

This is what happens in the lung: the surface tension changes to match the radius so that all alveoli contain about the same air pressure and the small do not tend to empty into the large (Fig. 3.13B). The air pressure inside an alveolus not only resists the effects of surface tension, causing the alveolus to collapse, but also resists the exudation of fluid from the pulmonary capillaries into the alveolar space. If the surface tension is reduced at any particular air pressure within an alveolus, more of that air pressure will be available to resist exudation and prevent pulmonary oedema.

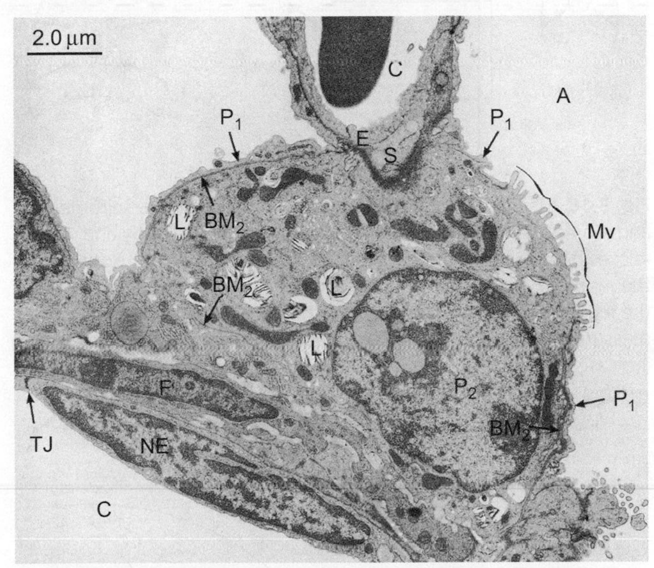

Fig. 3.14 Electron micrograph of an alveolar type II pneumocyte (P2). Most of the cell is surrounded by basement membrane (BM2). It is possible that surfactant from the lamellar bodies (L) is only secreted via the microvilli (Mv) into the alveolar space (A). C, capillary; P1, type I pneumocyte; TJ, tight junction.

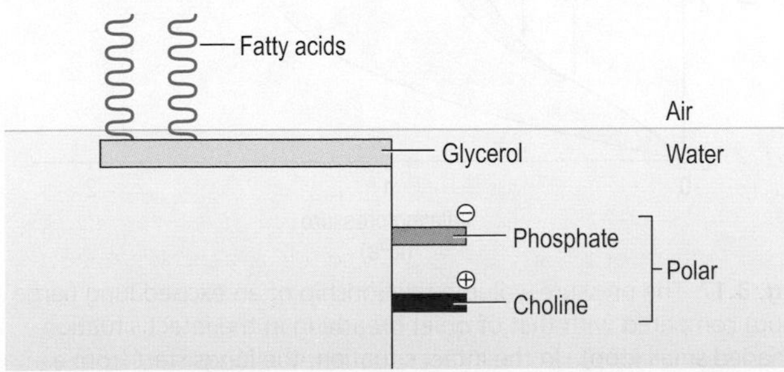

Fig. 3.15 The molecular structure of phosphatidylcholine and the way it orientates itself at an air–water interface.

The presence of surfactant is clearly important to normal lung function. It:

- reduces surface tension and therefore elastic recoil, making breathing easier and the alveoli less likely to collapse,
- reduces the tendency for pulmonary oedema to develop,
- equalises pressure in the large and small alveoli, and
- produces hysteresis, which 'props' alveoli open during exhalation.

Pulmonary surfactant appears rather late in human embryological development, at about 30 weeks. Women in preterm labour, between 24 and 34 weeks of gestation, are offered corticosteroids to promote the production of surfactant by their baby to reduce the incidence and severity of postnatal lung disease.

Opening and closing of alveoli

Even in an isolated lung, the relationship between pressure and volume is complicated by the interaction of the surface forces already discussed and the elastic tissue of the lung. One of the most important aspects of this is the tendency for alveoli to close at low lung volumes, despite assistance from the surfactant to stay open.

Range *1* of Figure 3.10 is the result of alveoli staying shut despite increased inflation pressure.

Range 2 begins at approximately 1 kPa when alveoli begin to pop open, and the lung inflates with very little increase in pressure.

Range 3 is where tissue elasticity, particularly from collagen fibres, stiffens the lung.

Range 4 is deflation, where surfactant hysteresis 'props open' the alveoli.

The lung volume at which the airways in the lower part of the lung begin to close (Range 1) is known as the 'closing volume'. This has considerable significance because regions of the lungs that are closed off from the atmosphere are functionally useless. In young people, the closing volume is less than the FRC. By an average age of 66 years, the closing volume equals the FRC, with the unfortunate consequence of increasing airway closure and reducing the ventilation of the lower lung.

Different functional units in the lungs may also have different **time constants**. These are sometimes termed 'fast' or 'slow' alveoli. A 'fast' alveolus has a low airway resistance (see Chapter 4) and a low compliance, therefore it reaches its maximal inflation more quickly. A 'slow' alveolus has a high airway resistance and a high compliance, therefore taking longer to reach its maximal inflation. If the lung consisted of tissues with similar time constants, then the distribution of ventilation (see Chapter 5) would be unaffected by the rate of inflation. If the lung is composed of tissues with variable time constants, the rate of inflation of the lung will affect the way ventilation is distributed within the lung. Under these circumstances, if an inflation breath was to be held, redistribution of ventilation from fast to slow alveoli would occur during this hold. Diseased lungs (e.g. chronic obstructive pulmonary disease) tend to demonstrate more heterogeneous time constants.

Measuring compliance

Static lung compliance

'Static conditions' are required to measure static compliance. These conditions are achieved when the subject breathes in a known volume of air relative to their baseline FRC (see Chapter 11) and relaxes against a closed airway. Changes in volume can be measured using a spirometer, body plethysmography, or integrated from the air flow determined using a pneumotachograph (see Chapter 4). The pressure change is equivalent to the unit change in the transmural pressure gradient, that is, the change in the pressure gradient from the alveoli to the intrapleural space. The change in pressure in the oesophagus as it passes through the thorax may be used as an indication of the change in pressure of the intrapleural space, which is otherwise difficult to measure directly. Intraoesophageal pressure is measured by introducing a catheter and small air-filled balloon, attached to a pressure transducer, into the oesophagus via the nose. Because intraoesophageal pressure rises as the balloon descends, the pressure reading is conventionally taken when the balloon has been passed 32–35 cm into the oesophagus from the tip of the nose. Alveolar pressure cannot be measured directly; however, when no gas is flowing, it is equal to the mouth pressure, which can be measured. The slope of the resultant pressure–volume graph is the total static compliance (Fig. 3.16).

Measuring C_{tot} (lungs *and* chest wall) is much easier because, in this case, the required measurement is simply the gradient between the alveoli (or mouth pressure under static conditions) and the atmosphere. These conditions are achieved when the subject breathes in a known volume, from their baseline FRC, and relaxes against a closed airway; the values are compared to the baseline values measured at FRC. The slope of the resultant pressure–volume graph is the total static compliance (Fig. 3.16).

The slopes of the lines making up the loops in Fig. 3.17 are a comparison of the compliance of lungs when intact in the body and their behaviour when excised. When excised, the loop describes the behaviour of the lung from total collapse to its maximum volume. During normal breathing, there are about 2.5 L of air left in the lungs at the end of expiration (the FRC) and we are seldom able to inhale to total lung capacity (TLC). Most quiet breathing takes place within the shaded area represented in Fig. 3.17, which shows less hysteresis than the total collapse to total volume manoeuvre. The representation still shows that compliance reduces (i.e. the curve flattens) due to airway collapse when the residual volume (RV) is approached.

The lung compliance of an average, healthy, young male is about 1.5 L kPa^{-1}. Because C_L depends on a change in volume, it also depends on lung and body size, and this effect is taken into account by measuring

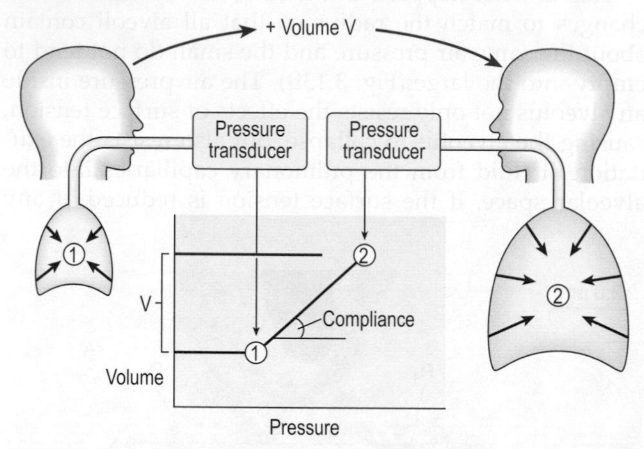

Fig. 3.16 Measuring total static compliance using only a spirometer and a pressure transducer. The subject breathes in slightly and relaxes his respiratory system while holding a pressure transducer in the mouth. He breathes in a further known volume (V), holds it in the lungs, and again relaxes against the transducer. This provides a measure of the increased lung recoil pressure associated with a known increase in volume.

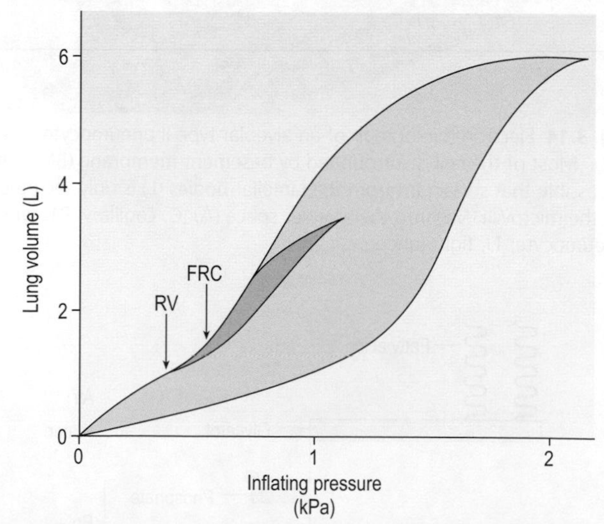

Fig. 3.17 The pressure–volume relationship of an excised lung (large loop) compared with that of quiet breathing in the intact situation (shaded small loop). In the intact situation, the lungs start from a partially inflated state at the functional residual capacity; there is little hysteresis. These curves were obtained under static conditions.

sC_L, which is compliance divided by the FRC. The nature of specific compliance can be visualised by considering the inflation of one or more balloons by a pump that provides as much air as you like, but only to a maximum pressure of 1 kPa above atmospheric pressure. If a single balloon is connected to the pump and is inflated to 2 L, the balloon has a compliance (volume increase/pressure) of 2 L kPa^{-1} (Fig. 3.18A). If two balloons are connected to the pump, they will both be subjected to a pressure of 1 kPa and increase in volume by 2 L, each (4 L, total), which gives the system a compliance (volume increase/pressure) of 4 L kPa^{-1} (Fig. 3.18B).

Dynamic lung compliance

Perhaps counterintuitively, dynamic compliance is also measured under static conditions, but the measurements are taken from a breathing subject. Two no-flow points occur in the respiratory cycle (at the end of inspiration and at the end of expiration) during which measurements are made. Measurements of dynamic compliance are therefore made 'on the fly', with less time for air to redistribute to the areas of the lung which fill more slowly. The change in the pressure gradient (intrapleural – alveolar pressure) and lung volume are measured (Fig. 3.19A), and the compliance is calculated as shown previously. Alternatively, the changes in P_{pl} and volume can be displayed as a loop (Fig. 3.19B). In this case, the angle of the long axis of the loop (volume/pressure) represents dynamic compliance. The area of the loop represents the work of breathing (see Chapter 4).

In a patient who is awake and spontaneously breathing, measuring compliance is difficult because of the need for intraoesophageal pressure measurements. However, in an intubated, anaesthetised patient on a ventilator, it is more straightforward because most ventilators are able to measure the volume of a breath (**tidal volume**) and the airway pressure.

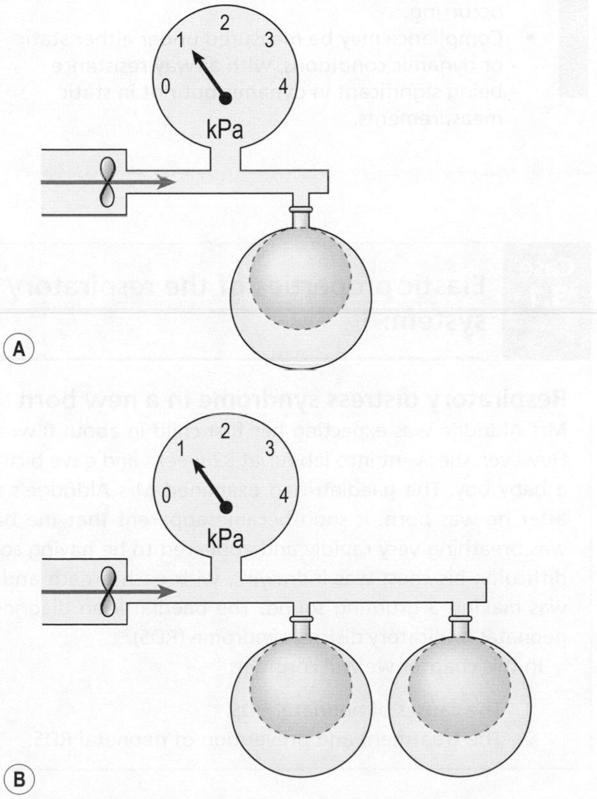

Fig. 3.18 The nature of specific compliance. A pump with an unlimited supply of air but delivering a fixed pressure will inflate (A) one or (B) any number of identical balloons, each to the same volume. The compliance (change in volume/change in pressure) of these two systems is very different.

Comparing static and dynamic compliance

Dynamic compliance reflects the overall impedance to a change in volume, and this takes into account both the elastic and resistance properties of the lung. In lungs in which all alveolar units inflate equally within a given timeframe, the ratio of dynamic compliance to static compliance is fairly constant at all respiratory rates. However, because measurements of dynamic compliance are made during short inspiratory or expiratory pauses in a breathing subject, when there is little time for the

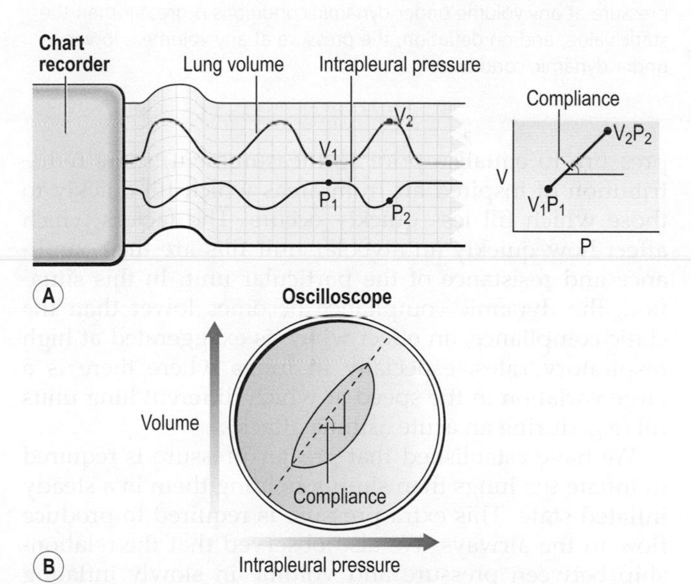

Fig. 3.19 Dynamic compliance. As with static compliance, we need to measure distending pressure and lung volume. The distending pressure is the *intrapleural pressure*. If this is displayed on a chart together with *lung volume*, points of zero flow can be detected at the peak of inspiration and at the end of expiration (A). *Compliance* is derived from these two conditions by the same method used for determining static compliance. Alternatively, *intrapleural pressure* (measured directly or using a balloon in the oesophagus) can be plotted against *lung volume* on what is known as a persistence *oscilloscope*; this draws a loop, the slope of which is proportional to *compliance* (B).

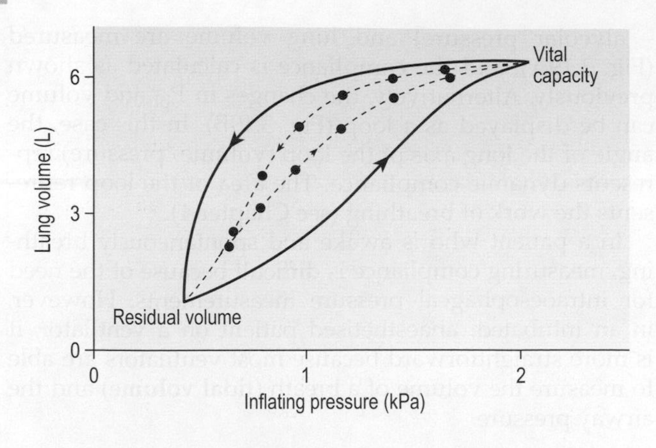

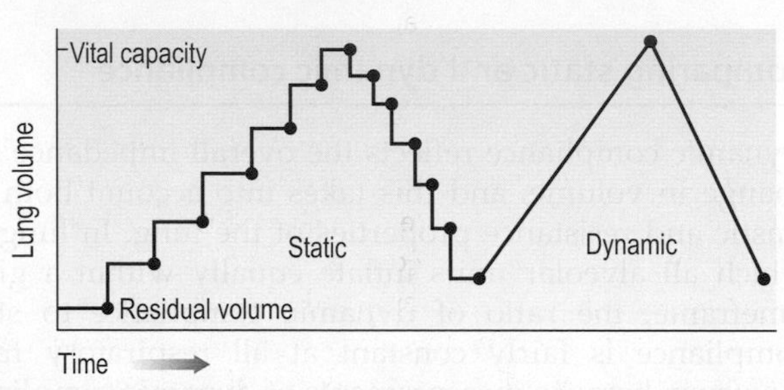

Fig. 3.20 Dynamic and pseudostatic lung inflation. The different relationships between volume and inflating pressure, in an excised lung, when inflation is in a series of steps (with pressure measured under static conditions after each step), or dynamically, with air flowing continuously into or out of the lung. During inflation, the pressure at any volume under dynamic conditions is greater than the static value, and on deflation, the pressure at any volume is lower under dynamic conditions.

pressure to equalise prior to measurement, some redistribution of inspired air from areas which fill quickly to those which fill less quickly occurs. The factors which affect how quickly an alveolar unit fills are the compliance and resistance of the particular unit. In this situation, the dynamic compliance becomes lower than the static compliance, an effect which is exaggerated at high respiratory rates, especially in lungs where there is a large variation in the speed at which different lung units fill (e.g. during an acute asthma attack).

We have established that greater pressure is required to inflate the lungs than simply holding them in a steady inflated state. This extra pressure is required to produce flow in the airways. We also observed that the relationship between pressure and volume in slowly inflating and deflating lungs is not a straight line, as you would get with a rubber balloon, but rather a loop, with a greater pressure needed to *inflate* the lungs to a given volume than that which exists at the same volume when they are allowed to deflate (Fig. 3.20). The small, dotted loop in Figure 3.20 was produced by inflating and deflating lungs slowly and stopping after each incremental inflation, a process called pseudostatic. If inflation and deflation are carried out at a normal respiratory rate (12 times per minute), the loop would be wider (solid line). **The inflation** pressures required for any given volume are greater under dynamic conditions than under static conditions, and **deflation** pressures are lower under dynamic conditions than under static conditions.

Summary 2

- Around half the elastic recoil of the lungs is due to their elastic properties, and the rest is due to their liquid lining.
- Air/liquid interfaces tend to contract, an effect known as the surface tension.
- Each lung is effectively made up of millions of bubbles. According to Laplace's law, because of radii differences, the small 'bubbles' should tend to collapse into the large ones.
- The lung is lined with a liquid that is similar to plasma, but with differences important to surface tension. Type II pneumocytes produce surfactants, which makes it easier to inflate the lungs and prevent this tendency of the alveoli to collapse from occurring.
- Compliance may be measured under either static or dynamic conditions, with airway resistance being significant in dynamic but not in static measurements.

Case 3.1 Elastic properties of the respiratory system: 1

Respiratory distress syndrome in a new born

Mrs Aldridge was expecting her first child in about 8 weeks. However, she went into labour at 32 weeks and gave birth to a baby boy. The paediatrician examined Mrs Aldridge's son after he was born. It soon became apparent that the baby was breathing very rapidly and appeared to be having some difficulty: his chest was indrawing with each breath and he was making a grunting sound. The paediatrician diagnosed neonatal respiratory distress syndrome (RDS).

In this chapter we will consider:

1. The causes of neonatal RDS.
2. The treatment and prevention of neonatal RDS.

Case 3.1 Elastic properties of the respiratory system: 2

Causes of RDS in new-borns

The principal cause of neonatal RDS is a deficiency of lung surfactant due to prematurity; the disease is also related to the general immaturity of a premature baby's respiratory system. The more premature an infant, the more likely it is to develop RDS.

The Type II pneumocytes that produce surfactant develop at about 24 weeks of gestation, although most fetuses do not start producing large amounts of surfactant until about 34 weeks (term babies are born at 40 weeks). Premature babies also have smaller lungs and alveoli than full-term babies. Remember Laplace's law, which states:

$$P = 2T/R$$

where P is the pressure inside a bubble, T is the surface tension, and R is the radius. In the alveoli of premature infants, T is greater than normal because of the lack of surfactant; R is also smaller than normal because the premature infant has smaller alveoli. For these reasons, high pressure (P) is needed to keep the alveoli open. This means that the neonate's lungs tend to collapse during expiration, and the effort of inspiration is very much increased. Furthermore, the lack of surfactant means that fluid tends to be drawn from the blood into the alveoli, which therefore become oedematous. All these things mean that the dynamic compliance of the lungs is very much decreased.

Because it has not developed fully, the compliance of a premature infant's chest wall is high, and this means that respiratory effort causes indrawing of the chest wall. Grunting in infants is thought to be an effort to increase airway pressure during expiration, which would tend to reduce airway collapse. Blood still flows through the collapsed areas of the lungs but remains deoxygenated. Without treatment, the baby's respiratory distress would become worse and would eventually lead to respiratory failure as the baby becomes increasingly hypoxic and exhausted by the effort of breathing.

The large number of collapsed alveoli leads to a characteristic chest X-ray appearance. Baby Aldridge's chest X-ray is shown in Figure 3.7. The collapsed alveoli give the chest X-ray a 'ground-glass' appearance. Against this are visible air bronchograms, which are the shadows of the gas within the bronchi. These are only visible on a chest X-ray if the lung tissue around them is unusually dense.

The lungs of infants who have died from RDS have a characteristic appearance under the microscope. The alveoli are collapsed, and they and the respiratory bronchioles appear to be lined with a membrane. This membrane is made up of proteinaceous exudates from the airways and can, in fact, be caused by many types of lung injuries, not only RDS. Because of its appearance with commonly used histological stains, the membrane is usually described as *hyaline*, meaning nearly transparent. For this reason, RDS was previously called 'hyaline membrane disease'.

Case 3.1 Elastic properties of the respiratory system: 3

Treatment and prevention of RDS in new-borns

Baby Aldridge was initially given oxygen by the paediatrician. An endotracheal tube was then inserted into his trachea and he was placed on a mechanical ventilator. Artificial surfactant was administered through the endotracheal tube in order to treat the natural surfactant deficiency. Mechanical ventilation was continued for 1 week, during which time Baby Aldridge continued to improve. After this time, the endotracheal tube was removed, and he was able to breathe by himself.

Mechanical ventilation is usually required for infants with RDS. However, the ventilation needs to be carried out very carefully. This is because of the low compliance of the infant's lungs, which means that relatively high airway pressures are needed to achieve adequate tidal and minute volumes. High airway pressures can cause trauma to immature lungs and airways, potentially causing a pneumothorax. Furthermore, high inspired oxygen concentrations (greater than 50% oxygen) can also cause lung damage. Such damage is caused by oxygen free radicals, which are toxic molecules. Reactive oxygen species include the hydroxide ion and the superoxide ion. These molecules have an unpaired electron, making them very reactive; high oxygen concentrations favour their production. The lung damage that can be caused by high airway pressures and high oxygen concentrations can lead to a chronic lung condition called 'bronchopulmonary dysplasia'.

In addition to artificial ventilation of the lungs, RDS is treated with exogenous surfactant, which is either an artificial preparation or obtained from the lungs of (mammalian) animals. One or two doses of artificial surfactant are administered to premature babies in order to try to prevent or treat RDS. Natural surfactant, obtained from animal lungs, or artificial surfactant containing dipalmitoyl phosphatidylcholine can be used. The administered surfactant acts in the same way as the endogenous surfactant to reduce the surface tension in the alveoli, stabilising them and increasing C_L.

It is also possible to try and prevent RDS, when a birth is expected to be premature (e.g. in the case of a foetus that is not growing adequately in the uterus and whose birth is to be induced). Administration of steroids to the mother increases the rate of foetal lung maturation and reduces the likelihood of RDS occurring in the neonate.

With modern treatment, survival rates in babies affected by RDS are good, particularly in older premature babies.

References and further reading

Chan R.Y., Pietzak M., Salazar A., 2019. Pediatrics Morning Report: Beyond the Pearls. Elsevier, Philadelphia.

Cotes, J.E., 1993. Lung Function: Assessment and Application in Medicine. Blackwell Science, Oxford.

De Troyer, 1997. Respiratory muscles. In: Crystal, R.G., West, J.B., Barnes, P.J., Weibel, E.R. (Eds.), The Lung: Scientific Foundation. New York Press.

Harris, R.S., 2005. Pressure-Volume Curves of the Respiratory System Respir Care, 50, pp. 78–98.

Jackson, 2012. Respiratory distress in preterm infants. In: Gleason, C.A., Devaskar, S.U. (Eds.), Avery's Diseases of Newborn. W.B. Saunders, Philadelphia, pp. 633–646.

Lumb, Thomas, 2020. Elastic forces and lung volumes. In: Lumb, A.B., Thomas, C.R. (Eds.), Nunn Applied Respiratory Physiology. Elsevier, London, pp. 14–26.

4

AIRFLOW AND RESISTANCE IN THE RESPIRATORY SYSTEM

Chapter objectives

After studying this chapter, you should be able to:

1. Define airway resistance.
2. State the relationship between airway radius and flow.
3. Describe laminar and turbulent flow and their significance.
4. Understand that airway resistance is a dynamic property.
5. Describe the distribution of airway resistance throughout the respiratory tract.
6. Outline the physiological factors that determine airway resistance.
7. Relate the concept of an equal pressure point to the collapse of airways, particularly in emphysema.
8. Explain how pattern of breathing relates to work of breathing.
9. List factors influencing bronchial smooth muscle tone.
10. Differentiate between reversible and nonreversible obstructive disease.
11. Explain the basis of clinical tests to evaluate airway resistance and differentiate between diseases.

Introduction

The lungs are blind-ended structures with only one entrance or exit, the trachea. Air is moved into the lungs and then removed when the exchange of gas between air and blood is complete; this movement of air takes place via the airways (see Chapter 2). Diseases of the airways include ***asthma*** and *chronic obstructive pulmonary disease* (COPD) which, together, account for the majority of respiratory diseases seen in clinical practice. Because of the association between smoking and air pollution and the development of COPD, this disease contributes significantly to the global health burden. The World Health Organisation reported that, in 2016, COPD was the third-ranked cause of death, worldwide, claiming 3 million lives.

There are many causes of obstructed or impaired airflow, including:

- obstruction of the airways (e.g. by foreign bodies, neoplasms, or secretions)
- reduction in diameter due to contraction of smooth muscle in the walls of the airway (e.g. asthma) or swelling due to inflammation (e.g. bronchitis)
- collapse of the airways due to disruption of the supporting parenchyma (e.g. emphysema) or changes in intrapleural pressure (e.g. coughing)

We saw, in the previous chapter, that negative intrapleural pressure holds the lungs 'stretched' against the chest wall. The degree of stretch, and therefore the lung volume, depends on the compliance of the lungs and the intrapleural pressure. We have also learned that movements of the lung are entirely passive and result from external forces. To breathe, intrapleural pressure is altered; it is lowered (becomes more negative) to bring about inspiration and increases (becomes less negative) during expiration.

The **impedance** of the respiratory system dictates the response of the lung to these changes. The elastic resistance of the lungs and thoracic cage and the resistance from surface forces at the large air–liquid interfaces of the lungs are discussed in Chapter 3. Additional important sources of impedance are known as nonelastic resistance. Nonelastic resistance is caused by frictional resistance to flow (**airway resistance**), resistance to thoracic tissue deformation, and inertia. These are relevant when air or gas is flowing in the airways. During breathing, intrapleural pressure can be considered to have two components: that which is required to hold the lungs open (the static component) *plus* a component to move the air in or out of the lungs. The latter component overcomes airway resistance. The pressure change required to overcome the resistance of the tissues and the inertia of the system is less significant.

Bringing about airflow

Our model from the previous chapter, in which the respiratory system is represented as a balloon inside a container, is often used to illustrate the two components of intrapleural pressure mentioned earlier and illustrated in Figure 4.1. The plunger of the syringe represents the diaphragm, the walls of the syringe represent the chest wall, the balloon represents the alveoli, and the narrow tube represents the airways of the lung. To hold the balloon inflated requires a certain effort; to draw air into the balloon (inspiration) requires more effort. There are three additional aspects which are, perhaps, not so obvious initially, but which can be deduced from this model of breathing; all have clinical relevance:

1. The changes in intrapleural pressure that bring about breathing can be superimposed on a small lung volume (the balloon being only slightly inflated) or on a large lung volume (the balloon being far more inflated). To hold the balloon at a large volume requires greater effort. During an asthma attack, the patient breathes with an increased lung volume due to bronchoconstriction and trapping of air in the lungs. This increased volume may be close to the total lung capacity, at which compliance is poor and leads to dyspnoea.
2. Airflow only occurs along an airway from a region of high pressure to a region of low pressure. Twice in each respiratory cycle (when inspiration has just ceased and expiration is yet to occur and when

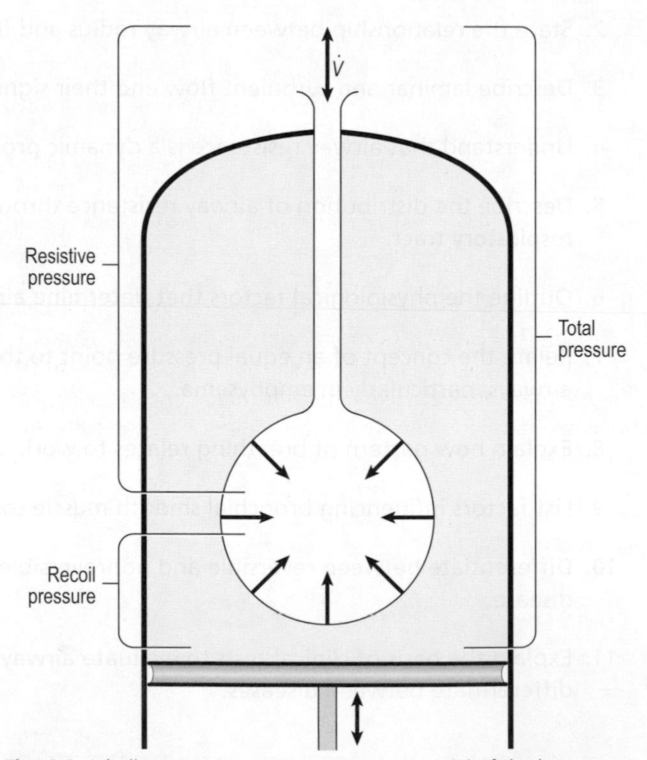

Fig. 4.1 A balloon inside a syringe is a good model of the human lungs and chest wall. To hold the 'lungs' stationary requires a certain negative pressure inside the syringe; to hold them at a larger volume requires a more negative pressure. These changes in intrapleural pressure bring about breathing and are themselves brought about by movement of the diaphragm.

expiration has just ceased and inspiration is yet to occur) there is no flow, and the pressure is equal from the lips to the alveoli. These points in the respiratory cycle can be used to measure dynamic lung compliance (see Fig. 3.19). It should also be noted that during quiet breathing at tidal volume, the pressure in the airway is much closer to atmospheric pressure than is the pressure in the intrapleural space.

3. The elastic recoil of the lungs produces a pressure which resists inspiration but *assists* expiration because potential energy is stored in the tissues. This is analogous to pushing a car up a hill: the weight of the car represents the recoil pressure and resists going uphill (inspiration). The weight of the car would, however, assist going downhill (expiration). This effect of assisting expiration and hindering inspiration is seen in the flow/volume loops used to test lung function (see Chapter 11).

Laminar and turbulent flow

Flow is the volume of air per unit time that passes a certain point or through an airway, and in respiratory physiology is usually expressed as either $L\ min^{-1}$ or $L\ s^{-1}$. The flow of fluids can be described as laminar, **turbulent**, or a mixture of the two. When discussing respiratory physiology, it is the nature of airflow through the airways being described, although these terms can also be applied to other occurrences, such as blood flow.

Laminar flow occurs when air moves smoothly and steadily in a series of concentric cylinders along a smooth, unbranched tube. The fastest moving air is at the centre, with the layers at the periphery moving more slowly (Fig. 4.2). Higher flow rates, and flow along irregular or branching tubes, favour the development of turbulent flow in which flow patterns are more complex and irregular. There is also greater airway resistance to turbulent flow. Parts of the respiratory system where turbulent flow is especially likely to develop include the nose, where turbulence causes inhaled particles to be thrown out of the airstream, and the larynx, where turbulence contributes to the production of sound. Due to the velocity of the air flow and the diameter of the airways, laminar flow does not consistently become established until division 11 of the airways.

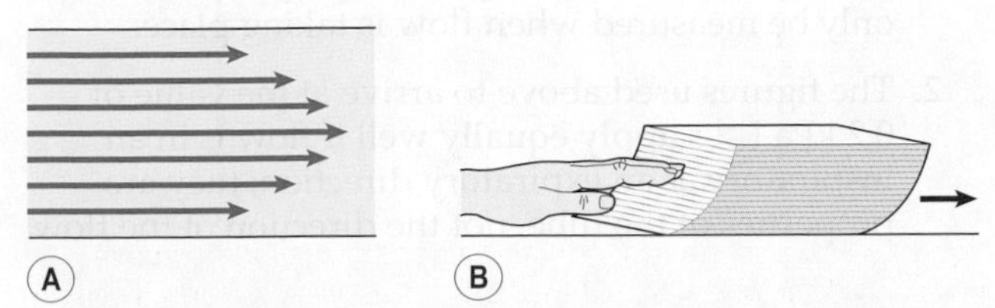

Fig. 4.2 A model of laminar flow. Laminar flow of air in a tube (A) involves very thin layers of air (laminae) sliding over each other, with the layer nearest the wall being stationary. It can be compared to a pile of paper on a surface being pushed along (B).

The ***Reynold's number*** (***Re***) tells us whether flow is likely to be laminar or turbulent. The Re does not have units; however, if the value is less than 2000, flow is more likely to be laminar, and if it is greater than 2000, flow is more likely to be turbulent.

The Re is calculated using the following equation, where ρ = density of the fluid, v = velocity of the fluid, d = diameter of the tube, and η = viscosity of the fluid:

$$Re = \frac{\rho v d}{\eta}$$

The variables related to the gas under consideration are its density and viscosity, specifically the ratio of its density to its viscosity. Whilst the viscosity of gases we breathe does not vary greatly, the density does. Because the density of helium is far lower than that of air, a mixture of 79% helium and 21% oxygen (Heliox) has a similar viscosity but a far lower density than air, and so promotes a greater proportion of laminar flow than turbulent flow and with this, lower airway resistance. This is beneficial in the temporary management of patients with some forms of partial large airway obstruction (e.g. a patient with a malignancy partially occluding an upper airway and awaiting placement of an airway stent).

Factors affecting flow

In 1828, Jean Poiseuille, a French physiologist, derived the equation to calculate pressure change from one end of a smooth, cylindrical pipe to the other, under laminar flow conditions. This was independently described by the German engineer Gotthilf Hagen, and they are jointly credited with the *Hagen–Poiseuille* equation. When the pressure change is known, the equation can be used to calculate flow.

The Hagen–Poiseuille equation is as follows, where ΔP = pressure drop or gradient along the tube (also called the driving pressure), r = radius of the tube, η = viscosity of the fluid, and l = length of the tube:

$$Flow = \frac{(\Delta P)\ \pi r^4}{8 \eta 1}$$

An important point to appreciate is the extent to which the radius of the tube affects flow. Because the radius of the tube is expressed in the equation as r^4, reducing the radius by half (keeping other parameters the same) reduces the flow to 1/16th of its original value. This is clinically relevant in conditions where narrowing of the airways occurs (e.g. asthma).

In practice, the flow of air along the airways displays complex calculation dynamics, compared with a purely laminar flow scenario. Due to the complexity of branching airways with different diameters, a mixture of laminar and turbulent flow exists, with laminar flow only becoming established in the lower airways where airway diameter and flow are both low and resulting in a low Re.

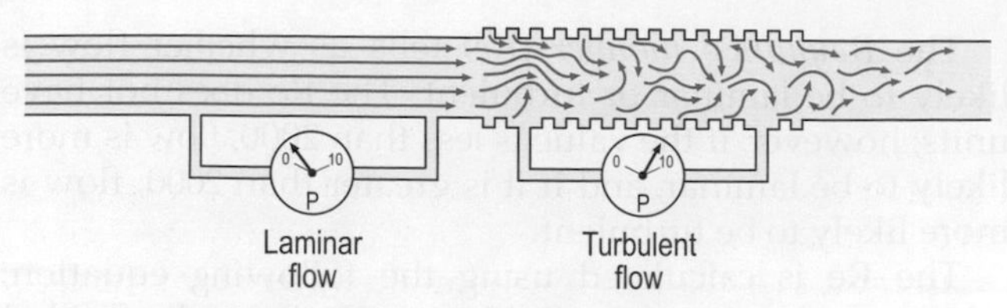

Fig. 4.3 Flow of gas in a tube, half of which is smooth and half of which is rough to produce turbulence. This demonstrates that the pressure gradient that exists when flow is turbulent is greater than when flow is laminar, although the flow in both tubes must be the same.

To double laminar flow (keeping other parameters the same), the driving pressure must be doubled. To double the flow under turbulent conditions, the driving pressure must be squared (Fig. 4.3). It is therefore important when designing a breathing apparatus to avoid turbulence, which would increase the subject's work of breathing.

Summary 1

- Flow takes place down a gradient from high to low pressure
- Radius is a significant determinant of flow in a tube
- Laminar flow can be calculated using the Hagen–Poiseuille equation; in practice, flow is a mixture of laminar and turbulent
- Airway resistance only exists when air is flowing

Respiratory system resistance

Resistance in the respiratory system originates from a number of sources. **Airway resistance** is due to frictional resistance during airflow and **tissue resistance** is caused by tissue deformation of the lung parenchyma and chest wall. A small contribution is also made by the **inertia** of gases and tissues. When adding resistances, normal integers are used.

Airway resistance

Energy is required to propel air along the airways and the airways can be said to resist flow; this is airway resistance. Airway resistance can be considered analogous to electrical resistance. The electrical resistance of a length of wire is calculated using the potential difference (voltage) between the two ends of the wire and the current flowing in the wire. Using currents in a range that do not overheat the wire, we find that the relationship between voltage (V) and current (I) is a straight line (Fig. 4.4). This is **Ohm's law**. The slope of the line (V/I) is the resistance of the wire in ohms (Ω):

$$\text{Resistance (ohms, } \Omega) = \frac{\text{Voltage (V)}}{\text{Current (I)}}$$

We can calculate airway resistance if we know the driving pressure (the difference in pressure between the two ends of the tube) and the airflow in the tube. Under laminar flow conditions, the resistance to gas flow can be

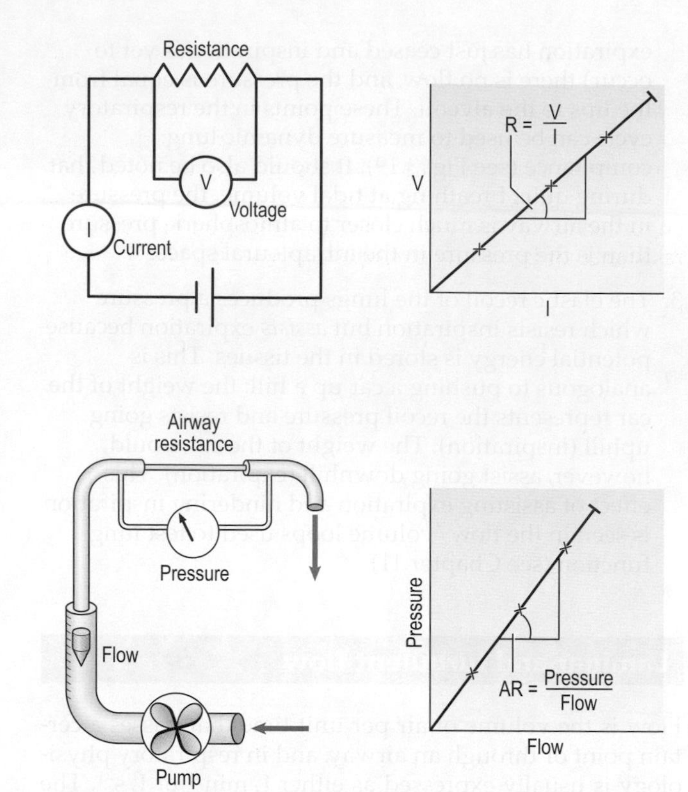

Fig. 4.4 The analogy between electrical and airway resistance, and how they are measured. R, resistance; I, current; V, voltage.

expressed as the ratio of pressure difference (ΔP) to flow rate ($\dot{V}$). The slope of the line is the airway resistance:

$$\text{Airway resistance} = \frac{\text{Pressure drop or gradient along the tube}}{\text{Flow } (\dot{V})}$$

(also called driving pressure, ΔP)

Airway resistance is usually expressed in cmH_2O per litre per second (cm H_2O L^{-1}·s) or kilopascals per litre per second (kPa L^{-1} s), where cm H_2O = cm of water, L = litre, kPa = kiloPascal, and s = second.

The airway resistance in an adult breathing quietly is about 0.2 kPa L^{-1}·s, which means that a normal flow rate of 0.5 L s^{-1} is brought about by a pressure difference of 0.1 kPa generated between the lips and the alveoli.

Two important points arise from this statement:

1. Airway resistance is a dynamic property and can only be measured when flow is taking place.
2. The figures used above to arrive at the value of 0.2 kPa L^{-1} s apply equally well if flow is in an inspiratory *or* an expiratory direction; they are properties of the tube, not the direction of the flow.

Sites of airway resistance

Airway resistance is not distributed uniformly along the respiratory tract. Almost half the total resistance resides in the *nose, pharynx,* and *larynx.* The vocal cords of the larynx open to allow inspiration and reduce resistance; they come close together, during expiration, to form an 'expiratory brake' and prevent a too-rapid collapse of the lungs. The significant resistance provided by the nose is a common experience, especially when the mucosa has become engorged because of the common cold. Even in health, the resistance of breathing through the nose is approximately twice that of breathing through the mouth, and we change to mouth breathing during exercise. In infants, the resistance when breathing via the nose is lower than when breathing via the mouth, which is of benefit when feeding.

Approximately half of the total airway resistance exists below the larynx and 80% of this is found in the *trachea* and *bronchi*. This is, at first, difficult to reconcile with Poiseuilles's law (see above) given that the airway resistance of a tube is proportional to the fourth power of its radius and that the trachea and main bronchi are the largest tubes in the bronchial tree. The explanation is that, at each generation, the airway divides into two; this doubles the number of airways at each branching. Therefore the number (N) at each generation (Z) (see Chapter 2) is N = Z2, beginning with the two main bronchi as generation 1 (Fig. 4.5). This rapid increase in number more than offsets

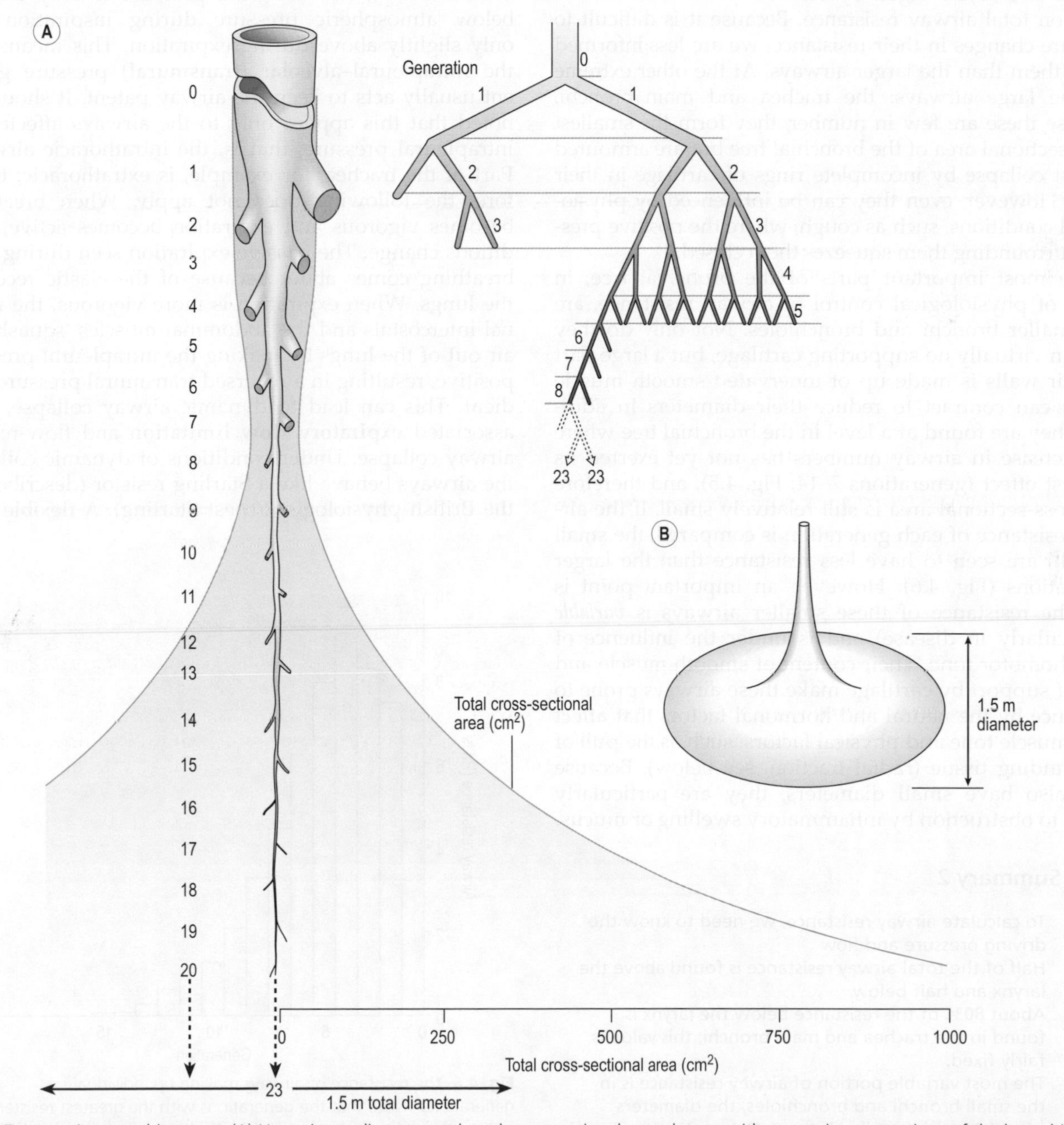

Fig. 4.5 Lung airway architecture. (A) How airway diameter and total cross-sectional area change with successive generations of the bronchial tree. (B) Change in *total cross-sectional area* represented three-dimensionally. (From E.R. Weibel, D.M. Gomez. Architecture of the Human Lung, 1962.)

the decrease in the diameters of the individual members of each generation; as a result, ***total*** cross-sectional area increases dramatically. The bronchi extend from generation 1–16, with the small bronchi (generations 5–11; 3.5–1 mm in diameter) not being directly attached to the lung parenchyma. They are supported against collapse by cartilage and the transmural pressure gradient, which it is now believed to rarely reverse sufficiently to cause complete collapse of these airways.

The bronchi give rise to such a great number of bronchioles that less than 20% of the total resistance to flow is attributable to airways less than 2 mm in diameter. For this reason, a considerable number of these smaller airways must be damaged by disease before there is any effect on total airway resistance. Because it is difficult to measure changes in their resistance, we are less informed about them than the larger airways. At the other extreme are the large airways: the trachea and main bronchi. Because these are few in number, they form the smallest cross-sectional area of the bronchial tree but are armoured against collapse by incomplete rings of cartilage in their walls. However, even they can be influenced by physiological conditions, such as cough, where the positive pressure surrounding them squeezes them closed.

The most important parts of the bronchial tree, in terms of physiological control of airway resistance, are the smaller bronchi and bronchioles. Not only do they contain virtually no supporting cartilage, but a large part of their walls is made up of innervated smooth muscle which can contract to reduce their diameters In addition, they are found at a level in the bronchial tree where the increase in airway numbers has not yet exerted its greatest effect (generations 7–14; Fig. 4.5), and therefore the cross-sectional area is still relatively small. If the airway resistance of each generation is compared, the small bronchi are seen to have less resistance than the larger generations (Fig. 4.6). However, an important point is that the resistance of these smaller airways is *variable* (particularly in disease) and is under the influence of bronchomotor tone. Their content of smooth muscle and lack of support by cartilage make these airways prone to influence by the neural and hormonal factors that affect their muscle tone and physical factors, such as the pull of surrounding tissue (radial traction, see below). Because they also have small diameters, they are particularly prone to obstruction by inflammatory swelling or mucus.

Summary 2

- To calculate airway resistance, we need to know the driving pressure and flow
- Half of the total airway resistance is found above the larynx and half below
- About 80% of the resistance below the larynx is found in the trachea and main bronchi; this value is fairly fixed.
- The most variable portion of airway resistance is in the small bronchi and bronchioles, the diameters of which are controlled by smooth muscle bronchomotor tone.

Other factors affecting airway resistance

Alterations to the airway diameters of the small bronchi and bronchioles affect airway resistance, but other factors, including lung volume, flow rate of air, and the rate of pressure drop along the airway, also have effects. Closed or compressed airways contribute to greater airway resistance.

Flow-related airway collapse

During tidal breathing, the intrapleural pressure is always considerably negative relative to the atmosphere. In the airway, however, the pressure is only slightly below atmospheric pressure during inspiration and only slightly above during expiration. This means that the intrapleural–alveolar (**transmural**) pressure gradient usually acts to keep the airway patent. It should be noted that this applies only to the airways affected by intrapleural pressure, that is, the intrathoracic airways. Part of the trachea, for example, is extrathoracic; therefore, the following does not apply. When breathing becomes vigorous and expiration becomes active, conditions change. The passive expiration seen during tidal breathing comes about because of the elastic recoil of the lungs. When expiration is more vigorous, the internal intercostals and the abdominal muscles 'squash' the air out of the lungs by making the intrapleural pressure positive, resulting in a reversed transmural pressure gradient. This can lead to dynamic airway collapse, with associated **expiratory flow limitation** and flow-related airway collapse. Under conditions of dynamic collapse, the airways behave like a Starling resistor (described by the British physiologist Ernest Starling). A flexible tube

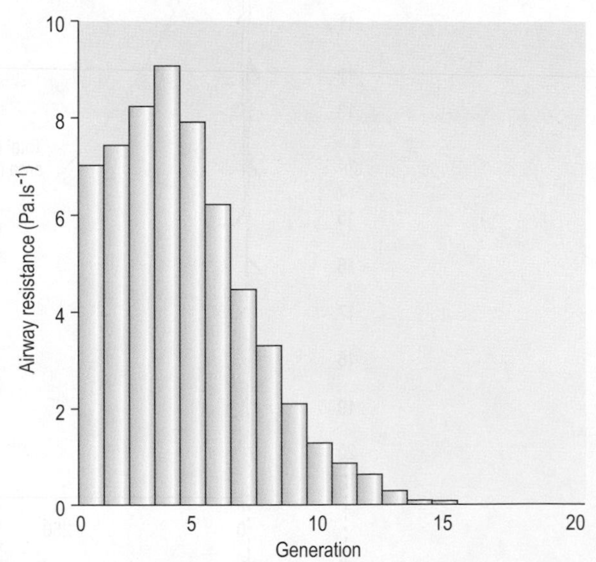

Fig. 4.6 The resistance of airways making up individual generations. Note that the generations with the greatest resistance are not those made up of airways with the smallest diameters. (From T.J. Pedley, R.C. Schroter, M.F. Sudlow. Respiration Physiology, 1970.)

runs through an area of constant surrounding pressure, and a pressure gradient drives air through the tube (Fig. 4.7). The pressure inside the tube falls as air flows from left to right, whilst the external pressure does not change. At one point along the tube, the inside pressure falls below the outside pressure and the tube collapses. Equal pressure point is the term used to describe the point where the pressures inside and outside the airway are equal. At the equal pressure point, the rigidity of the wall and surrounding parenchyma are the only factors holding the airway open. As the lung volume decreases during expiration, the equal pressure point moves progressively towards the smaller airways, as the contribution to the pressure within the airways from elastic recoil is reduced (Fig. 4.8).

Volume-related airway collapse

At lower lung volumes, airway resistance is greater. This is because there is a reduction in all aspects of the lung volume, including the airway diameter, and because the more distal airways have no structural support within their walls. At low lung volumes, where the transmural pressure gradient is small, airway collapse in these regions is promoted. This is termed 'volume-related

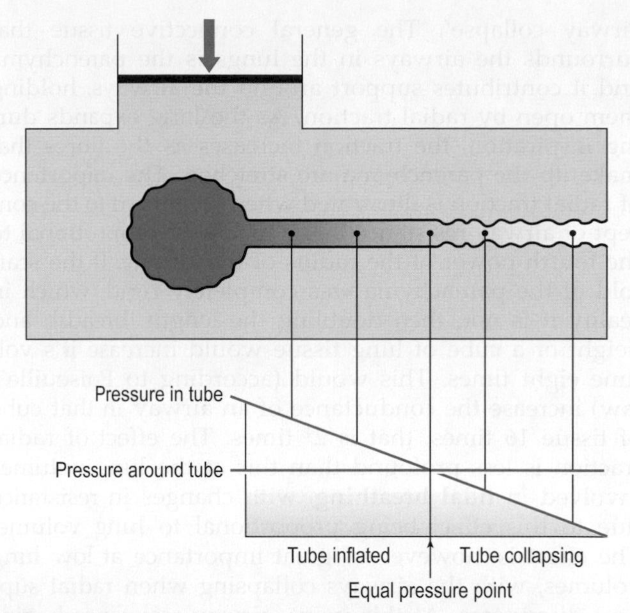

Fig. 4.7 A Starling resistor. In this, a flexible tube is surrounded by a uniform pressure. Pressure drives air along the tube. As this driving pressure is used up, it falls until an equal pressure point is reached, where the internal and external pressures are equal. Downstream from that point the pressure around the wall of the tube is greater than the pressure inside, causing it to collapse, frequently in an unstable vibrating manner.

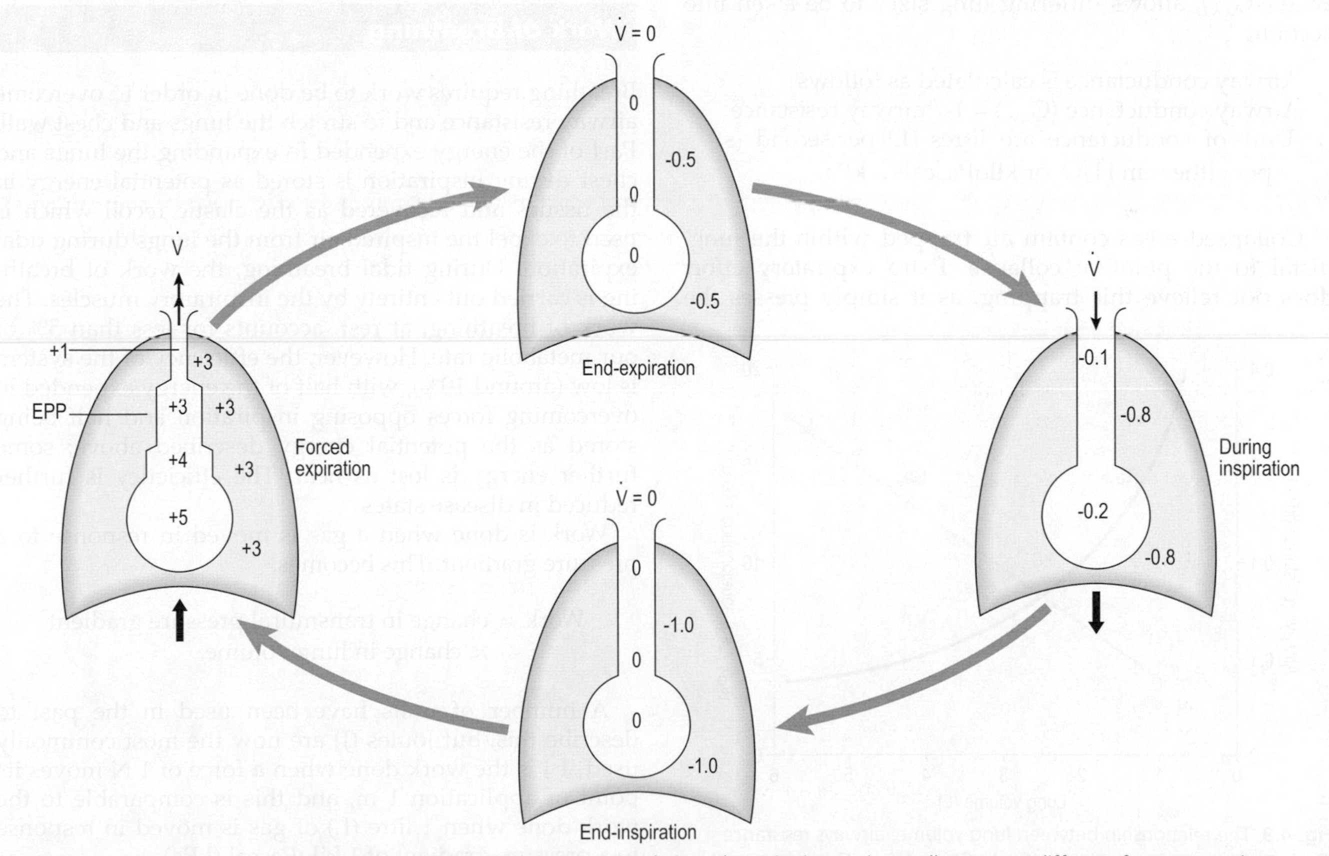

Fig. 4.8 Transmural pressure in intrathoracic airways. The pressure inside intrathoracic airways is usually not very different from atmospheric pressure, which tends to keep them open because the pressure around the airways is usually negative (subatmospheric). During a forced expiration, however, the pressure may become positive and equal to that within the airway (an equal pressure point, EPP). The pressure within the airway downstream of the EPP is less than the intrapleural pressure, and the airway there tends to collapse.

airway collapse'. The general connective tissue that surrounds the airways in the lungs is the parenchyma and it contributes support around the airways, holding them open by radial traction. As the lung expands during inspiration, the traction increases as the fibres that make up the parenchyma are stretched. The importance of radial traction is illustrated when we return to the concept of airway resistance being inversely proportional to the fourth power of the radius of the airway. If the scaffold of the parenchyma was completely rigid, which in reality it is not, then doubling the length, breadth and height of a cube of lung tissue would increase it's volume eight times. This would (according to Poiseuille's law) increase the conductance of an airway in that cube of tissue 16 times, that is 2^4 times. The effect of radial traction is less profound than this at the lung volumes involved in **tidal breathing**, with changes in resistance due to this effect being proportional to lung volume. The effect is, however, of great importance at low lung volumes, with the airways collapsing when radial support disappears. At this point, airway resistance begins to increase dramatically (Fig. 4.9). Figure 4.9 illustrates airway **conductance** (G_{aw}). Conductance is the reciprocal of airway resistance, and it may be used to describe the resistance at varying volumes because it forms a straight line rather than a hyperbola. Specific airway conductance (sG_{aw}), allows differing lung sizes to be taken into account.

Airway conductance is calculated as follows:
Airway conductance (G_{aw}) = 1 / airway resistance
Units of conductance are litres (L) per second (s) per either cm H_2O or kiloPascals, kPa.

Collapsed areas contain air trapped within the lung, distal to the point of collapse. Extra expiratory effort does not relieve this trapping, as it simply presses the collapsed area more firmly shut. In healthy lungs, these conditions do not occur at volumes above the **functional residual capacity** (FRC). In lungs affected by damage to the airway wall or when the supporting parenchyma has been destroyed (e.g. in obstructive lung diseases), this collapse takes place at greater volumes. During expiration, the collapsing segment vibrates and is a major source of the wheeze heard in many lung diseases. In emphysema, the destruction of the supporting parenchyma is the cause of airway loss of support. In asthma, it is the high bronchomotor tone and oedema of the airways that augments collapse and increases the rate of pressure drop along the airway.

Because of the weight of the overlying tissue, this closure begins first in the lower lobes of the lungs at closing capacity. In young people, closing capacity is less than the FRC and so airway closure does not occur during normal breathing. With advancing age, it becomes greater than the FRC, initially when lying down (around the age of 44) and then greater than the FRC when upright (around the age of 66). Under these conditions, blood is shunted (see Chapter 7) through the lungs without coming into contact with air, and this is an important aspect of the desaturation of arterial blood with increasing age.

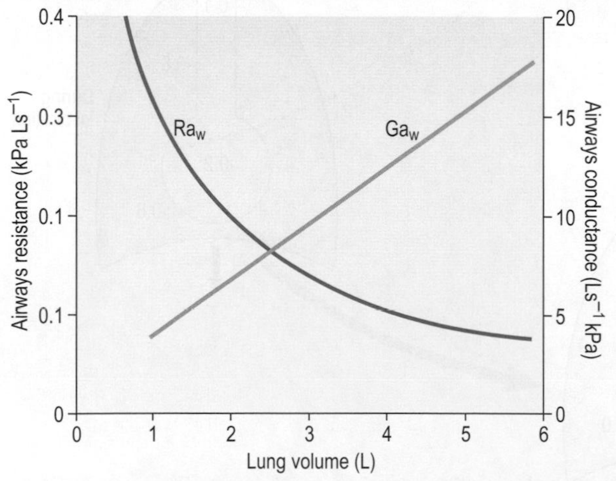

Fig. 4.9 The relationship between lung volume, airways resistance (R_{aw}), and airways conductance (G_{aw}). G_{aw} is $1/R_{aw}$; G_{aw} is frequently used clinically in the form of specific conductance (sG_{aw}), which takes into account the different lung sizes of different subjects.

Work of breathing

Breathing requires work to be done in order to overcome airway resistance and to stretch the lungs and chest wall. Part of the energy expended in expanding the lungs and chest during inspiration is stored as potential energy in the tissues and recovered as the elastic recoil which is used to expel the inspired air from the lungs during tidal expiration. During tidal breathing, the work of breathing is carried out entirely by the inspiratory muscles. The work of breathing, at rest, accounts for less than 5% of our metabolic rate. However, the efficiency of the system is low (around 10%), with half of the energy expended in overcoming forces opposing inspiration and half being stored as the potential energy described above; some further energy is lost as heat. The efficiency is further reduced in disease states.

Work is done when a gas is moved in response to a pressure gradient. This becomes:

$$\text{Work} = \text{change in transmural pressure gradient} \times \text{change in lung volume}$$

A number of units have been used in the past to describe this, but Joules (J) are now the most commonly used. 1 J is the work done when a force of 1 N moves its point of application 1 m, and this is comparable to the work done when 1 litre (L) of gas is moved in response to a pressure gradient of 1 kiloPascal (kPa)

This is illustrated in Figure 4.10. In panel A, if there is no change in either volume or pressure, no work is

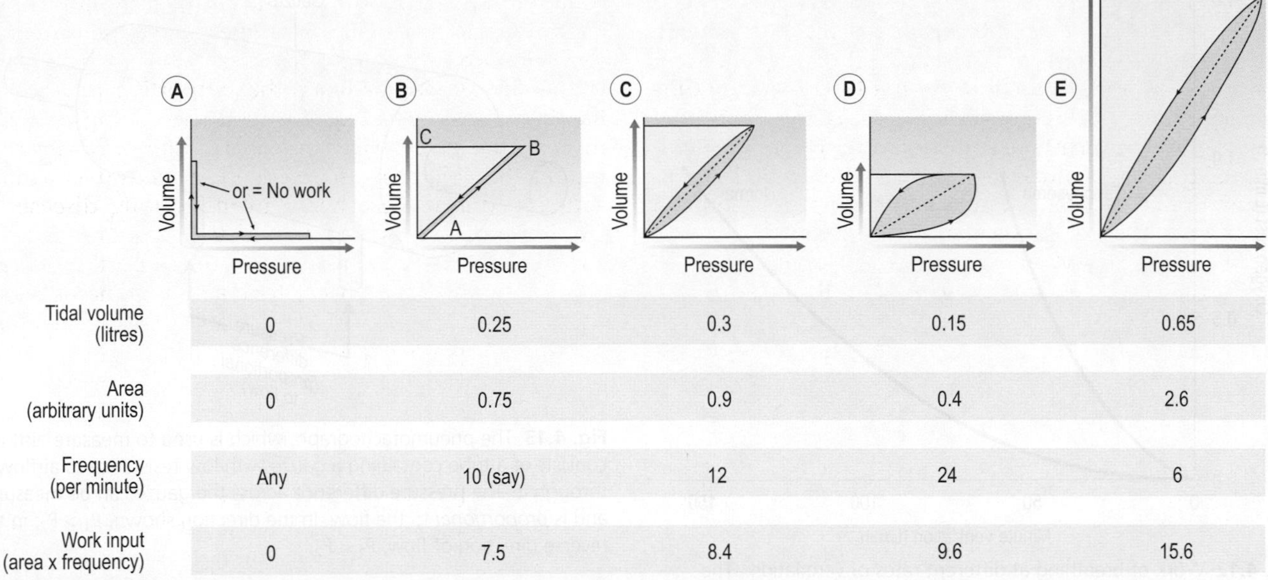

	A	B	C	D	E
Tidal volume (litres)	0	0.25	0.3	0.15	0.65
Area (arbitrary units)	0	0.75	0.9	0.4	2.6
Frequency (per minute)	Any	10 (say)	12	24	6
Work input (area x frequency)	0	7.5	8.4	9.6	15.6

Fig. 4.10 The work of breathing. This is pressure change × volume change. If either of these remains the same (A), no work of breathing is done. Panel B is an artificial situation used to demonstrate how work of breathing is calculated: if the lung is completely nonelastic and is inflated from A to B, it will stay there (like a piece of putty which has been stretched) and the work put into it will be the area ABC. If the lung is *perfectly* elastic, once the inflating pressure is released it will return from B to A, giving up all the energy that has been put into it. The total work of breathing is represented by the area ABC. The straight diagonal line (shown dotted in subsequent panels) is the energy required to overcome simple elastic forces within the lung. In normal quiet breathing (C), the work done during inspiration, which is *not* recovered during expiration, is lost in overcoming the frictional forces of the tissues and airways and is represented by the area to the right of the diagonal line. The area shown from the diagonal line to the y-axis represents the work required to overcome elastic forces. The sum of the two areas is the total work of breathing. If breathing is made either rapid and shallow (D), or deep and slow (E), more work than normal is required to achieve the same ventilation as in C.

done. In panel B, a perfectly elastic lung is very slowly (pseudostatically) inflated. Here, the work of inflation is the *area* of the figure ABC. In panels C, D and E, different patterns of breathing are shown to require different amounts of work to produce the same ventilation. This is because the work of breathing is made up of work against the:

1. elastic resistance of the tissues
2. frictional resistance of the airway and tissues.

Deep, slow breathing, described in E, requires the most work to be done against elastic resistance, whereas rapid shallow breathing, described in D, works largely against airway resistance. If breathing is commenced slowly and deeply, then the frequency increases whilst reducing the volume, the work against elastic resistance decreases and work to produce airflow increases (Fig. 4.11). Humans are efficient at minimising the expenditure of energy by the respiratory muscles (as a fraction of our total energy use) and, in healthy subjects, the work done in breathing provides 'good value' in providing extra oxygen. For example, exercise is rarely limited by the respiratory system using too much energy. In diseased lungs, however, the airway resistance, elastic properties, or control system may be compromised and the

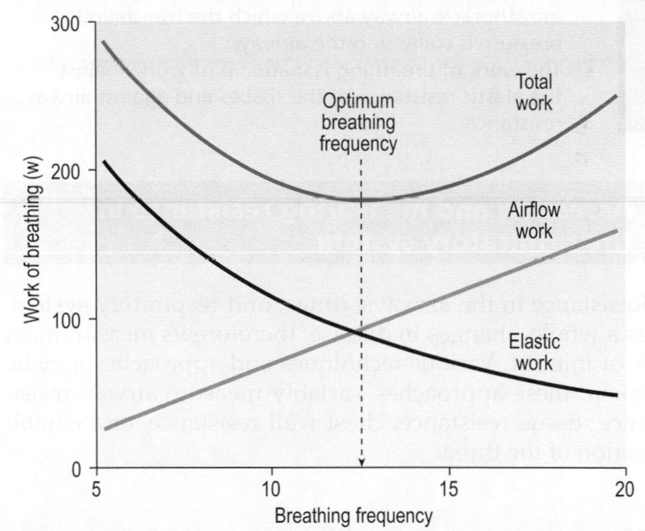

Fig. 4.11 Total work of breathing. This is effectively the sum of work done against the elastic recoil of tissue plus the work to produce airflow. These change with frequency of breathing, shown with the sum reaching a minimum at the frequency where the two lines intersect.

extra work done by the respiratory muscles to provide extra oxygen to the rest of the body, during exercise, demands more oxygen than it provides (Fig. 4.12), which is clearly an untenable situation that limits exercise.

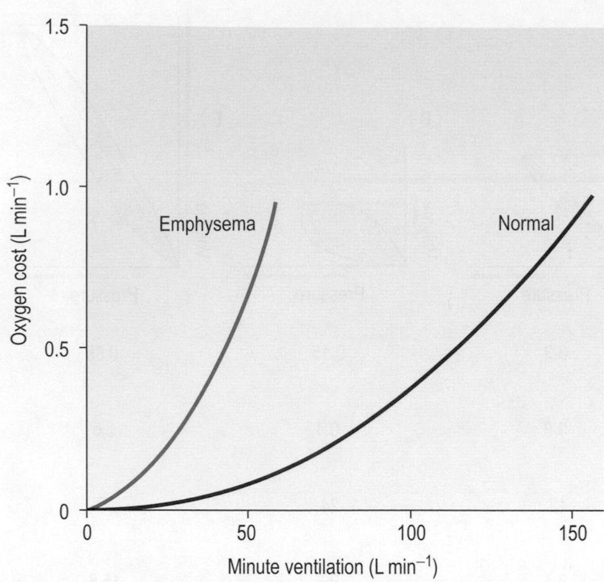

Fig. 4.12 Work of breathing at different rates of ventilation. The work of breathing in a normal individual is low until high levels of ventilation are reached, and then it begins to rise steeply. Diseased lungs consume more energy at low ventilation, and their requirement increases more rapidly than normal.

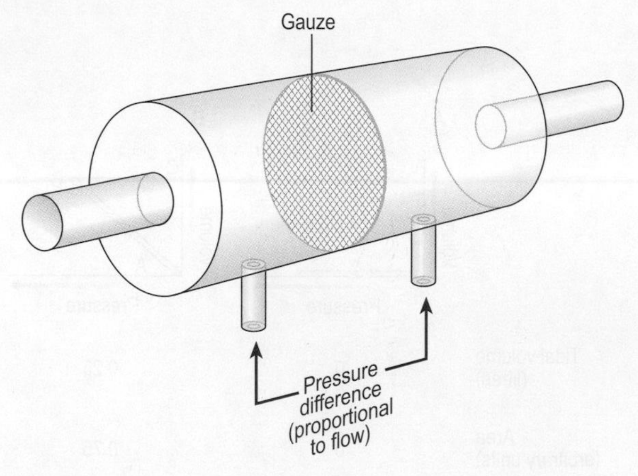

Fig. 4.13 The pneumotachograph, which is used to measure airflow, consists of a tube containing a *gauze* with low resistance to airflow through it. The pressure difference across the gauze can be measured and is *proportional* to the flow. In the direction shown, $P_1 > P_2$; in the reverse direction of flow, $P_1 < P_2$.

Summary 3

- Forced expiration (e.g. a cough) makes the normally negative intrapleural pressure positive.
- When intrapleural pressure is positive, there is an 'equal pressure point' somewhere along the intrathoracic airway above which the transmural pressure is collapsing the airways.
- The work of breathing is made up of work against the elastic resistance of the tissues and against airway resistance.

Assessing and measuring resistance in the respiratory system

Resistance in the airways, lungs, and respiratory system, as a whole, changes in disease; therefore its measurement is of interest. Various techniques and approaches may be taken; these approaches variably measure airway resistance, tissue resistance, chest wall resistance, or a combination of the three.

Measuring pressure and flow

To measure airway resistance, we need to measure the driving pressure gradient and the flow. Measurement of airflow may be carried out using an instrument known as a pneumotachograph, which itself illustrates the principle of airway resistance. The pneumotachograph consists of a tube through which the subject breathes (Fig. 4.13); the tube also contains a resistance to flow. The pressure difference across the resistance is measured and is proportional to the flow, which can then be integrated to give the volume. Laminar flow conditions must be met in order for this to be accurate.

Measurement of the driving pressure in a subject is more difficult. Consider the changes in the intrapleural pressure and compliance of the lungs during a single respiratory cycle (Fig. 4.14). If the pressure component used to overcome elastic forces is subtracted, the pressure required to overcome flow resistance can be determined. By subtracting the changes in recoil pressure from the changes in intrapleural pressure, we are left with the changes in alveolar pressure that produce changes in airflow. By measuring changes in the pressure inside the oesophagus, as it passes through the thorax, continuous measurement of resistance can be obtained. Oesophageal pressure changes may be used as an indicator of the change in pressure in the intrapleural space, which is otherwise difficult to measure directly. The technique of measuring intraoesophageal pressure is described in Chapter 3. By including the changes in the intrapleural pressure, the chest wall part of resistance is excluded and the measurement obtained is therefore airway and lung tissue resistance.

The interrupter technique

This technique measures airway resistance but excludes tissue resistance. It is based on using a single manometer to measure mouth and alveolar pressure by interrupting the flow of air out of the lungs using a rapidly closing shutter in the tube through which the subject is breathing. The principle is that during the interruption, the mouth pressure very rapidly rises to equal the alveolar pressure; the pressure measured at the lips is the pressure in the alveoli a fraction of a second before the shutter closes and is the pressure that was producing flow just before the shutter closed. Using these values of

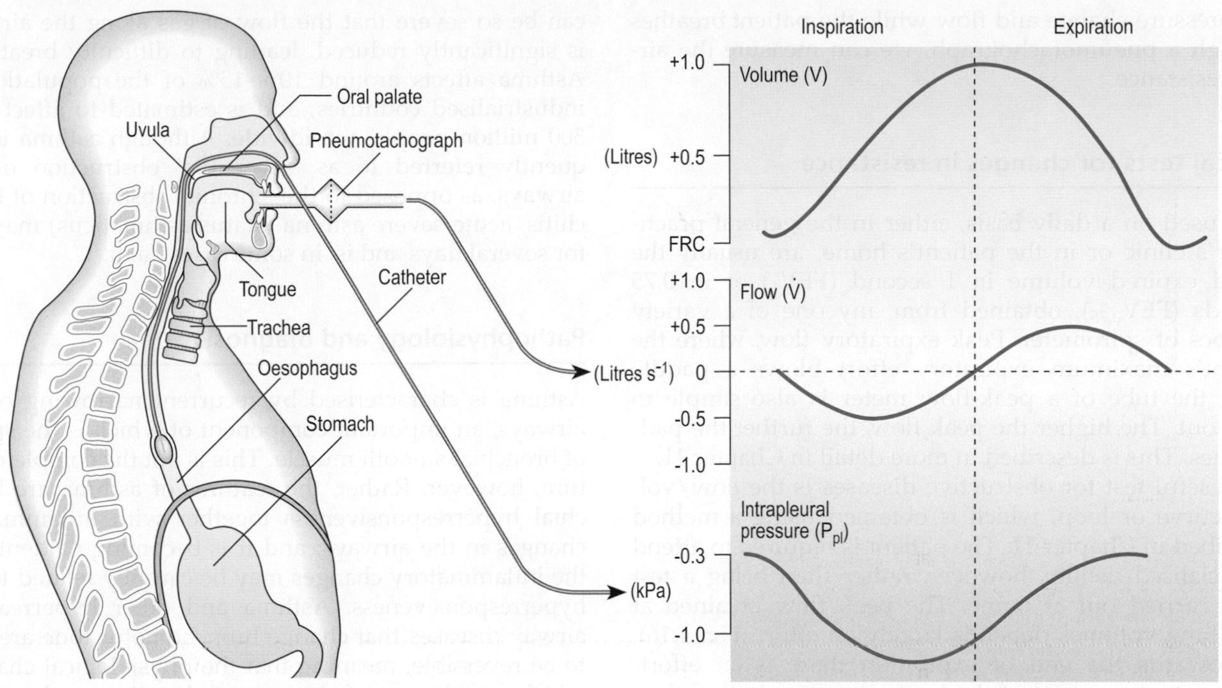

Fig. 4.14 Determination of airway resistance (R_{aw}) by measuring airflow and the intrapleural pressure, which is measured using an intraoesophageal catheter. The changes in measured pressure can be taken as a surrogate for changes in intrapleural pressure.

pressure and flow, airway resistance is calculated. This technique is accepted as being fairly accurate in a subject with healthy lungs, but in subjects with lung disease, the equilibration may not take place rapidly enough to give an accurate measurement.

Whole-body plethysmography

This approach measures airway resistance and requires an airtight box in which the subject sits. This is further described in Chapter 11. During inspiration, alveolar volume increases due to lung expansion and the intra-alveolar pressure decreases slightly, relative to atmospheric pressure, facilitating air to be drawn into the lungs. The total quantity of air in the box (inside the patient's lungs and around them in the box) is the same throughout the measurement because the box is airtight. The patient first pants against a closed shutter while the pressure changes in the mouth and in the box are measured simultaneously. The pressure changes in the mouth are assumed to be the same as those in the alveoli (by the same arguments as in the interrupter technique, above). The pressure changes in the box while the patient is panting because they are compressing and decompressing the air in the lungs and therefore changing the volume of the chest in the closed box. Consider the subject like the syringe in Figure 4.15: when air is compressed in the chest, the air in the box is decompressed; when air is decompressed in the chest, the air in the box is compressed.

The pressure changes in the box are therefore related to pressure changes in the alveoli, and so by measuring

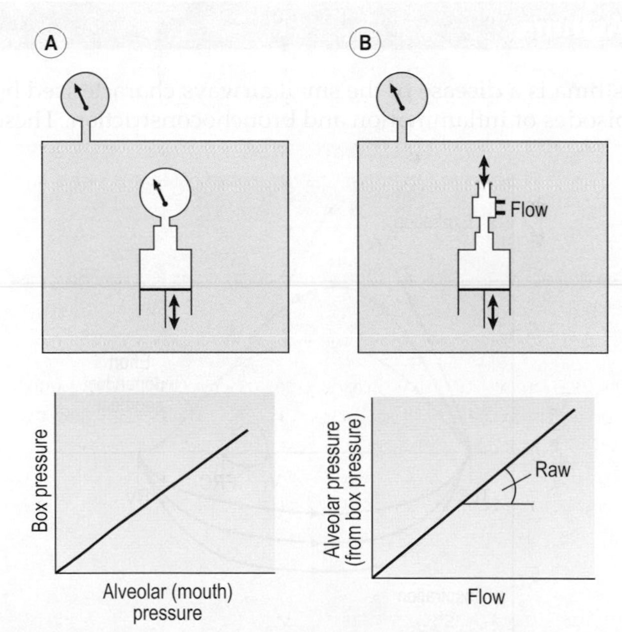

Fig. 4.15 Measurement of airway resistance using a whole-body plethysmograph (body box). Calibration of the relationship between the alveolar pressure and box pressure is being determined in (A), where the subject pants against a closed shutter. Because there is no airflow while the shutter is closed, changes in pressure measured at the mouth are the same as the changes in pressure in the alveoli. (B) Airway resistance (R_{aw}) is being measured while the subject breathes through a pneumotachograph, which measures flow, while changes in box pressure are converted into changes in alveolar pressure.

box pressure change and flow while the patient breathes through a pneumotachograph, we can measure the airway resistance.

Clinical tests for changes in resistance

Tests used on a daily basis, either in the general practitioner's clinic or in the patient's home, are usually the forced expired volume in 1 second (FEV_1) or in 0.75 seconds ($FEV_{0.75}$), obtained from any one of a variety of types of spirometer. Peak expiratory flow, where the patient's maximum expiratory effort blows a paddle along the tube of a peak-flow meter is also simple to carry out. The higher the peak flow, the further the paddle goes. This is described in more detail in Chapter 11.

A useful test for obstructive diseases is the flow/volume curve or loop, which is obtained using a method described in Chapter 11. The patient is required to attend a specialised facility, however, rather than being a test to be carried out at home. The peak flow obtained at large lung volumes depends largely on effort (Fig. 4.16), but towards the end of expiration there is an effort-independent segment of the loop where expiratory flow is determined by airway collapse below the equal pressure point. The alteration in the shape of this loop caused by disease is also dealt with in Chapter 11.

Asthma

Asthma is a disease of the small airways characterised by episodes of inflammation and bronchoconstriction. These can be so severe that the flow of gas along the airways is significantly reduced, leading to difficulty breathing. Asthma affects around 10%–15% of the population of industrialised countries, and is estimated to affect over 300 million people, worldwide. Although asthma is frequently referred to as 'reversible' obstruction of the airways, as opposed to the 'chronic' obstruction of bronchitis, acute severe asthma (status asthmaticus) may last for several days and is, in some cases, fatal.

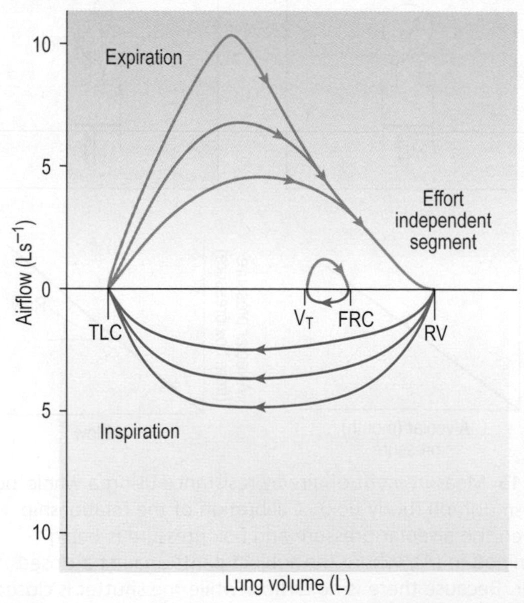

Fig. 4.16 Normal flow–volume loops. These were obtained using three different expiratory efforts. Note that all three loops meet in an *effort-independent segment*. Flow in this condition is being limited by airways collapse. A normal tidal volume breath is shown for comparison.

Pathophysiology and diagnosis

Asthma is characterised by recurrent narrowing of the airways, an important component of which is the spasm of bronchial smooth muscle. This is not the complete picture, however. Rather, the features of asthma are bronchial hyperresponsiveness together with inflammatory changes in the airways, and it is becoming evident that the inflammatory changes may be causally related to the hyperresponsiveness. Asthma and other hyperreactive airway diseases that change bronchomotor tone are said to be reversible, meaning that the physiological changes which are the manifestations of the disease should be reversed spontaneously or as a result of treatment. Bronchial smooth muscle can contract in all individuals; hence the diameters of the airways change but the effect on ventilation is usually negligible. In asthmatics, the hyperresponsiveness of the airways often extends to non-specific irritants, such as cold air, smoke, and exercise, which would not provoke an individual unaffected by asthma. Between attacks, the patient frequently has no symptoms, although the inflammation persists.

Bronchial hyperreactivity is related to an underlying inflammation of the bronchial mucosa. The mucosa of asthmatics is thickened and infiltrated with inflammatory cells. During an asthma attack, chemical mediators released by the inflammatory cells cause contraction of the underlying bronchial smooth muscle. In addition, these secretions may also cause thickening of the mucosa, and excessive mucous secretions in the airways can lead to plugging of the smaller airways. In many asthmatics, bronchial hyperreactivity is closely associated with an increased sensitivity of the immune system to everyday substances in the environment. This increased sensitivity is called atopy and is also associated with conditions such as eczema. Asthma related to atopy is particularly common among children. Clinically, this sensitivity may be demonstrated by a characteristic skin-wheal reaction to common environmental substances.

Atopic individuals readily produce antibodies of the IgE class against a variety of environmental allergens. It is thought that these antibodies attach to mast cells in the airways. Mast cells are part of the immune system; when an antigen binds to IgE on their surface, they release a range of substances, including prostaglandins, leukotrienes, and histamine. It is thought that these substances are responsible for triggering bronchoconstriction in susceptible individuals. Asthma is not confined to atopic individuals and is not necessarily provoked by environmental antigens. This is particularly the case in asthmatics who are diagnosed later in life. Asthmatics who respond to environmental stimuli are sometimes referred to as having nonallergic or intrinsic asthma, whereas those who do not are described as having allergic or extrinsic asthma.

Asthma is diagnosed on the basis of symptoms of episodic wheeze, breathlessness, and cough. These symptoms are often worse at night and may be brought on by triggering agents, as described above. Diagnosis is also facilitated by lung function tests, particularly forced expiration spirography and measurement of peak expiratory flow. A fall in FEV_1, FEV_1/forced vital capacity (FVC) ratio, and peak flow are all indicative of an asthma attack. The patient may be dyspnoeic, with breathing laboured and involving the accessory muscles of respiration. Any sputum produced is usually scant and viscid. Most asthma attacks can be divided into two phases:

- *the **immediate phase**,* due mainly to spasms of the bronchial smooth muscle
- *the **late phase**,* an acute inflammatory reaction

Early bronchoconstriction is a particular feature of allergic asthma that leads to wheezing within minutes of exposure to the allergen. Bronchoconstriction occurs variably throughout the lungs, with some patients developing marked ventilation-perfusion mismatch (see Chapter 7). This has implications for the delivery of drugs by inhaler or nebuliser as they may not be able to reach the areas where they are required. As a result of bronchoconstriction, gas trapping occurs, and the lungs become hyperinflated. During severe attacks, an individual may be attempting to breathe at almost total lung capacity, with the associated feeling of dyspnoea.

Factors affecting bronchomotor tone

The tension in the walls of the bronchi is the major determinant of their diameter. This tension is, in turn, determined by bronchial smooth muscle tone. Physiological control of airway smooth muscle involves several mechanisms (Fig. 4.17). Disordered physiological control of airway smooth muscle represents a major feature of asthma and other pathological conditions where the airways are hyperreactive. Multi-unit smooth muscle controls the tension in the walls of the bronchi, and therefore, in many cases, their diameter. These muscle fibres are, in turn, controlled by:

- ***Parasympathetic nerves.*** The efferent preganglionic fibres of this system run in the vagus nerve to ganglia located in the walls of the small bronchi. Postganglionic fibres release acetylcholine, which stimulates muscarinic receptors on the smooth muscle fibres, causing them to contract. Atropine blocks these receptors; injections of atropine in a normal individual

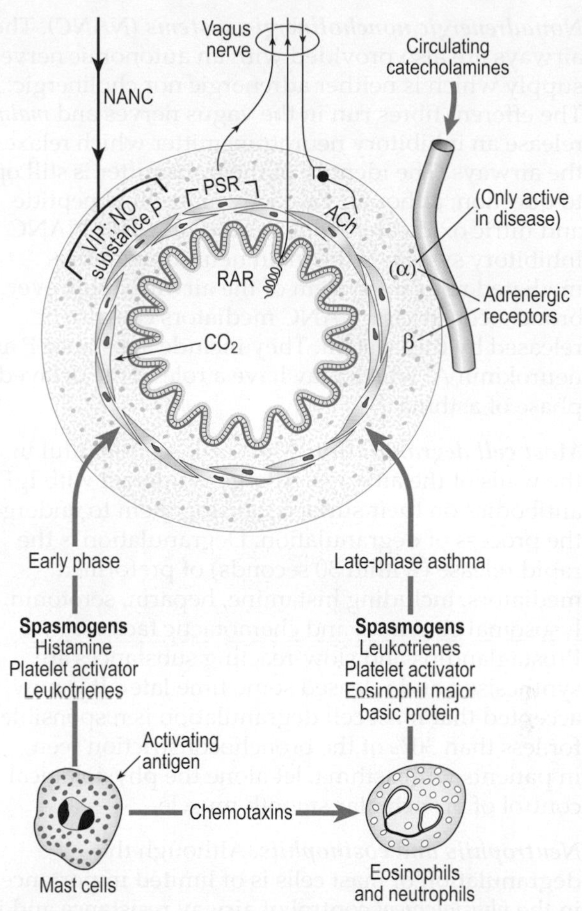

Fig. 4.17 Factors that affect bronchomotor tone. These are implicated in early- and late-phase asthma. NANC, nonadrenergic noncholinergic systems; NO, nitric oxide; PSR, slowly adapting pulmonary sensory receptor; RAR, rapidly adapting pulmonary sensory receptor; VIP, vasoactive intestinal peptide.

can reduce airway resistance by about 30%. This limited response demonstrates that parasympathetic nerves, though important, are not the only method of bronchomotor control.

- ***Sympathetic nerves.*** Most organs with a parasympathetic nerve supply also have a sympathetic input. In the case of the lungs, this nerve supply does ***not*** extend as far as the bronchial smooth muscle, and its effect in the lung, in general, is thought to be minimal. Any sympathetic effects seen in the lung are due to circulating catecholamines.
- ***Circulating catecholamines.*** The membrane of airway smooth muscle carries β_2 receptors which, when stimulated by the naturally occurring catecholamine, adrenaline (epinephrine), or drugs such as salbutamol, relax smooth muscle, inhibit the action of mast cells, and improve mucociliary activity. Therefore, they form an important treatment for asthma. α-Adrenergic agents only cause contraction of bronchial smooth muscle in diseased states.

- ***Nonadrenergic noncholinergic systems (NANC)***. The airways are also provided with an autonomic nerve supply which is neither adrenergic nor cholinergic. The efferent fibres run in the vagus nerves and *mainly* release an inhibitory neurotransmitter which relaxes the airways. The identity of the transmitter is still open to question, although vasoactive intestinal peptide and nitric oxide are strong candidates. This NANC inhibitory system is the main neurotransmitter-mediated relaxant system of the airways. However, bronchoconstrictor NANC mediators can also be released by this system. They include substance P and neurokinin A, which may have a role in the delayed phase of asthma.
- ***Mast cell degranulation***. Mast cells are plentiful in the walls of the airways. Allergens interact with IgE antibodies on their surface, causing them to undergo the process of degranulation. Degranulation is the rapid release (within 30 seconds) of preformed mediators, including histamine, heparin, serotonin, lysosomal enzymes, and chemotactic factors. Prostaglandins and slow-reacting substances are synthesised and released some time later. It is now accepted that mast cell degranulation is responsible for less than 30% of the bronchoconstriction seen in patients with asthma, let alone the physiological control of bronchiolar smooth muscle.
- ***Neutrophils and eosinophils***. Although the degranulation of mast cells is of limited importance in the *physiological* control of airway resistance and its role is restricted to the immediate phase of asthma, neutrophil and eosinophil chemotactic factors are of such importance during the late (inflammatory) phase that is has been suggested that it has been suggested asthma should be called 'chronic desquamating eosinopilic bronchiolitis'.
- ***Rapidly adapting pulmonary receptors*** *(irritant and cough receptors)*. Stimulation of these airway receptors by inhalation of particles, chemicals, or by disease provokes contraction of airway smooth muscle by a reflex that has both its arms in the vagus nerves. This contraction of the airways may improve the efficiency of coughing but is not helpful in conditions of asthma.
- ***Slowly adapting pulmonary receptors***. These receptors also have their afferent nerves in the vagus nerves. Their activity reduces bronchomotor tone. They are stimulated by stretching the lungs. Thus a large breath dilates the airways both by passive stretch and by this reflex effect.
- ***Carbon dioxide***. This gas causes bronchodilation by its direct relaxing action on the bronchial smooth muscle. In those parts of the lung that are underventilated, carbon dioxide will build up, dilate the airways, and improve local ventilation.

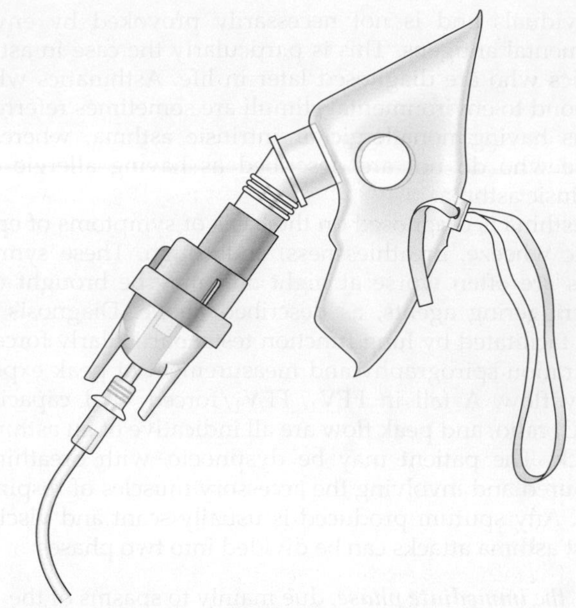

Fig. 4.18 A nebuliser. The flow of oxygen picks up droplets of the drug in the chamber of the nebuliser. Larger droplets are removed by directing the aerosol stream against a buffer. This leaves only fine droplets behind, which are able to reach the airways when inhaled from the mask.

Principles of treatment of asthma

National guidelines on the management of asthma are published, frequently updated, and should be referred to for clinical management. The following outlines the principles of management.

The treatment of asthma may address the early (bronchoconstrictor) or late (inflammatory) phases of the disease, frequently involving drugs delivered directly to the airway (e.g. as droplets produced by a nebuliser). One of the many types of nebulisers used in hospitals is shown in Figure 4.18.

Treatments for asthma are aimed at:

1. relieving bronchoconstriction,
2. reducing airway inflammation, and
3. influencing the immune system.

Relief of bronchoconstriction

Drugs that relieve bronchoconstriction act either to ***stimulate*** β_2 adrenoceptors or to ***block*** cholinergic receptors on the membranes of bronchial smooth muscle cells.

- *β_2-Adrenergic agonists.* Activation of these receptors causes an increase in cyclic adenosine monophosphate (cAMP) in the cell cytoplasm, which triggers muscle relaxation. Drugs in this class include salbutamol and terbutaline; they can be administered during attacks of bronchoconstriction or can be taken regularly to prevent attacks from occurring. They are generally administered with an inhaler or a nebuliser directly into the airways, although they may also be administered orally or even intravenously. In severe asthma attacks, they are regarded as the first line of treatment.

• *Anticholinergic drugs.* These drugs act by blocking the muscarinic acetylcholine receptors on the bronchial smooth muscle, reversing the bronchoconstriction produced by activation of these receptors. They may also reduce bronchial secretions by blocking the parasympathetic innervation of the submucosal glands in the bronchial tree. Drugs in this class include ipratropium. They are usually administered with an inhaler or a nebuliser and are usually regarded as being more effective in older patients with asthma.

• *Aminophylline/theophylline.* These drugs act on the bronchial smooth muscle. They increase the levels of cAMP in the cytoplasm by blocking the enzyme phosphodiesterase, which is responsible for breaking down cAMP. A rise in cAMP levels in the smooth muscle cells causes them to relax.

• *Leukotriene receptor antagonists.* An example of this class of drug is montelukast. These drugs act as bronchodilators by inhibiting leukotriene receptors on bronchial smooth muscle. Leukotrienes are potent bronchoconstrictors and these drugs may be especially useful in those with exercise-induced asthma.

Drugs that relieve airway inflammation

• *Corticosteroids.* Steroids have an anti-inflammatory effect and are more effective in the prevention of asthma than in the treatment of an acute attack. They reduce the inflammation in the airways and also modulate the immune response to allergens. Steroids can be administered via an inhaler. In this way, an effective dose is administered but many of the side effects of steroids can be avoided, as the blood concentration of the drug remains low. However, some patients need to take steroids orally. Whichever route is used, it is important that steroids are taken regularly to be effective. Although steroids are usually given during an acute attack, it probably takes some considerable time for them to have an acute effect.

Drugs that influence the immune system

• *Sodium cromoglicate.* The exact mode of action of this drug is not known, but it is thought that one of its actions is to 'stabilise' mast cells and prevent them from releasing bronchoconstrictor mediators. Like steroids, cromoglicate must be taken regularly and is a drug which is used to prevent asthma rather than to treat an acute attack.

Chronic obstructive pulmonary disease

Chronic obstructive pulmonary disease (COPD) is a term used to describe a disease which comprises bronchitis and emphysema. Often, patients have a greater contribution to their symptoms from one of these than the other.

Bronchitis

The airways, from nose to alveoli, are lined with a watery layer containing mucus. The normal mucus film within the lungs is approximately 5–10 μm thick and consists of two layers. The layer next to the airway wall is the waterier one that allows the cilia of the ciliary escalator to work, brushing the overlying, more viscous layer and any foreign particles it contains towards the mouth. Mucus is produced by ducted seromucous glands deep in the bronchial walls and by goblet cells in the bronchial epithelium. The accumulation of mucus results from excess production, drying of the surface, failure of the ciliary escalator to clear it, or infection making it too viscous to be moved. This effectively results in a narrowing or total blockage of the airways (Fig. 4.20). The secretion of mucus is normally controlled by vagal reflexes and local chemical stimulation. Curry and other spicy foods provoke the vagal reflex, and tobacco smoke stimulates both mechanisms. In extreme cases of bronchitis, mucus can solidify into tiny, solid casts of the small airways; chronic bronchitic patients may expectorate these casts.

Bronchitis is clinically defined by an excessive production of lung mucus. Diagnosis is based on expectoration, on most days, for at least 3 months during two successive years. The pathology that produces this excessive mucus is hypertrophy of the mucous glands of the large bronchi. Airway wall structure was described in Chapter 2. The **Reid Index** (Fig. 4.21) describes the ratio of bronchial glands to total wall thickness. In health, this is ≤0.4, but in chronic bronchitis it may exceed 0.7 due to hyperplasia of the glands. The smaller airways, which may undergo the initial pathological changes, are narrowed, inflamed, and show oedematous changes in their walls. The pathogenesis of bronchitis is clearly linked to tobacco smoking; air pollution also plays a role.

Emphysema

The support provided to the airway by **radial traction** is diminished in patients with emphysema. Emphysema is anatomically defined as an irreversible loss of parenchyma and an increase in the size of the air spaces distal to the terminal bronchioles. The destruction of lung parenchyma that brings about this increase in size is now generally agreed to be due to the uncontrolled action of proteolytic enzymes from leucocytes associated with pulmonary inflammation (Fig. 4.22). Cigarette smoke is often the cause, as it stimulates the release of elastase from neutrophils. Lung elastase is normally inhibited by antiprotease enzymes, the most important of which is **α_1-antitrypsin**. About 1 in 4000 people have a genetic α_1-antitrypsin deficiency, and therefore have a predisposition towards developing emphysema. Airway collapse, owing to loss of radial traction, is exacerbated by changes in transmural pressure, which brings about flow-related airway collapse. Closure of the airways can be prevented

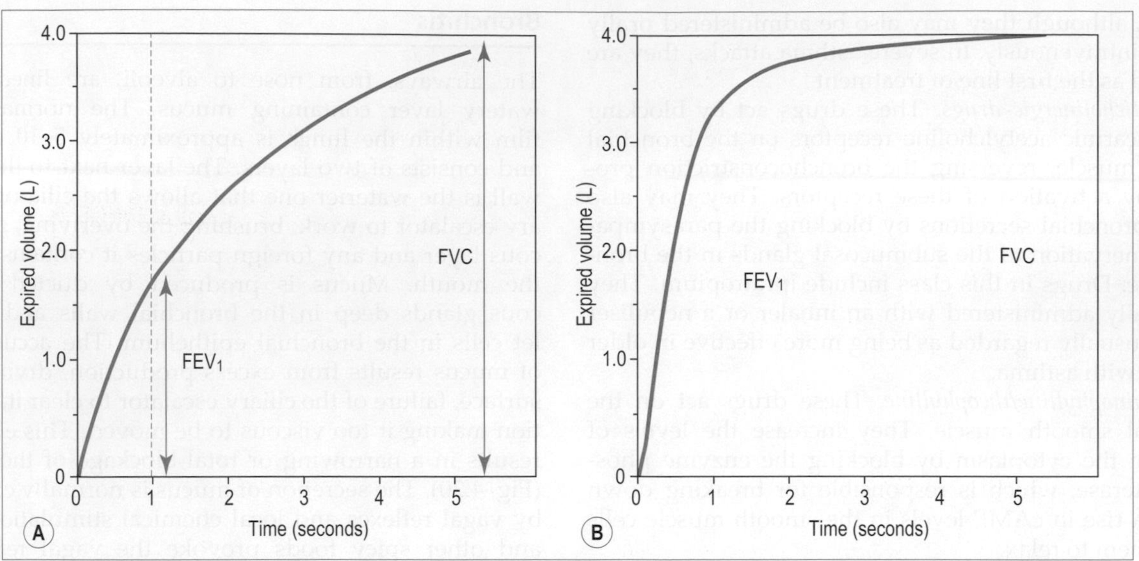

Fig. 4.19 Forced expiratory spirograms recorded from Mr Graham. Recording A was made while Mr Graham was feeling a bit wheezy. Recording B was made after Mr Graham had taken a dose of salbutamol from his inhaler. In recording A, the FEV_1 is very much reduced, although the FVC is essentially little different from normal. This means that the FEV_1/FVC ratio is reduced, indicating an obstructive respiratory defect. FEV_1, forced expiratory volume in 1 s; FVC, forced vital capacity.

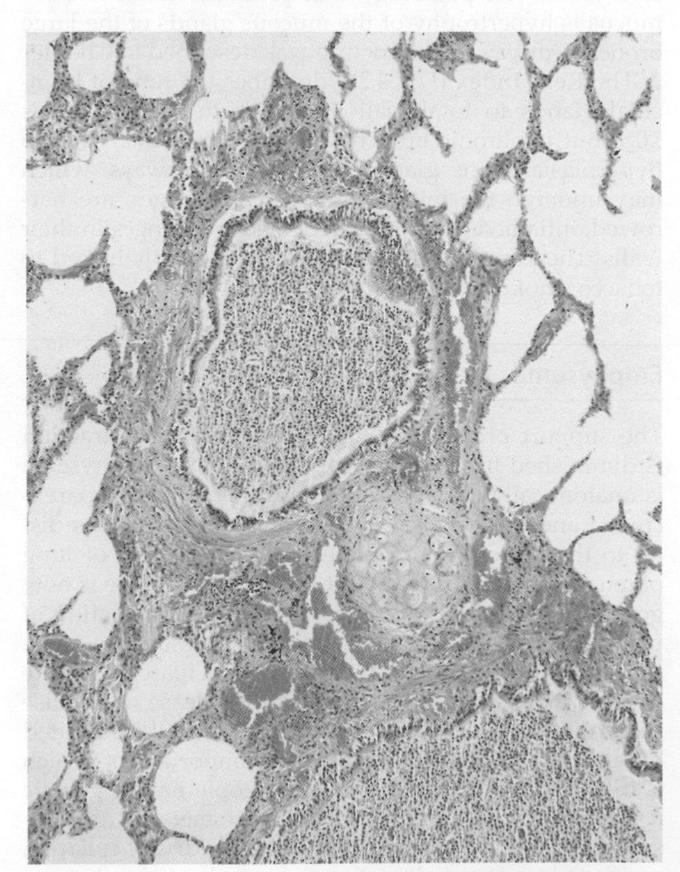

Fig. 4.20 Bronchitis with mucus totally blocking the airway lumen. (Source: Stevens, A., Lowe, J.S., Young, B., 2002. Wheater's Basic Histopathology. Churchill Livingstone.)

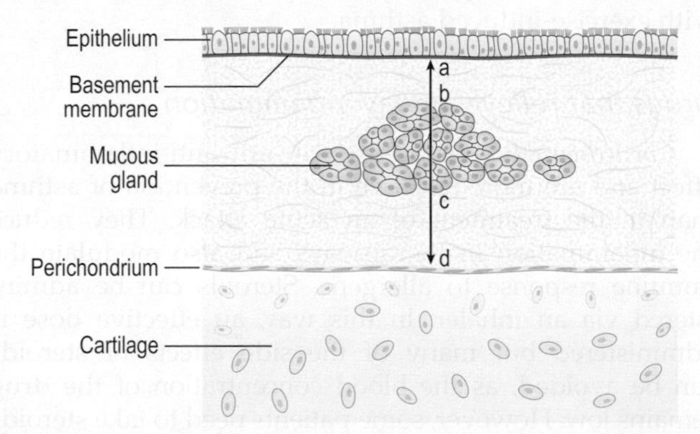

Fig. 4.21 The Reid Index. The percentage of bronchial wall thickness occupied by gland tissue is known as the Reid Index, and is used as a measure of chronic bronchitis.

by increasing the pressure within them, and many patients with emphysema whose airways are closing in this way intuitively exhale through pursed lips; the positive pressure within the airway generated by this 'pursed lip breathing' helps to keep their airways open.

Summary 4

- Asthma is characterised by an immediate bronchoconstrictive phase and a late inflammatory phase; both are targeted in treatment.
- Bronchomotor tone is controlled by parasympathetic nerves, sympathetic nerves, circulating catecholamines, NANC nerves, mast cells, neutrophils, pulmonary stretch, and rapidly adapting receptors.
- Reduced FEV_1, FEV_1/FVC ratio, and peak flow are indicative of an asthma attack.
- Emphysema is associated with airway collapse distal to the equal pressure point.

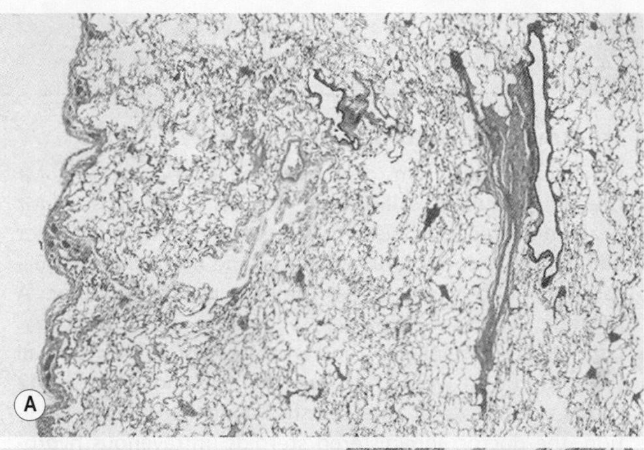

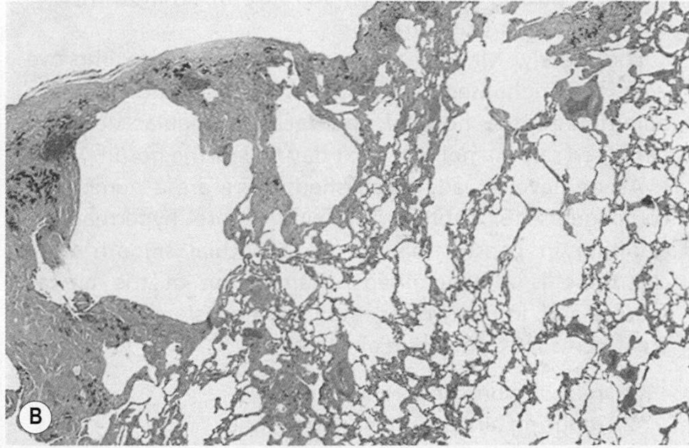

Fig. 4.22 Normal (A) and emphysematous lungs (B). (Source: Stevens, A., Lowe, J.S., Young, B., 2002. Wheater's Basic Histopathology. Churchill Livingstone.)

Case 4.1 Airflow in the respiratory system

Asthma

Mr Graham is a 25-year-old man who suffers from asthma. He has had the condition since he was a boy. He finds that his asthma is brought on by domestic animals (e.g. cats and dogs), cold or windy weather, and if he exercises too hard. However, his condition is kept under control with inhalers. Twice a day, he takes two inhaled doses of beclometasone, and he always keeps a salbutamol inhaler with him, which he uses when he gets wheezy. The salbutamol inhaler nearly always relieves his asthma.

We will consider:

1. The pathophysiology of asthma.
2. What provokes an asthma attack?
3. The drug treatment of asthma.

Case 4.1 Airflow in the respiratory system

The pathophysiology of asthma

Mr Graham attended a routine clinic appointment feeling a little wheezy. Figure 4.19A shows the forced expiratory spirogram which Mr Graham made at that appointment. After making the recording, Mr Graham used his salbutamol inhaler, which relieved his wheeziness. He then made a second forced expiratory spirogram, shown in Figure 4.19B. The principle behind measuring forced vital capacity (FVC) and forced expiratory volume in one second (FEV_1) is explained in Chapter 11. The spirogram in Figure 4.19A shows a reduced FEV_1, although the FVC is not particularly abnormal. In other words, the FEV_1/FVC ratio is reduced, indicating an obstructive abnormality. Following the administration of salbutamol, the airway narrowing reversed and the obstructive pattern on the spirogram improved. This reversibility of airway narrowing is characteristic of asthma.

Case 4.1 Airflow in the respiratory system

What provokes an asthma attack in patients with nonallergic or extrinsic asthma?

One day, Mr Graham suffered a particularly bad attack of asthma. He had had a cold for a week or so, but apart from that there did not seem to be any particular trigger for his attack. However, he became increasingly wheezy and found it more and more difficult to breathe. He found it especially difficult to exhale. He used his salbutamol inhaler several times but did not get any relief from it. Mr Graham's wife became increasingly worried about him and decided to call an ambulance. In the ambulance, Mr Graham was given oxygen to breathe; he was taken to the hospital where he was examined by the emergency doctor. The doctor noted that Mr Graham's respiratory rate was over 30 breaths per minute and that his chest was very expanded. Upon auscultation, the air entering into Mr Graham's lungs was reduced and there were wheezes throughout his chest. The doctor asked Mr Graham to perform a peak expiratory flow test. Mr Graham's peak expiratory flow was about two-thirds of his normal value. In most patients with asthma, a range of 'triggers' provoke attacks of bronchoconstriction. Such triggers include specific allergens, other nonspecific substances, exercise, and some drugs.

Allergens

Allergens are foreign substances that are able to provoke an immune response in susceptible individuals. In patients with extrinsic or allergic asthma, an attack of bronchoconstriction may be provoked by exposure to a specific allergen or to a range of allergens. The most common allergen responsible

Case 4.1 Airflow in the respiratory system – cont'd

for provoking asthma is a protein derived from the faeces of the house dust mite, which lives in warm locations, such as bedding, and feeds on scales of shed human skin. For many asthmatic patients, the presence of animals, such as cats, dogs, and birds, can provoke bronchoconstriction. In these cases, the allergen responsible is derived from animal skin, fur, feathers, or excreta. Allergens derived from pollen, particularly grass pollen, can provoke asthma as well as cause hay fever. In such cases, asthma may be confined to certain seasons of the year. Although the allergen normally has to be inhaled to provoke bronchoconstriction, in a small number of patients, an attack of asthma may be provoked by eating specific foods or chemicals.

Nonspecific provokers of asthma

In addition to reacting to specific allergens, the hyperreactive airways of asthmatic patients may also respond to a wide range of substances, including strong smells, dusts, vapours, smoke (including tobacco smoke), and airborne chemicals. These agents are thought to act directly on the airway itself, and an immune response is not provoked.

Exercise

In many patients, asthma may be provoked by exercise. The exact mechanism by which this occurs is not clear, but it is likely that cooling of hyperreactive airways may have an important role to play, as exercise-induced asthma often occurs more readily during cold weather. Drying of the airway mucosa may also play a role, as many asthmatics report that swimming is less likely to induce bronchospasms than other forms of exercise.

Drugs

A variety of drugs are known to induce asthma. Aspirin and other anti-inflammatory drugs can provoke bronchoconstriction in a small proportion of asthmatics. This action is probably brought about because these drugs affect the production of prostaglandins and leukotrienes; an imbalance of these substances in the airway may cause bronchoconstriction. β-Blocking drugs are also prone to producing bronchoconstriction in asthmatic patients, presumably by blocking β2 receptors on the bronchial smooth muscle; however, these drugs may also influence cells of the immune system.

Emotions

In many patients, strong emotional responses may result in attacks of bronchoconstriction. This is most probably mediated by a central neural mechanism.

Case 4.1 Airflow in the respiratory system

Treatment of asthma

After examining him, the emergency doctor gave Mr Graham nebulised salbutamol, the same drug as in Mr Graham's inhaler. However, whereas Mr Graham's inhaler administers a dose of 100 μg, each time it is used, the doctor prescribed 5 mg of salbutamol via the nebuliser. A nebuliser produces a fine aerosol of drug in a flow of oxygen. Mr Graham inhaled the aerosol, although only a small proportion of it would have reached his lungs. Figure 4.12 shows a nebuliser of the type that might be used. In addition, the doctor administered steroids (intravenous hydrocortisone) to Mr Graham.

Fortunately, Mr Graham's condition began to improve with the nebulised salbutamol. He was, nevertheless, admitted to the hospital and received regular doses of nebulised salbutamol. The next day he left the hospital.

As we have already established, there are a number of components to asthma. The airways are hyperreactive, resulting in constriction of the bronchial smooth muscle; there is a generalised inflammation of the airway mucosa and, in many cases, the immune system is involved. Treatments for asthma are aimed at:

1. relieving bronchoconstriction,
2. reducing airway inflammation, and
3. influencing the immune system.

References and further reading

Busse, W., Kraft, M., 2005. Cysteinyl leukotrienes in allergic inflammation: strategic targets for therapy. Chest 127, 1312–1326.

Healthcare Improvement Scotland, SIGN and British Thoracic Society, 2019. British Guideline on the Management of Asthma. Available at: sign158-updated.pdf (Accessed 31 December 2020).

Lumb, A.B., Thomas, C.R., 2020. Respiratory system resistance. In: Lumb, A.B., Thomas, C.R. (Eds.), Nunn Applied Respiratory Physiology. Elsevier, pp. 27–41.

Stevens, A., Lowe, J.S., Young, B., 2002. Wheater's Basic Histopathology. Churchill Livingstone.

Viegi, G., Pistelli, F., Sherrill, D.L., et al., 2007. Definition, epidemiology, and natural history of COPD. Eur. Respir. J. 30, 993–1013.

World Health Organization, 2007. Asthma and chronic obstructive pulmonary disease. In: Bousquet, J., Khaltaev, N. (Eds.), Global Surveillance, Prevention, and Control of Chronic Respiratory Diseases: A Comprehensive Approach. WHO Press, pp. 15–31.

5

PULMONARY VENTILATION

Chapter objectives

After studying this chapter, you should be able to:

1. Define ventilation.
2. Define the common lung volumes and capacities and how they are changed by restrictive and obstructive diseases.
3. Explain the importance of the structure of the respiratory system (as blind-ended tracts in parallel) on ventilation.
4. Differentiate between physiological and anatomical dead space and relate increased dead space to disease states.
5. Explain the composition of the parts of a single exhaled breath and why these are changed by disease.
6. Understand the alveolar gas equation.
7. Describe the physiological factors influencing the distribution of ventilation.

Introduction

In respiratory medicine, the term ventilation is used to describe the rate of flow of air into or out of the lungs. This results from the expansion and contraction of the lungs caused by changes in intrapleural pressure. These are described in Chapter 4 and illustrated in Figure 5.1. 'Normal' breathing consists of about 12 breaths per minute, each breath being around 0.5 litres (L) L.

The symbol for ventilation, $\dot{V}$, has a dot over the V to indicate that it is a *rate*. Because the volume expired is approximately equal to the volume inspired (tidal volume, V_T), the net flow over a complete cycle is zero. This is not a very helpful way of expressing ventilation if we want to express changes in breathing as a result of exercise or disease. Flow is therefore measured in one direction only, and this is conventionally the volume expired per minute ($\dot{V}_E$) to give us **minute ventilation**, as below:

$$\text{respiratory rate}\left(\sim 12\ \text{min}^{-1}\right) \times \text{tidal volume}\ (\sim 0.5\ \text{L}) = \text{minute ventilation}\left(\sim 6.0\ \text{L min}^{-1}\right)$$

Alveolar ventilation is a part of the V_T which ventilates the alveoli, where gas exchange with the blood takes place. Alterations in alveolar ventilation occur in many lung pathologies.

Lung volumes, capacities and spirometry

In respiratory physiology, capacity is the sum of two or more volumes. We can consciously alter the volume of our lungs by breathing in or out more deeply than normal, but we cannot completely empty our lungs. At the end of a normal quiet expiration, the average intrapleural pressure is approximately −0.5 kPa (i.e. below atmospheric pressure) and the lung volume is around 2.5 L. This volume represents the functional residual capacity (FRC). When a subject inhales as much as they can and then holds their breath, *intrapleural pressure* decreases to −2 kPa and lung volume increases to about 6 L. After exhaling as much as possible, the intrapleural pressure will increase to −0.2 kPa and the lung volume will decrease to 1.0 L. This is the residual volume (RV) that cannot be expelled.

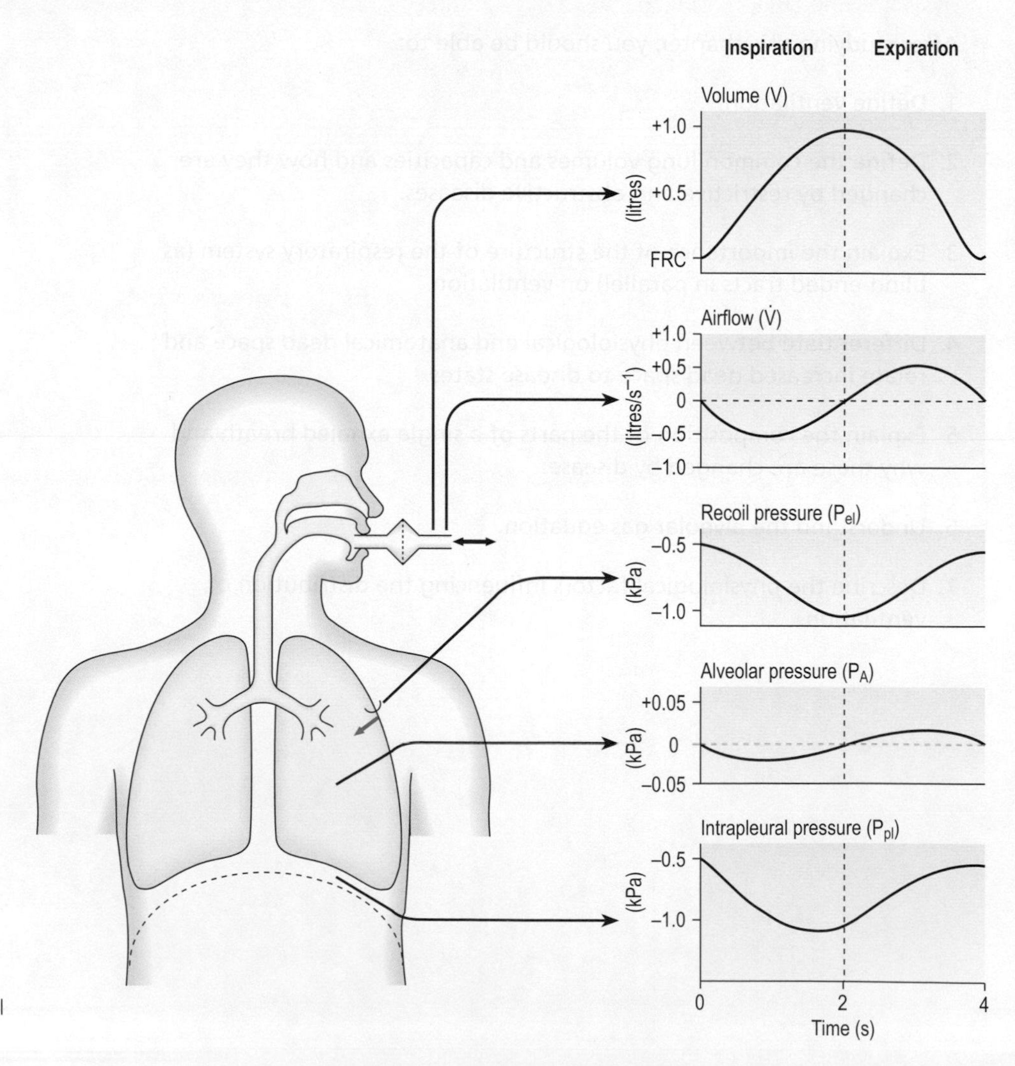

Fig. 5.1 A single respiratory cycle. Airflow is measured using a pneumotachograph and integrated to give tidal volume. *Recoil pressure* has a negative sign because it is the difference between *alveolar* and *intrapleural pressure*, relative to atmospheric pressure. FRC, functional residual capacity.

The size of an individual's chest, the elasticity of the lungs and chest wall, and the strength of the respiratory muscles determine these volumes. Changes in lung volume can be measured using a spirometer, as illustrated in Figure 5.2. This instrument, which comes in many forms, consists of a closed space from which the subject breathes. In the type illustrated, a hollow bell is supported in a trough of water. As the subject inspires, air is drawn from the bell, and it sinks slightly; upon expiration, the bell rises. Movements of the bell are recorded as changes in the lung volume on a moving chart. Information about lung properties and the diagnosis of diseases can be obtained by measuring changes in lung volume.

Static lung volumes are those which are independent of the rate of flow. Five of these can be measured using the spirometer technique described above. These are the V_T, **inspiratory reserve volume** (IRV), **expiratory reserve volume** (ERV), **vital capacity** (VC) and inspiratory capacity which is the sum of the V_T and IRV. To ascertain the RV, FRC and **total lung capacity** (TLC), an alternative methodology is required (see below).

When maximum inspiration is taken, the increase in lung volume (IRV) to reach the TLC is about 3 L. A maximal expiration from TLC will expel the IRV, V_T, and ERV, the total of all these volumes being the VC. If the lungs are taken out of the body, postmortem, and allowed to collapse, there will still be a little air left in them. This is called minimal air (see Chapter 2, 'Lights').

The changes in intrapleural pressure that bring about these volume changes do not vary much between individuals in health or disease. However, a number of factors lead to greater or smaller lung volumes. These factors include:

- *Body size.* All are linearly related to height. Obesity causes a reduction in static lung volumes, except for V_T.
- *Age.* Volumes are smaller in children, only partially due to their smaller body size. With increasing age, VC decreases, but both FRC and RV increase because of degenerative changes in the tissues, leading to a reduced **recoil pressure.**
- *Sex.* Volumes are smaller in females (e.g. the FRC of females is 10% less than that of males of the same height). This is due to the more muscular chest of males.
- *Posture.* FRC is reduced in the supine position compared with measurements made when a subject is upright because the diaphragm is displaced cephalad by the abdominal contents.
- *Muscle training.* This increases all lung volumes and allows greater maximal ventilation during exercise.
- *Disease.* Changes in lung volumes from the normal values are used in the diagnosis of many diseases of the lungs and respiratory system.

Because the RV cannot be expired, the RV, FRC and TLC (the latter two include the RV) cannot be directly measured using a spirometer. If one of these is measured, the others can be derived, and the capacity most usually measured is the FRC. Three techniques can be used to measure FRC. A gas dilution technique may be used, whereby a subject inhales a known volume of a non-absorbable tracer gas, such as helium, and its concentration is then measured, allowing the volume to be calculated. Alternatively, a nitrogen washout technique may be used. Here, the subject begins from the FRC and breathes from a bag containing a known volume of 100% oxygen. Then, they breathe out into the bag. Because the air in the FRC contained approximately 80% nitrogen, the dilution of this by the known volume of pure oxygen in the bag enables the volume to be calculated. The third method uses body plethysmography (see Chapter 11, 'Helium Dilution Method and Plethysmography'), which is the only technique that accounts for gas trapping in the lung beyond closed airways.

Spirometric abnormalities in disease

Lung disease changes many lung volumes, as shown in Figure 5.2. Dynamic studies can be performed to assist diagnoses; the patient breathes in as deeply as possible and out as hard as possible to obtain data from a single breath. Measurements made under these circumstances

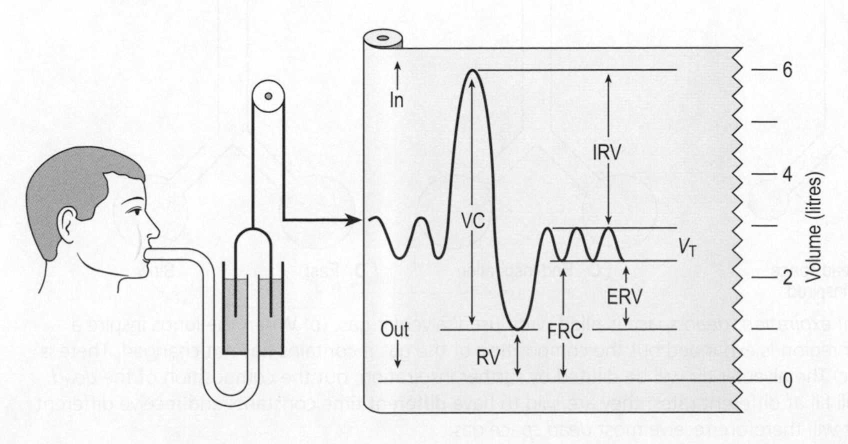

Fig. 5.2 A spirometer record of breathing. Average adult volumes are shown. Because the lungs cannot be completely emptied, RV and FRC cannot be measured by direct spirometry. ERV, expiratory reserve volume; FRC, functional residual capacity; IRV, inspiratory reserve volume; RV, residual volume; VC, vital capacity; V_T, tidal volume.

include the forced expiratory volume in 1 second (FEV_1) and forced vital capacity (FVC), which is the total volume of air a patient can breathe out after maximal inspiration. It is usual to express FEV_1 as a percentage of FVC. This takes into account the fact that taller people normally have larger lungs and therefore a greater FVC. Much careful work has gone into preparing tables that relate spirometric measurements to a normal subject's height and weight. Deviations from the values predicted by these tables are diagnostic of lung diseases.

Diseases of the thoracic cage (such as ankylosing spondylitis), diseases of the nerves and muscles of respiration (such as poliomyelitis), diseases that restrict expansion of the lungs (such as fibrosis) and diseases that cause airway collapse during expiration limit these spirometric measurements. The spirometric trace changes produced by lung diseases can be summarised in a general way as follows (see Chapter 11):

Variable	*Restrictive disease*	*Obstructive disease*
FVC	–	–
FEV_1	–	–
FEV_1/FVC	0	–
FRC	–	+
RV	–	+
TLC	–	+

0, no change; +, increase; –, decrease.

FEV_1, forced expiratory volume in 1 second; FRC, functional residual capacity; FVC, forced vital capacity; RV, residual volume; TLC, total lung capacity.

NB: Some of these changes are not observed to any degree until the disease is very advanced.

Dead space

The distribution of ventilation within the lungs is not uniform. In Chapter 2, the anatomy of the bronchial tree was described as blind-ended sacs connected to the outside environment through a system of tubes. The composition of gas may be different at the entrance to the respiratory system (the lips or nares) from that at the end (the alveoli), and these can be considered differences in series. The composition of gas in different alveoli may also vary, and this variation can be considered differences in parallel. In addition, a combination of both variations may exist. Differences in the composition of air in different parts of the lung depend largely on how well that part is ventilated and the extent to which gas exchange between the air and blood takes place. In the ideal situation, just the right amount of both air and blood are supplied to a particular region so that there is no 'waste' or under-delivery of either. One particular example of inequality between air (ventilation) and blood supply (perfusion) is known as **the dead space**.

Anatomical and alveolar dead space

The exchange of gases between air and blood occurs only at the alveolar surface. The conducting airways, connecting this surface to the atmosphere, do not participate in gas exchange and comprise the **anatomical dead space**. It is called 'anatomical' because it is equivalent to the anatomical volume of the conducting airways. Anatomical dead space may be considered as the volume of an inspired breath which does not mix with the gas in the alveoli. To understand anatomical dead space, the lungs must be understood to fill and empty in a sequential fashion (Fig. 5.3). At the end of inspiration, the contents of the alveoli have been diluted by inspired air, which now also fills the anatomical dead space (see Fig. 5.3C). As the lungs then empty during expiration, the rule of 'last in first out' applies, and the dead space containing unmodified air is exhaled first. At the end of expiration, the anatomical dead space is filled with alveolar air, and this is then inhaled first in the next inspiration (see Fig. 5.3A and B). Healthy lungs are generally composed of tissues which inflate and deflate at similar rates. However, if some regions of the lung have different **time constants** and expand more quickly than others during the process of inspiration (see Chapter 3), they will receive an inappropriately large part of this dead space gas, and the regions receiving air later in inspiration will receive more fresh air (see Fig. 5.3 C and D). The timing of the inflation of a part of the lung during inspiration affects the composition of the gas it receives.

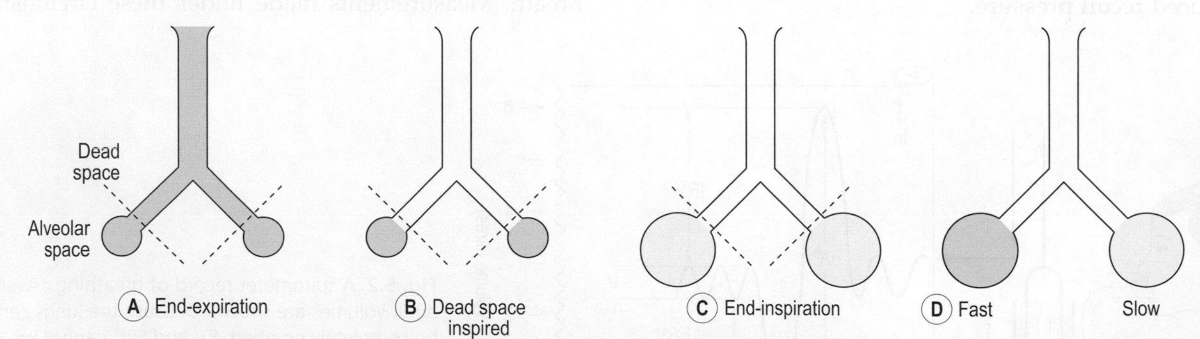

Fig. 5.3 Distribution of dead space gas. (a) At the end of *expiration, dead space* is filled with 'used' alveolar gas. (b) When the lungs inspire a volume of fresh air equal to the *dead space*, the alveolar region is expanded but the composition of the gas it contains has not changed. There is fresh air in the *dead space* and 'used' air in the alveoli. (c) The alveolar air will be diluted by further inspiration, but the composition of the *dead space* air will remain that of the fresh air. (d) If the alveoli fill at different rates, they are said to have different time constants and receive different amounts of *dead space* gas. The alveoli that expand first will therefore receive most *dead space* gas.

In healthy subjects, the anatomical dead space is all dead space, but with ageing and/or lung disease, alveolar dead space begins to appear. Alveolar dead space is the volume of inspired air which reaches the respiratory surfaces of the alveoli, which then have insufficient blood supply to act as effective respiratory membranes. Anatomical and alveolar dead spaces, together, constitute a physiological dead space. A 'rule of thumb' is that a healthy subject's weight, in pounds (1 lb = 0.45 kg), is numerically equal to their dead space, in millilitres, or around 150 mL in a 70-kg adult.

The alveolar dead space is not a fixed volume. In Chapter 7, we will see that the body is generally effective at promoting blood flow to regions of the lung that are well ventilated and supplying relatively less blood to poorly ventilated regions. This matching of ventilation and perfusion is very important and is a major defect in a wide variety of diseases.

Measuring and calculating dead space

Fowler's method

Because gas exchange occurs effectively only in the alveoli, there is no carbon dioxide (CO_2) excreted by the dead space. In 1948, a physiologist named W.S. Fowler described how anatomical dead space could be measured as the volume of gas expired prior to CO_2 appearing at the lips (Fig. 5.4). However, there may be a considerable slope, particularly when the subject is breathing vigorously or when alveoli empty at different rates, making it difficult to decide where to draw the vertical line. This can be a particular issue if a patient has, for example, chronic obstructive pulmonary disease and has rather varied time constants across different functional lung units.

Bohr equation

The physiological dead space is the volume of inspired air which has not taken part in gas exchange and includes both the anatomical and alveolar dead space. In 1891, Carl Bohr developed an equation to calculate the ratio of physiological dead space volume to V_T:

$$\frac{V_D}{V_T} = \frac{(Pa_{CO_2} - PE_{CO_2})}{Pa_{CO_2}}$$

where V_D is the volume of the physiological dead space, V_T is the tidal volume, PE_{CO2} is the partial pressure of CO_2 in expired air and Pa_{CO2} is the partial pressure of CO_2 in the arterial blood. The volume of gas expired in a single breath (V_T) is the sum of the volume from the physiological dead space (V_D) plus the volume taking part in alveolar ventilation (V_A):

$$V_T = V_D + V_A$$

$$V_A \text{ is therefore } V_T - V_D$$

The other terms which appear in the derivation of the equation are those used to describe the fractional CO_2 concentrations in inhaled, exhaled and alveolar gas, which are F_I, F_E and F_A, respectively. The CO_2 in an expired breath is the volume of that breath (V_T) multiplied by the fractional concentration (%) of the CO_2 (F_E) in the whole breath, that is, $F_E \times V_T$. This total is made up of alveolar gas (F_A [$V_T - V_D$]) and dead space gas ($F_I \times V_D$).

The Bohr equation is derived as follows:

$F_E \times V_T = (F_I \times V_D) + (F_A [V_T - V_D])$,

The F_I is 0, so $(F_I \times V_D)$ is eliminated.

$F_E \times V_T = F_A (V_T - V_D)$ which can be rearranged to

$F_E \quad V_T = (F_A \times V_T) - (F_A \times V_D)$. This is rearranged to give

$(F_E \times V_T) + (F_A \times V_D) = F_A \times V_T$. Then,

$F_A \times V_D = (F_A \times V_T) - (F_E \times V_T)$. This is simplified to

$F_A \times V_D = V_T (F_A - F_E)$ and rearranged to

$V_D / V_T = (F_A - F_E) / F_A$

Because, as above, the F_A is the PA_{CO2}, and F_E is PE_{CO2}, the Bohr equation is

$$\frac{V_D}{V_T} = \frac{(Pa_{CO_2} - PE_{CO_2})}{Pa_{CO_2}}$$

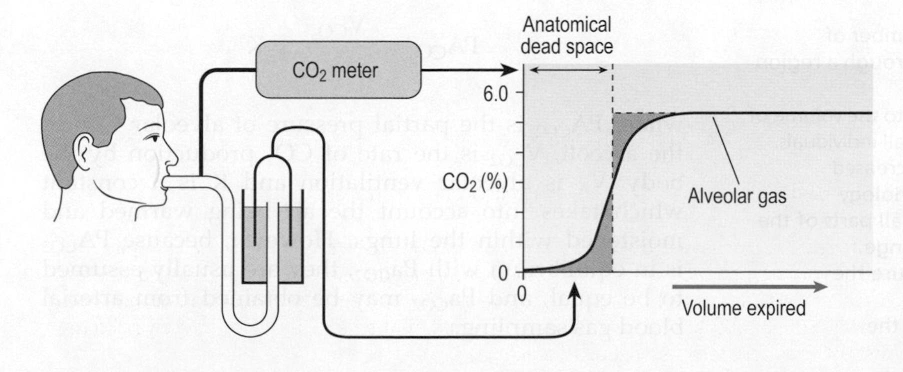

Fig. 5.4 Estimating *dead space* volume. Carbon dioxide concentrations rise rapidly in the expired air when the *dead space* has been expired. The volume at the midpoint of this rapid rise is taken as *dead space* volume. The flat part of the curve is called the alveolar plateau.

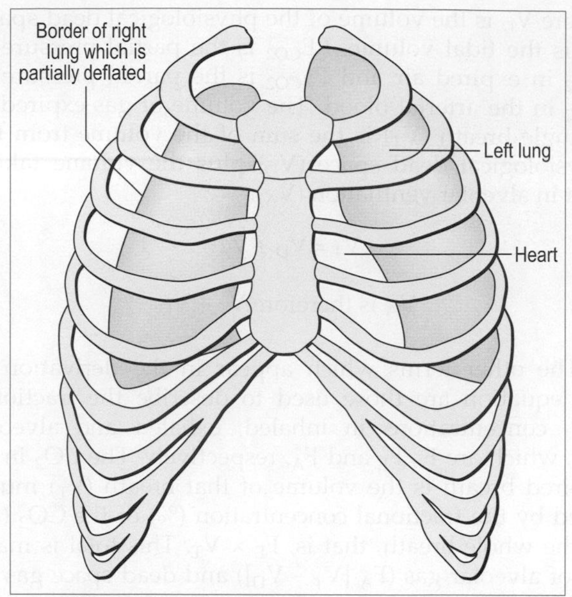

Fig 5.5 A right-sided pneumothorax. There is no space between the left lung and the chest wall whereas the right lung is partially collapsed and there is air in the intrapleural space.

The partial pressure of arterial CO_2 (Pa_{CO2}) is almost identical to the partial pressure of alveolar CO_2 (PA_{CO2}); therefore, the equation is written as

$$\frac{V_D}{V_T} = \frac{(Pa_{CO_2} - PE_{CO_2})}{Pa_{CO_2}}$$

In health, the dead space volume is around 30% of the V_T, and the normal ratio is 0.3.

Factors affecting dead space

Because the alveolar dead space is small in health, the anatomical and physiological dead spaces are very similar at around 150 mL. Like other lung volumes, this varies with the height of the individual. Posture, age and sex also affect the physiological dead space, with males having a larger dead space than females. Changes in dead space are a feature of lung diseases, including pulmonary embolus (see Chapter 7), where ventilation is maintained in the presence of restricted perfusion due to the embolus.

Summary 1

- Ventilation can be measured as the number of changes in air or the rate of airflow through a region of the lung per minute.
- The anatomical dead space is equivalent to the volume of the conducting airways and is present in all individuals.
- Alveolar dead space is variable, and increased alveolar dead space occurs in lung pathology
- Physiological dead space is the sum of all parts of the V_T that do not participate in gas exchange.
- Fowler's method may be used to measure the anatomical dead space.
- The Bohr equation is used to calculate the physiological dead space.

Alveolar ventilation and respiratory exchange

Gas exchange only takes place in the alveoli, and only takes place efficiently in alveoli that are both ventilated and perfused. Dead space increases in disease when regions of the lung receive too little blood to carry out adequate gas exchange, which may adversely affect lung function. In a subject breathing with a V_T of 0.5 L and a respiratory rate of 12 min^{-1}, the flow of O_2 into and CO_2 out of the body is carried by a minute ventilation of 6 L min^{-1}. If V_D = 0.15 L, the effective ventilation that brings about the exchange of O_2 and CO_2 ventilation of the alveoli is

$$6 - (12 \times 0.15) = 4.2 \text{ L min}^{-1}$$

Room air contains virtually no CO_2, and the alveolar gas contains 5.5%, giving an output of

$$4.2 \times \frac{(5.5 - 0)}{100} = 231 \text{ mL min}^{-1}$$

Oxygen, on the other hand, forms 21% of the atmosphere, and alveolar gas contains about 14%; therefore, the uptake of oxygen is:

$$4.2 \times \frac{(21 - 14)}{100} = 294 \text{ mL min}^{-1}$$

The ratio of CO_2 output divided by O_2 uptake is called the respiratory exchange ratio (or respiratory quotient, when used to describe the exchange in tissues or cells). It is given the symbol R and can range from 1, when only carbohydrates are being metabolised, to 0.7, when only fats are being used. In a subject with a mixed diet, it is around 0.8. The ratio depends on the amount of oxygen already in the molecule being oxidised; the more oxygen the molecule contains, the less has to be 'brought in' to complete the oxidation. For the figures above:

$$R = \frac{231}{294} = 0.79$$

The partial pressure of oxygen or CO_2 in the alveoli depends on the rate at which it is supplied (oxygen) or removed (CO_2) by ventilation. For CO_2 this is:

$$PA_{CO_2} = \frac{\dot{V}_{CO_2}}{\dot{V}_A} \times K$$

where PA_{CO2} is the partial pressure of alveolar CO_2 in the alveoli, $\dot{V}_{CO2}$ is the rate of CO_2 production by the body, $\dot{V}_A$ is alveolar ventilation and K is a constant which takes into account the air being warmed and moistened within the lungs. However, because PA_{CO2} is in equilibrium with Pa_{CO2}, they are usually assumed to be equal, and Pa_{CO2} may be obtained from arterial blood gas sampling.

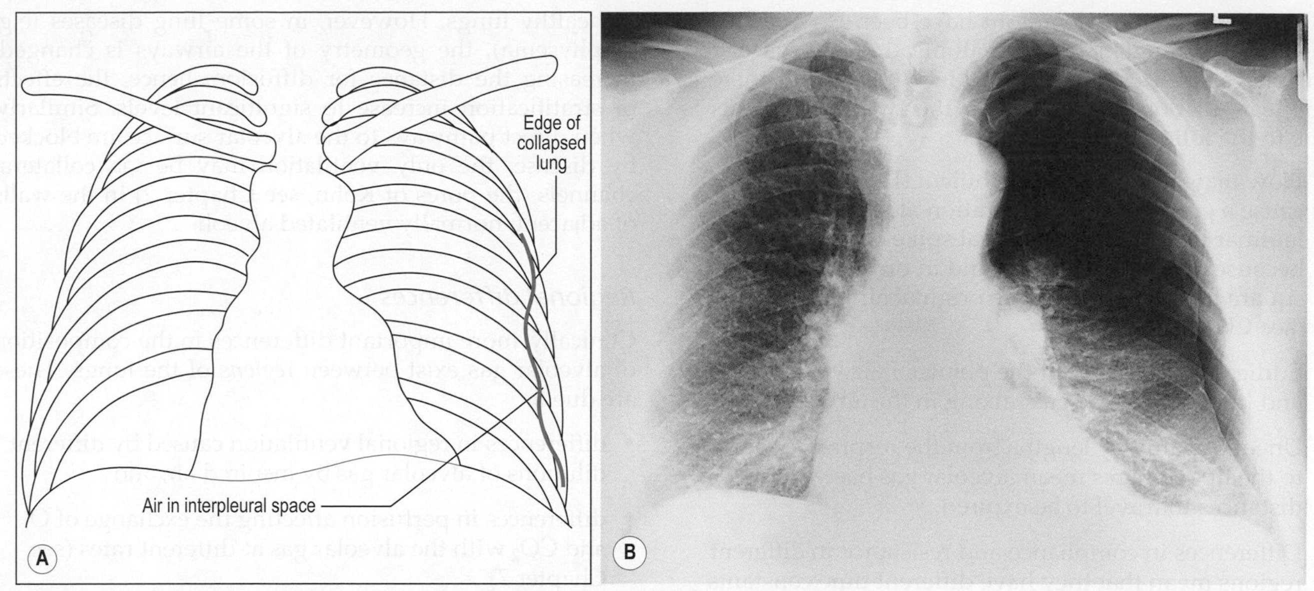

Fig. 5.6 Small left-sided pneumothorax. (A) Diagram showing that the left lung has partially *collapsed* and there is air between it and the inside of the right chest wall. (B) Chest X-ray of a patient with a left-sided pneumothorax. This chest X-ray is similar to the diagram in (A). The border of the left lung is clearly visible, and the air-filled space between the lung margin and the chest wall appears darker than the adjacent lung on the X-ray.

Alveolar gas equation

The **alveolar gas equation** can be used to find the partial pressure of oxygen in an alveolus (PA_{O2}) when supplied with a varying fraction of inspired oxygen:

$$PA_{O_2} = [FI_{O_2} \times (P_{ATM} - P_{H_2O})] - (PA_{CO_2}/R)$$

where FI_{O2} is the fraction of inspired oxygen (e.g. 0.21) in the case of room air with an oxygen content of 21%, P_{ATM} is atmospheric pressure in kPa, P_{H_2O} is the standard vapour pressure (SVP) of water at 37°C in kPa and R is the respiratory exchange ratio or quotient, as described above. The SVP of water is subtracted because the fractional concentration of oxygen only applies to the dry gas component.

A worked example to demonstrate the situation under normal conditions is therefore:

$$\begin{aligned} PA_{O_2} &= [0.21 \times (101 - 6.3)] - 5.3/0.8 \\ &= (0.21 \times 94.7) - 6.6 \\ &= 19.88 - 6.6 \\ &= 13.3 \text{ kPa} \end{aligned}$$

The effect of changing alveolar ventilation on the alveolar partial pressures of oxygen and CO_2 is shown graphically in Figure 5.7. Increased or decreased ventilation have opposite effects on the alveolar concentrations of these two gases. You will see later (see Chapter 8) that this does not mean that the amount of oxygen carried into the circulation can increase or decrease in a linear fashion, as with CO_2, because in the case of oxygen, carriage is limited by the capacity of its carrier rather than by the amount flowing into the lungs.

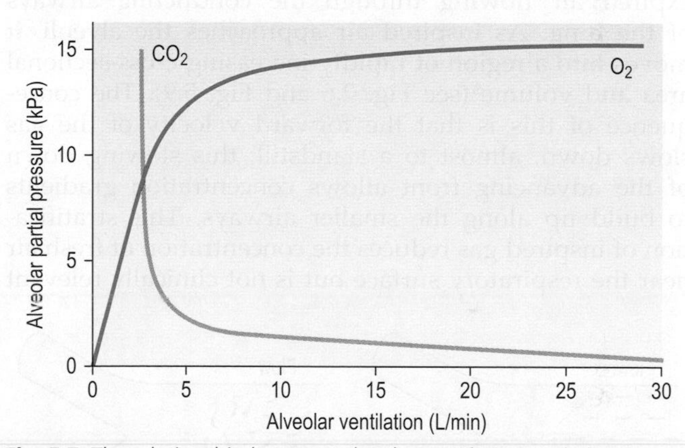

Fig. 5.7 The relationship between alveolar ventilation and alveolar partial pressures of O_2 and CO_2. The alveolar partial pressure of CO_2 (PCO_2) varies inversely with ventilation in an asymptotic fashion. The alveolar partial pressure of O_2 (PO_2) rises with increasing ventilation and reaches a plateau.

Variations in the composition and distribution of inspired air

Because the bronchial tree consists of a large number of paths in parallel, differences in the composition of the air exist both in series (along any path from the atmosphere to the alveoli) or between regions (e.g. between the right and left lungs or between functional units within the same lung). These differences can become so significant that they interfere with gas exchange.

Differences along the airway from atmosphere to alveoli

It can be seen from Figure 5.4 that the concentration of CO_2 in an expired breath does not rise as a sudden step to its alveolar value, as might have been expected from the serial arrangement of anatomical dead space and alveolar space described so far. In other words, there is no clear-cut boundary between the two spaces. This is due to the following factors.

- Flow may be laminar or turbulent (Fig. 5.8), and both cause a gradient of concentration along the tube. In laminar flow, there is a central spike of faster flow because of axial streaming, and in turbulent flow, the square front mixes with the original air as it advances (see Chapter 4).
- Eddies of turbulence at the points of airway branching and heartbeat cause gas mixing in the airways.
- Unequal pathway lengths from the respiratory surface to the lips or nares mean alveolar gas has varying distances to travel to be expired.
- Differences in compliance and resistance in different regions mean that they have different time constants and take different lengths of time to fill and empty.

These considerations apply to both the inspired and expired air flowing through the conducting airways of the lung. As inspired air approaches the alveoli, it moves into a region of rapidly increasing cross-sectional area and volume (see Fig. 2.6 and Fig. 5.9). The consequence of this is that the forward velocity of the gas slows down, almost to a standstill; this slowing down of the advancing front allows concentration gradients to build up along the smaller airways. This stratification of inspired gas reduces the concentration of fresh air near the respiratory surface but is not clinically relevant in healthy lungs. However, in some lung diseases (e.g. emphysema), the geometry of the airways is changed, increasing the distance for diffusion; hence, the effects of stratification increase to significant levels. Similarly, when direct pathways to the alveolar surface are blocked by disease, the only ventilation may be via collateral channels (the pores of Kohn, see Chapter 2) in the walls of adjacent, normally ventilated alveoli.

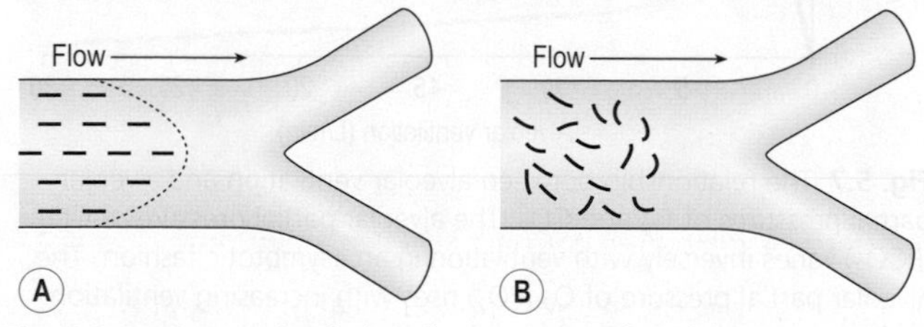

Fig. 5.8 Laminar and turbulent flow. Laminar flow (A) moves in organised layers parallel to the sides of the airway, with the maximum velocity at the centre. Turbulent flow (B) is disorganised, and the velocity profile is flat.

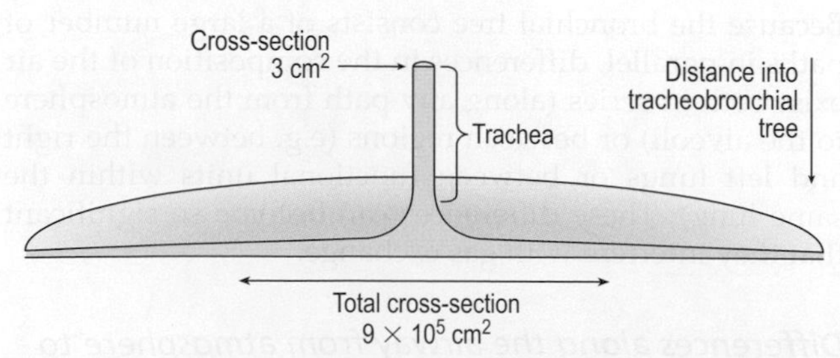

Fig. 5.9 Airway cross-sectional areas. The total cross-sectional area increases as you penetrate deeper into the bronchial tree. The area of the alveolar respiratory surface, represented by the horizontal line, is 300 000 times greater than the cross-sectional area of the *trachea*.

Regional differences

Clinically, more important differences in the composition of alveolar gas exist between *regions* of the lungs. These are due to:

- differences in regional ventilation caused by different dilutions of alveolar gas by inspired air, and
- differences in perfusion affecting the exchange of O_2 and CO_2 with the alveolar gas at different rates (see Chapter 7).

The greatest difference in regional ventilation in a healthy, standing subject is between the apex (top) and the base of the lungs; ventilation in a horizontal plane is similar in different regions. To explain this vertical difference in regional ventilation, we must remember:

- Ventilation is the amount of gas moved into and out of a region, irrespective of the initial volume of that region.
- The motive force which brings about ventilation is the change in the intrapleural pressure around the

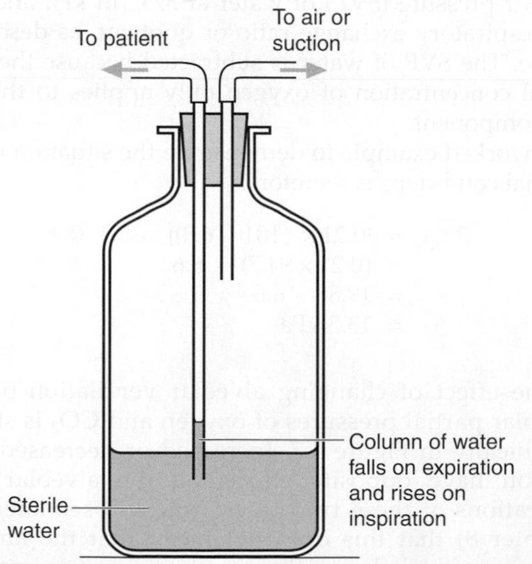

Fig. 5.10 An underwater seal. Gas from the pneumothorax passes from the chest drain and bubbles through the water in the seal. The water prevents gas passing from the atmosphere into the intrapleural space and also collects blood and other liquid secretions, which might block a mechanical valve (Gardner, 2010).

lungs, which becomes more negative with respect to the atmosphere during inspiration and leads to the expansion of the lungs (see Chapter 3).

- The effect of gravity on the contents of the chest is to cause the intrapleural pressure to be less negative at the base of the lungs than at the apex. It increases (becomes less negative) by about 0.025 kPa for every centimetre closer to the base of the lung (see Chapter 3).

The effect of this gravity-induced gradient of intrapleural pressure is clearly seen if the structure of the lungs in the upright position at the end of expiration (i.e. at FRC) is viewed under a microscope (Fig. 5.11) or via imaging modalities. We see that the alveoli at the top are expanded to nearly their full size, whereas those at the bottom are only slightly expanded. What happens during inspiration was investigated in a series of experiments using the radioactive gas Xenon (^{133}Xe). The radioactive gas was used to inflate isolated lungs suspended in a pressure gradient that mimicked that found in the upright human chest, i.e. increasing by 0.025 kPa for every centimetre moved towards the base. This can be achieved by placing the lungs in a foam of appropriate density. The amount of radioactive gas in a region at any time during inflation can be measured by radioactivity counters placed over the surface of the lungs (Fig. 5.12).

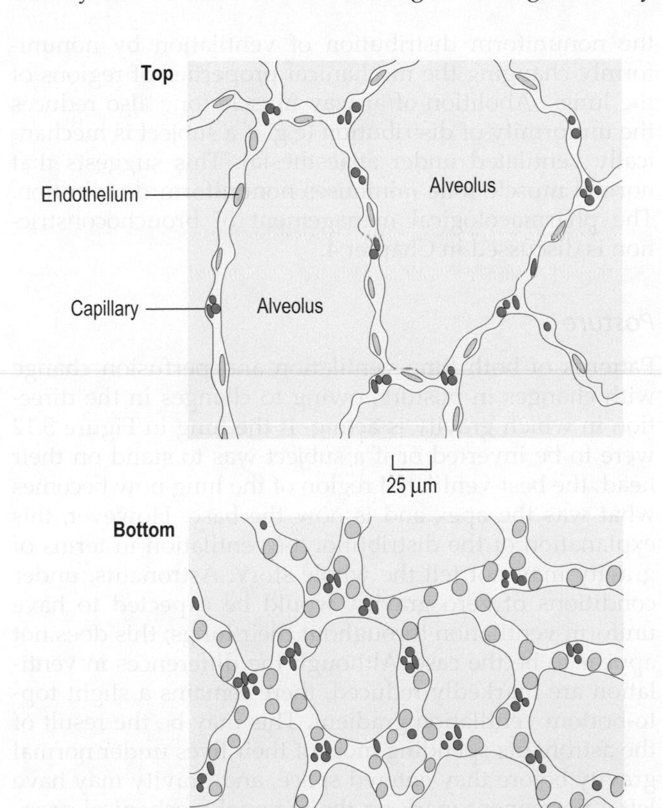

Fig. 5.11 Alveolar dimensions at the top and bottom of an upright lung. These are images of the alveolar regions at the top and bottom of a lung frozen in the upright position. In the top of the lung the *alveoli* are distended, and the *capillaries* empty of blood, compared with those in the bottom of the lung. This effect is due largely to gravity.

Although these effects apply in a continuous fashion from apex to base, for now we will treat the lungs as if they were just two regions, upper and lower. The vertical axis of Figure 5.12 shows the volumes of the upper and lower regions of the isolated lungs as a percentage of their ultimate volume when fully inflated. The horizontal axis gives the volume of the whole lung (i.e. that of all regions). If the lungs were free of any pressure gradient, the upper and lower regions would both expand at the same rate, and the points representing these volumes would fall along the same line, as shown by the dotted line in Figure 5.12. With a pressure gradient applied over the lungs, the two regions behaved differently. The slope of the lines in Figure 5.12 represents the rate of change in volume: the steeper the slope, the greater the rate of inflation. The cubes represent the fraction of the maximum achievable volume that a sample of lung from the top or bottom has achieved at that moment.

It can be seen that:

- The lower lobe starts at a smaller percentage of the maximal volume because it is compressed by the greater pressure.
- The ventilatory capacity of the upper region is smaller than that of the lower region (i.e. it operates in the range of 40%–100% of its total volume range), whereas the lower lobe operates in the 15%–100% range. This is because the upper region is initially more inflated.
- At volumes well below the FRC, there is proportionally more rapid inflation of the upper regions (compare the slopes of the lines in Fig. 5.12). This is because at these volumes, some of the airways to the lower lobes close, and it takes a greater pressure to re-expand them.
- At greater lung volumes, the situation reverses, and there is more ventilation in the lower region.
- Upon deflation of the lungs, the points in Figure 5.12, representing the volumes of the two lung regions described, move down the two curves, reversing the effects.

It should also be remembered that human lungs are roughly cone shaped, with more tissue at the base than at the apex; this amplifies the effect of greater ventilation on the base of the lung.

Other factors affecting regional variation in ventilation

Age

The degenerative changes of ageing produce differences in the mechanical properties of the lung regions. These cause ventilation to become increasingly nonuniform.

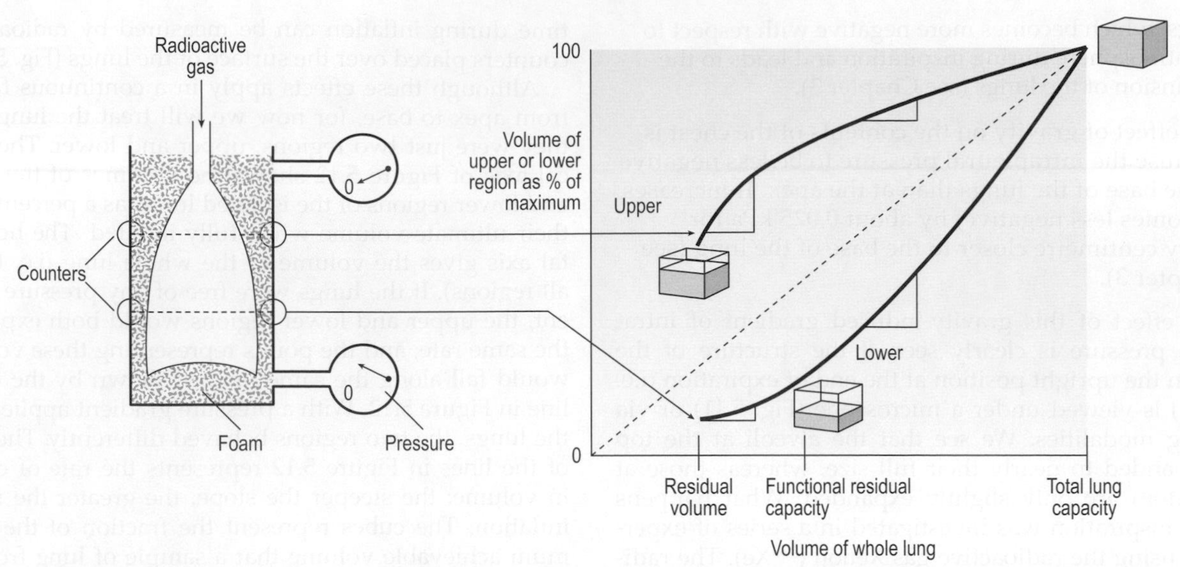

Fig. 5.12 The effect of gravity on ventilation. An excised lung is surrounded by foam, to mimic the gradient of pleural pressure that exists due to gravity and caused to 'breathe' *radioactive gas*. Ventilation in different areas is measured as the amount of radioactivity that goes to those areas with 'inspiration'. The graph shows the volumes of the upper and lower parts of the lungs as the total lung volume increases from *residual volume* to *total lung capacity*. The cubes illustrate the fraction of its potential volume that each lung unit, at the top or bottom, contains at different total lung volumes.

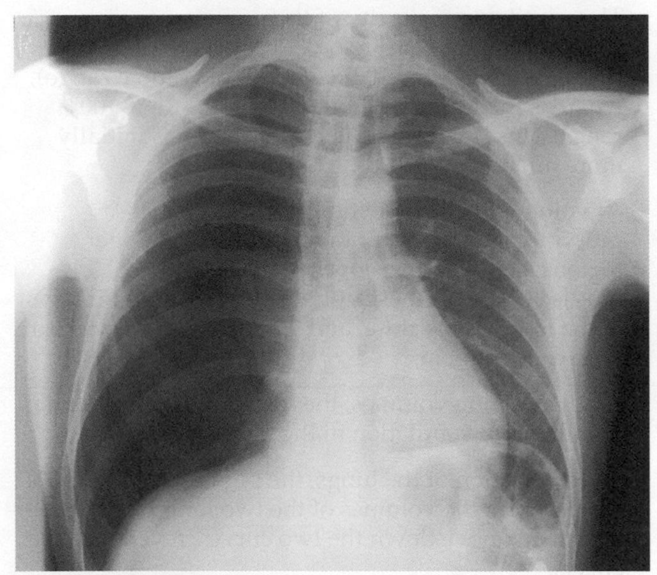

Fig. 5.13 Chest X-ray of a patient with a right tension pneumothorax. The air in the pneumothorax is under pressure and the heart and other structures are pushed *away* from the affected side.

The critical closing volume of the airways (the lung volume at which airways start to close) increases with age, and this becomes important when some airways remain closed throughout the whole of a normal breath, making parts of the lung useless for gas exchange.

Airway smooth muscle tone

Substances that increase airway smooth muscle tone and cause bronchoconstriction (e.g. histamine) act to increase the nonuniform distribution of ventilation by nonuniformly changing the mechanical properties of regions of the lungs. Abolition of airway muscle tone also reduces the uniformity of distribution (e.g. if a subject is mechanically ventilated under anaesthesia). This suggests that normal muscle tone minimises nonuniform distribution. The pharmacological management of bronchoconstriction is discussed in Chapter 4.

Posture

Patterns of both lung ventilation and perfusion change with changes in posture, owing to changes in the direction in which gravity is acting. If the lung in Figure 5.12 were to be inverted or if a subject was to stand on their head, the best-ventilated region of the lung now becomes what was the apex and is now the base. However, this explanation of the distribution of ventilation in terms of gravity may not tell the whole story. Astronauts, under conditions of zero gravity, would be expected to have uniform ventilation throughout their lungs; this does not appear to be the case. Although the differences in ventilation are markedly reduced, there remains a slight top-to-bottom ventilation gradient. This may be the result of the astronauts spending most of their lives under normal gravity before they entered space, and gravity may have left a permanent mark on the regional mechanical properties of their lungs.

Pathological changes

Acute changes, such as pneumothorax, affect the distribution of ventilation between and within the lungs;

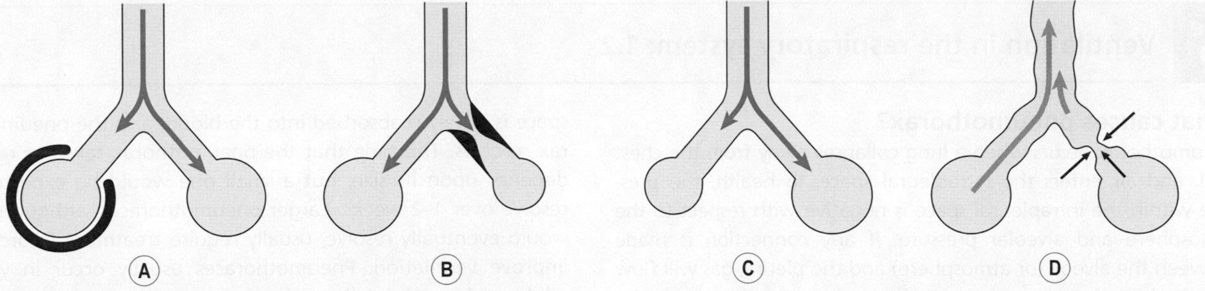

Fig. 5.14 Some pathological changes affecting distribution of ventilation. (A) Restriction; (B) obstruction; (C) change in compliance; (D) airway collapse.

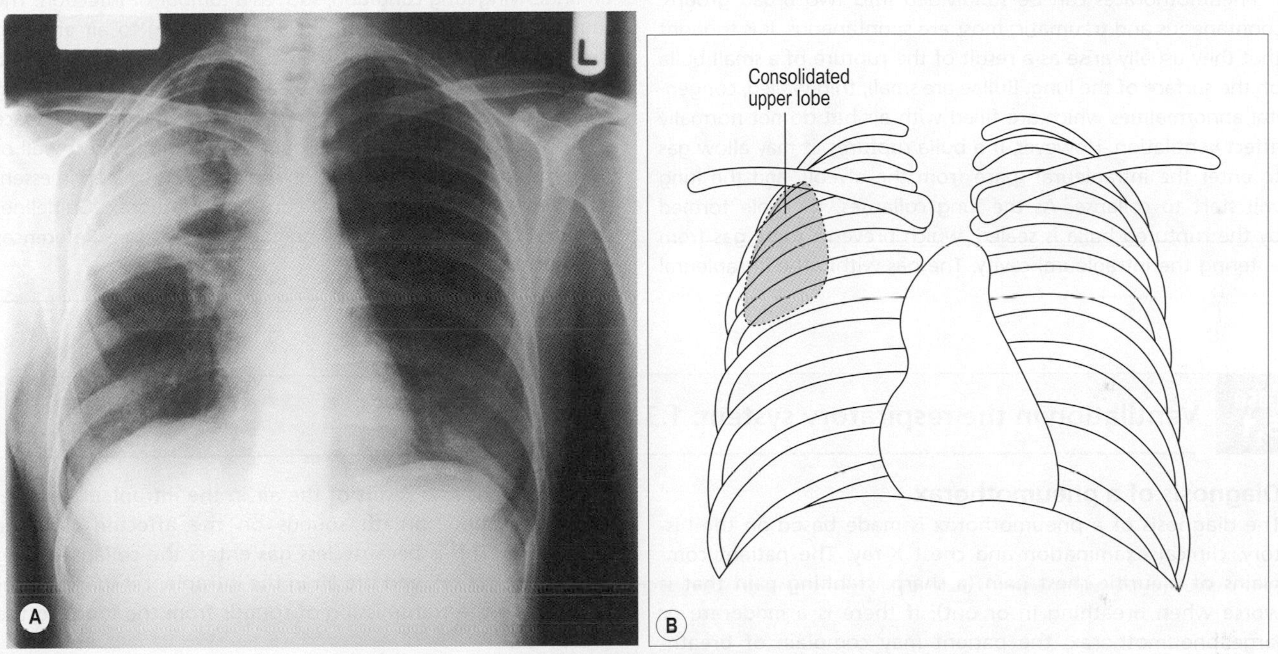

Fig. 5.15 Chest X-ray showing consolidation in the right upper lobe.

in the case of pneumothorax, this effect is mediated by limiting the expansion of one lung (Fig. 5.14A). Normal ageing and other less acute conditions alter the distribution of ventilation and, to a greater or lesser extent, perfusion. Airway obstruction (see Fig. 5.14B) in asthma and bronchitis restricts supply to the region served by the airway, and diseases such as emphysema change the compliance (see Fig. 5.14C) and lead to collapse of the airways (see Fig. 5.14D).

Summary 2

- The respiratory exchange ratio (R) is the CO_2 output divided by oxygen uptake.
- The ventilation of a region is independent of its size.
- Stratification of gas concentration is not as important as regional differences in concentrations for determining uneven distribution.
- The effect of gravity means that the base of the lung is better ventilated than the apex.

Case 5.1 Ventilation in the respiratory system: 1.1

Pneumothorax: a failure of lung ventilation

Mr. Price is a 21-year-old man who presented to the Accident and Emergency Department of his local hospital complaining of chest pain. The pain had come on suddenly while he was playing football. The pain was right sided, stabbing in nature, and was very much worse when he took a breath. He also felt rather short of breath.

After taking a history, performing a physical examination and taking a chest X-ray, the doctor in the emergency department diagnosed a pneumothorax.

In this chapter we will consider:

1. What causes pneumothorax?
2. Diagnosis of pneumothorax.
3. Treatment of pneumothorax.
4. Tension pneumothorax: a medical emergency.

Case 5.1 Ventilation in the respiratory system: 1.2

What causes pneumothorax?

Pneumothorax occurs when a lung collapses away from the chest wall, and air enters the intrapleural space. In health, the pressure within the intrapleural space is negative with respect to the atmosphere and alveolar pressure. If any connection is made between the alveoli (or atmosphere) and the pleura, gas will flow into the intrapleural space. As gas flow occurs, the pressure in the intrapleural space approaches atmospheric pressure. The lung partially collapses, and the chest wall expands slightly (Fig. 5.5).

Pneumothoraces can be subdivided into two broad groups: spontaneous and traumatic; most are spontaneous. It is thought that they usually arise as a result of the rupture of a small bulla on the surface of the lung. Bullae are small, thin-walled, congenital abnormalities which are filled with air but do not normally affect ventilation. However, if a bulla ruptures, it may allow gas to enter the intrapleural space from the alveoli, and the lung will start to collapse. As the lung collapses, the hole formed by the ruptured bulla is sealed, which prevents more gas from entering the intrapleural cavity. The gas within the intrapleural space is slowly reabsorbed into the blood, and the pneumothorax resolves. The time that the pneumothorax takes to resolve depends upon its size, but a small one would be expected to resolve over 1–2 weeks. Larger pneumothoraces, although they would eventually resolve, usually require treatment in order to improve ventilation. Pneumothoraces usually occur in young adults and are about three times more common in men than in women. They also seem to be more common in tall, thin individuals. So-called *secondary pneumothoraces* are the result of an underlying lung condition, such as a tumour or infection. The tumour or infected lung breaks down, leading to air entering the intrapleural space. As its name suggests, a traumatic pneumothorax is caused by trauma to the chest wall (e.g. following a stabbing to the chest). Gas may enter the intrapleural space either from the atmosphere through a hole in the chest wall or from the alveoli through a hole in the lung. It is treated in essentially the same way as spontaneous pneumothorax. Guidelines exist for the management of pneumothoraces (see **References and further reading**).

Case 5.1 Ventilation in the respiratory system: 1.3

Diagnosis of a pneumothorax

The diagnosis of a pneumothorax is made based on the history, clinical examination and chest X-ray. The patient complains of pleuritic chest pain (a sharp, stabbing pain that is worse when breathing in or out); if there is a moderate or large pneumothorax, the patient may complain of breathlessness as the affected lung is not well ventilated. Because the affected lung has partially collapsed away from the chest wall, the trachea may appear deviated towards the affected side. Air in the intrapleural space allows the ribcage to expand outward. For this reason, the affected side of the chest may appear expanded, and its movement during respiration may appear to be reduced compared with the normal side. On percussion, the affected side of the chest sounds hyperresonant as a result of the air in the intrapleural space. On auscultation, breath sounds on the affected side are diminished. This is because less gas enters the collapsed lung during inspiration, and the air in the intrapleural space acts as a barrier to the transmission of sounds from the lungs to the chest wall.

The definitive diagnosis of pneumothorax is made with a chest X-ray. A chest X-ray of a healthy individual does not reveal a gap between the lung fields and the inside of the chest wall. Fig. 5.6B is a chest X-ray of a patient with a left-sided pneumothorax. On the right, the lung field fills the space within the ribcage, but on the left-hand side, the border of the partially collapsed lung is clearly visible and there is a dark gap between the lung and the rib cage caused by air in the intrapleural space.

Case 5.1 Ventilation in the respiratory system: 1.4

Treatment of a pneumothorax

Mr Price's pneumothorax was treated using a chest drain. This consisted of a length of plastic tubing inserted into the intrapleural space through a small incision, made under local anaesthesia, between two of Mr Price's ribs. The chest drain allows air to escape from the intrapleural space so that the underlying lung can reinflate.

Therefore, the chest drain removes air from the intrapleural space rather than allowing more air to enter, and a one-way valve must be placed at the end of the drain. This takes the form of an underwater seal (Fig. 5.10). An underwater seal consists of a container of water with a tube extending below the surface of the water. Gas can pass from the tube into the atmosphere by forming bubbles in

Case 5.1 Ventilation in the respiratory system: 1.4 – cont'd

the water, but no gas can pass back up the tube, and the water effectively acts as a one-way valve at the end of the tube.

As the pressure in the intrapleural space becomes positive (e.g. during coughing or forced expiration), air passes along the chest drain and out to the atmosphere through the underwater seal, and the pneumothorax is drained. If additional air enters the intrapleural space from the defect in the visceral pleura, air is drained from the pneumothorax. Bubbles appear in the underwater seal until the hole in the pleura has sealed. After the hole has healed, the chest drain can be removed. In addition to draining air from the intrapleural space, the underwater seal also collects blood and other secretions, which would otherwise clog up a mechanical valve, that pass along the chest drain.

Chest drains may also be used to drain blood (a haemothorax) or fluid (a pleural effusion) that has accumulated in the intrapleural space as a result of chest trauma or disease.

Case 5.1 Ventilation in the respiratory system: 1.5

Tension pneumothorax - a medical emergency

As we have seen, pneumothoraces are caused when gas enters the intrapleural space. In the majority of cases, gas flow stops when the pressure in the intrapleural space reaches atmospheric pressure. Very rarely, the pressure within the intrapleural space continues to rise above the atmospheric pressure. This is usually because the defect in the lung wall behaves like a valve, allowing gas to enter the intrapleural space without allowing it to leave. Gas enters the intrapleural space when the pressure within the alveoli is positive, this is a particular problem in patients whose lungs are being artificially ventilated, either in an intensive care unit or in an operating theatre.

As the pressure within the intrapleural space rises, the mediastinum is pushed *away* from the affected side (remember that in a pneumothorax that is not under tension, the mediastinum is deviated *towards* the affected side). Pressure on the heart and major vessels within the mediastinum results in cardiac output being reduced, and the displacement of the other lung may result in gas exchange being compromised. In severe cases, cardiovascular collapse occurs. Figure 5.13 shows an X-ray of a tension pneumothorax. The right lung is almost completely collapsed, and the heart and mediastinum have deviated away from the affected side. A tension pneumothorax is a condition which can quickly become fatal, and a clinical decision must be made as to whether or not imaging is obtained prior to decompression of the pneumothorax.

A tension pneumothorax is a medical emergency and urgent release of the trapped gas is necessary. This is achieved by the prompt insertion of any available cannula through the chest wall into the intrapleural space. In most cases, intravenous cannulas are readily available and are usually used for this purpose. Gas escapes under pressure with an audible hiss, and the cardiorespiratory status rapidly improves. Once the patient has been stabilised, a formal chest drain must be inserted, as the cannula is only a temporary measure. Cannulae are of a far finer bore than a chest drain and are easily occluded and displaced; thus, they are not considered definitive management.

Case 5.1 Ventilation in the respiratory system: 2.1

Pneumonia

Mrs O'Donnell is a 70-year-old, retired woman who lives alone. She has been troubled for some years with a chronic cough and has a history of smoking 20 cigarettes per day for over 50 years. She often finds that, after a cold, for example, she develops a worsening cough that produces green sputum.

On one occasion, however, after what seemed to be a relatively minor cold, she developed worsening respiratory symptoms. Her cough became much worse than usual and was productive of large volumes of sputum. She felt very unwell and was hot but shivery. She also felt quite breathless and tired and was finding it increasingly difficult to cope at home.

She called her general practitioner who came out to see her. He examined Mrs O'Donnell and decided that she should be admitted to a local hospital. In the hospital, Mrs O'Donnell was examined by the doctors, a chest X-ray was performed, and blood was collected. A sample of the sputum that Mrs O'Donnell was coughing up was also sent for analysis. A diagnosis of pneumonia was made on the basis of Mrs O'Donnell's symptoms, signs, chest X-ray appearance, and laboratory results.

We will consider:

1. The diagnosis and aetiology of pneumonia.
2. How pneumonia is treated.

Case 5.1

Ventilation in the respiratory system: 2.2

Diagnosis of pneumonia

Pneumonia essentially means an infection of the lung. It is a common condition affecting about two adults per 1000 people in the community. It is responsible for far more deaths than all other types of infections. Pneumonia is usually caused by bacterial infections, and the most common bacterium to cause pneumonia outside hospitals is *Streptococcus pneumoniae*, which causes about half of all such pneumonias. Other bacteria that cause pneumonia include:

- *Haemophilus influenzae*, which is particularly common in patients with pre-existing lung diseases, such as chronic bronchitis
- *Staphylococcus aureus*, which is more common in children and intravenous drug abusers.

About one-fifth of pneumonia cases are caused by unusual agents, and pneumonia caused by these agents may be termed 'atypical pneumonia'. Examples of these agents include:

- *Mycoplasma pneumoniae*, the second most common bacterial cause of pneumonia
- *Chlamydia psittaci*, which causes psittacosis, a pneumonia associated with proximity to caged birds
- *Coxiella burnetti*, which causes Q fever, a pneumonia acquired from animal hides
- *Legionella pneumophila* causes Legionnaire's disease, a pneumonia which was first identified in 1976. The disease was caught by several members of the American Legion (an ex-servicemen's association) who were attending a conference at a hotel in Philadelphia. The causative bacteria, which had not been previously identified, infected the water in the hotel's air-conditioning unit. Droplets of infected water in the air in the hotel were inhaled by the legionnaires, causing the disease.

Pneumonia may also be caused by viruses (most commonly by the influenza A virus) and *Mycobacterium tuberculosis*, which causes tuberculosis. A much wider spectrum of agents causes pneumonia in patients in hospitals. Pneumonia acquired in hospitals is sometimes called hospital-acquired pneumonia.

The term lobar pneumonia refers to the infection of one lobe of the lung, whereas bronchopneumonia refers to a more widespread infection. Infection causes accumulation of fluid and pus in the alveoli and airways. This means that there is reduced or no ventilation in the affected areas. The blood that continues to flow through these areas remains deoxygenated. Patients with pneumonia usually complain of fever and cough, although cough is not always productive at the start of the illness. If the area of infection extends to the pleura, the patient may complain of pleuritic chest pain over the infected area.

Upon examination, the patient usually has a fever and may have reduced air entry on the affected side. If the patient is suffering from lobar pneumonia, the chest wall over the area of infection may be dull to percussion, and auscultation may reveal bronchial breath sounds over the affected lobe. Bronchial breath sounds are harsher than normal because the fluid in the affected lobe conducts sound from the trachea better than air.

Mrs O'Donnell's chest X-ray is shown in Figure 5.15, and shows an area of right upper lobe consolidation caused by right upper lobe pneumonia. Note that the infection has a clearly defined lower border. This is because the area of the infection lies completely within the upper lobe. The lower border of the opacification in the chest X-ray is the lower border of the upper lobe.

Blood tests often show a raised white cell count (often greater than $15 \times 10^9\ L^{-1}$). In the microbiology laboratory, the causative agent may be identified from sputum samples and its sensitivity to a range of antibiotics may be ascertained to guide the best choice of antimicrobial therapy.

Case 5.1

Ventilation in the respiratory system: 2.3

Treatment of pneumonia

Mrs O'Donnell was initially treated with supplemental oxygen, via a facemask, and started on a course of penicillin. Laboratory tests confirmed that her pneumonia had been caused by *S. pneumoniae* and that it was sensitive to the penicillin she was receiving. Her condition improved over the next few days, and she was allowed to return home.

The mainstay of treatment for pneumonia is antibiotic therapy. Treatment can be tailored to the particular infective agent that is causing the pneumonia, after it has been identified from sputum samples in the microbiology laboratory. However, antibiotics are usually started before these results are available, on the basis of a 'best guess' as to the likely infective organism, as was done for Mrs O'Donnell. The choice of antibiotic can later be modified, based on laboratory data.

Other supportive measures may include supplemental oxygen to help maintain oxygenation of the patient's blood, paracetamol to relieve the fever, fluids to keep the patient well hydrated and analgesics to relieve the pleuritic chest pain.

References and further reading

S. Eccles, et al., 2014. Diagnosis and management of community and hospital acquired pneumonia in adults: summary of NICE guidance. BMJ. 349, g6722.

W.S. Fowler, 1948. Lung function studies. II. The respiratory dead space. Am. J. Physiol. 154, 405–416.

E. Gardner, 2010. Care of the patient requiring thoracic surgery. In: Pudner R. (Ed), Nursing the Surgical Patient, Third Edition. Elsevier, Oxford.

H.J. Guy, et al., 1994. Inhomogeneity of pulmonary ventilation during sustained microgravity as determined by single breath washouts. J. Appl. Physiol. 76, 1719–1729.

A.B. Lumb, C.R. Thomas, 2020. Elastic forces and lung volumes. In: Lumb, A.B., Thomas, C.R. (Eds.), Nunn's Applied Respiratory Physiology. Elsevier, London, pp. 14–26.

A. MacDuff, A. Arnold, J. Harvey, 2010. Management of spontaneous pneumothorax: British Thoracic Society pleural disease guideline. Thorax. 65, ii18–ii31.

K. Suga, 2002. Technical and analytical advances in pulmonary ventilation SPECT with xenon-133 gas and Tc-99m-Technegas. Ann. Nuc. Med. 16, 303–310.

6

DIFFUSION OF GASES BETWEEN AIR AND BLOOD

Chapter objectives

After studying this chapter, you should be able to:

1. Explain the 'series' nature of diffusion in the lungs.
2. Understand the importance of the partial pressure gradient.
3. State and understand Fick's law of diffusion.
4. Define diffusing capacity.
5. Relate the properties of oxygen and carbon dioxide to the influence of pathology on their transfer.
6. Explain why the equilibrium for oxygen is established at about the same rate as that for carbon dioxide.
7. Outline the important components limiting diffusing capacity and how they are affected by disease.
8. Explain the rationale behind the selection of carbon monoxide as a gas to measure diffusing capacity.
9. Explain why ventilation, rather than diffusion, is the most important factor in the diffusion of carbon dioxide.

Introduction

This chapter focuses on the transfer of the respiratory gases oxygen (O_2) and carbon dioxide (CO_2) between the alveoli and the haemoglobin in red blood corpuscles (RBCs). Once thought to be an active process in which the lungs extract O_2 from the air, it is now known that the process is passive and relies entirely on the diffusion of both O_2 and CO_2 along their **partial pressure** gradients, from an area where the gas exerts a high partial pressure to an area where the exerted partial pressure is lower.

For O_2 to transfer between the alveolus and the haemoglobin in the RBCs, it must diffuse across the alveolar and capillary walls, through the plasma, and across the RBC membrane to combine with haemoglobin. CO_2 takes this route in the opposite direction. The evaluation of the efficiency of the transfer of the respiratory gases is undertaken to investigate pathology, but the terminology can be confusing. Commonly used terms include 'transfer factor' and '**diffusing capacity**', the latter being the standard term and the term used preferentially, here. It should be noted that factors other than diffusion itself affect the efficiency with which gases are transferred across the alveolar membrane to haemoglobin. These include pulmonary blood flow and the time taken for the reaction between haemoglobin and oxygen to take place.

Diffusion and the significance of partial pressure

In Chapter 5, we looked at the way in which the ventilation of different regions of the lung results in different compositions of gas in the alveoli. To understand the next step in the journey from air to blood or blood to air, it is important to clearly differentiate between the *amount* of a gas present in a mixture and the fraction of that gas, frequently expressed as ***partial pressure** (P)*. Partial pressure is applicable to a gas in a gas mixture and is the pressure the gas would exert if it occupied the volume alone. This concept is important because it is only the difference in partial pressures that drive diffusion from one area to another. To use an analogy, the pressure across the enormous lock gates holding the Atlantic Ocean out of a dock in which the water is 10 cm lower than the ocean is the same as that across the walls of a child's paddling pool containing water 10 cm deep. The amount of water either side (or gas in the case of the lung) has nothing to do with the driving pressure: the difference in *the depth* of water (or the difference in *the partial pressure of gas*) provides the motive force. It is useful to use the term partial pressure gradient rather than concentration gradient when describing the movement of gases from one part of the body to another; a gas in solution in one liquid exerts a partial pressure which is directly proportional to its concentration but inversely proportional to its solubility in that liquid. When a dissolved gas diffuses into another liquid in which its solubility is different, it may move against its concentration gradient, but will always move with the partial pressure gradient.

Diffusion, alone, leads to the movement of gas between air and blood in the lungs and between blood and cells in the tissues; it is the circulation of blood that effectively links the two sites. In the case of O_2 (Fig. 6.1), diffusion in the lungs is sufficient to reduce any difference in partial pressure between alveolar air and pulmonary blood to virtually zero, whereas in tissues, a large difference in the partial pressures between arterial blood and the mitochondria ensures a vigorous flow into these organelles of oxidative metabolism. The single step of O_2 diffusing from air to blood in Fig. 6.1 is, in fact, a series of steps through components which will be considered, in detail, hereafter. The important thing to remember is that they are in series (i.e. one after another), like a hosepipe that is made up of a number of sections joined together, and where *constricting one segment reduces flow in all.*

Factors affecting the rate of diffusion

Fick's law of diffusion (see 'The Gas Laws', Appendix) describes the factors affecting the rate of diffusion of a gas across a membrane and is useful when we consider the movement of gas across the alveolar and capillary walls:

$$\text{Rate of diffusion} = \frac{A \times S\ (\Delta C)}{t\sqrt{MW}}$$

where A is the area of the membrane available for diffusion, S is the solubility of the gas in the membrane, ΔC is the concentration gradient brought about by the differences in partial pressures on either side of the membrane, t is the thickness of the membrane, and MW is the molecular weight of the gas (Fig. 6.2). The solubility of a gas determines the rate of diffusion of a gas in solution. The gases that we are particularly interested in are CO_2 and O_2. CO_2 is 24 times more soluble in tissue fluid than O_2 but has a higher molecular weight; it will therefore diffuse from blood to air 20 times more readily, with the same partial pressure gradient, than O_2 moving in the opposite direction. However, the equilibrium for CO_2 is established at about the same rate as that for O_2 because:

1. the reaction releasing CO_2 from blood is relatively slow
2. the partial pressure gradient driving CO_2 from blood to alveolar air is only 0.8 kPa, whereas that driving O_2 in the opposite direction is 8 kPa.

Although the process of diffusion is a physical one, chemical reactions also exert their influence on this process in the lungs. In particular, the rate at which O_2

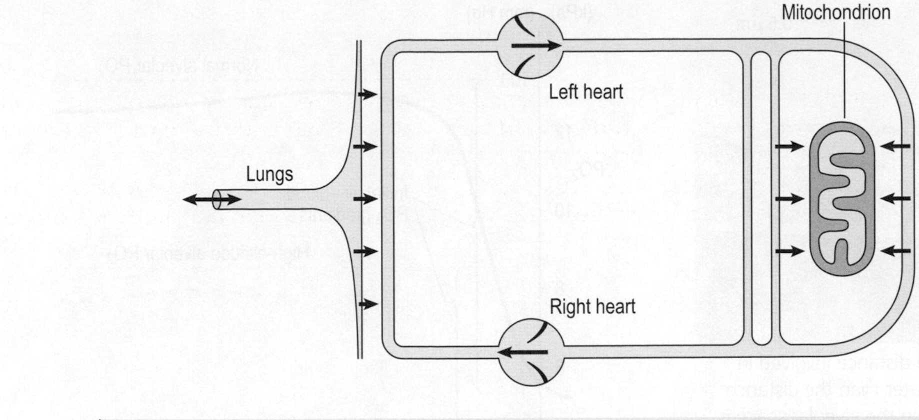

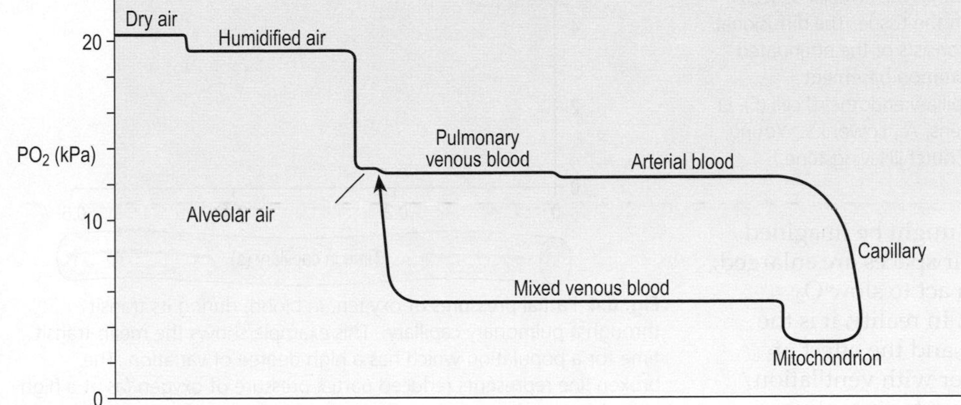

Fig. 6.1 The path of oxygen (O_2). The physical path is shown in the upper diagram. The partial pressures of O_2 in air, blood, and tissue fluids at different points along its journey are shown in the lower diagram.

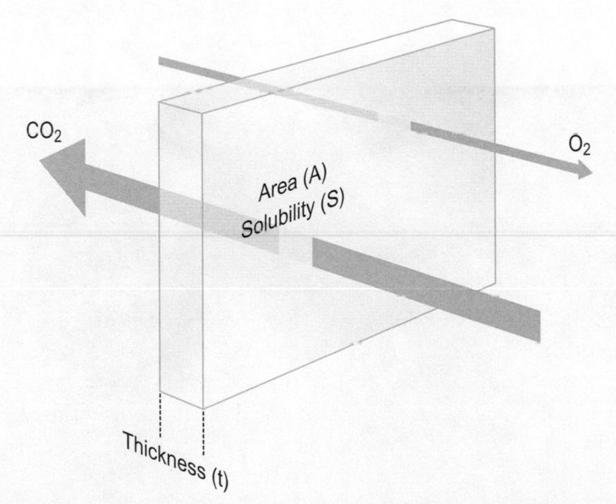

Fig. 6.2 Diffusion through a membrane. Gas will diffuse more quickly if the area is great, the thickness is small, and the partial pressure gradient of the gas across the membrane is high.

can be taken up or released by haemoglobin in the RBC acts as a rate-limiting step, reducing its overall rate of transfer. There are situations in which the lung can be so damaged as to restrict the diffusion of CO_2, but it is usually O_2 that is first affected by diffusion difficulties. The rate of removal of CO_2 is governed primarily by alveolar ventilation (see Chapter 5 and below).

In Figure 6.1, it can be seen that there are three places where diffusion is the major transport mechanism and where this transport can effectively be impeded by the failure of diffusion:

1. within the alveoli
2. from the alveolar air to the RBCs
3. from the RBCs to the tissue mitochondria.

As this is a textbook on the respiratory system, we will concentrate on the first two. The anatomical sites of these two sources of impedance to diffusion are shown in Fig. 6.3.

Factors affecting diffusing capacity

The major factors affecting diffusing capacity are the surface area available for gas exchange, the physical properties of the membrane over which gas exchange takes place, and the ability for gas uptake by the RBC.

Surface Area Available for Gas Exchange

- In healthy lungs at functional residual capacity, the average diameter of the alveoli is about 200 μm. Any differences in the concentrations of the respiratory gases at different points within the alveolus will be overcome by diffusion across these tiny distances in less than 10 ms. Therefore alveolar gas is considered

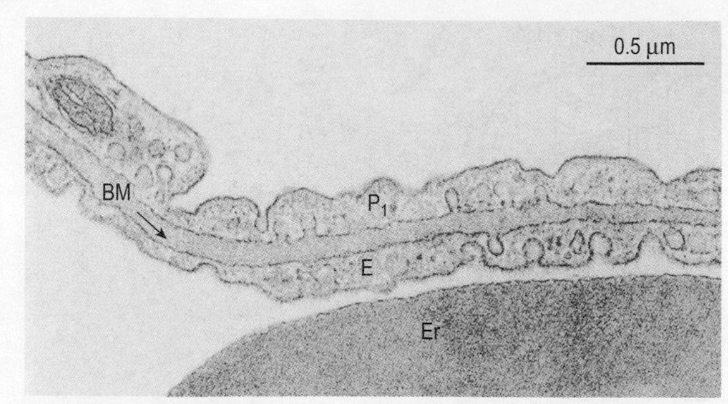

Fig. 6.3 The site of diffusion in the lungs. The distance involved in diffusion within the alveolar space is much greater than the distance within the lung tissue. However, diffusion within the alveolar space is in air and therefore much more rapid than in the tissue. The diffusional barrier between the blood and alveolar air consists of the attenuated cytoplasm of a type 1 pneumocyte (P_1), a common basement membrane (BM), and the cytoplasm of a capillary endothelial cell (E). Er is an erythrocyte in a capillary. (Source: Stevens, A., Lowe, J.S., Young, B., 2002. Wheater's Basic Histopathology. Churchill Livingstone.)

to be of uniform composition. It might be imagined that, in emphysema where the air spaces are enlarged, increased distances for diffusion act to slow O_2 transport to unacceptable levels. In reality, it is the destruction of the alveolar septa and the effect of the reduced surface area, together with ventilation/perfusion mismatching, which exerts a negative influence on diffusing capacity.

- Lung volume increases with height, so taller people generally have greater diffusing capacities than shorter people, and the diffusing capacity is also greatest within an individual at total lung capacity.
- Ventilation/perfusion ($\dot{V}/\dot{Q}$) mismatch results in an effectively reduced area over which gas exchange can take place, as ventilated alveoli with good blood supplies are required for an efficient process. Blood takes, on average, 0.8 seconds to transit the pulmonary capillary. The changes in concentration and, hence, in the partial pressure of O_2 in the blood during transit along the capillary are shown in Fig. 6.4. Consideration of Fig. 6.4 reveals a number of potential complications which can arise; there are great variations in transit time through different regions of the lung. Transit times less than 0.2 seconds do not allow sufficient time for equilibration and capillaries with these short transit times pass deoxygenated blood to the pulmonary veins. This is functionally equivalent to a spread of $\dot{V}/\dot{Q}$ ratios contributing to an increased $\dot{V}/\dot{Q}$ mismatch (see Chapter 7). During heavy exercise, cardiac output increases and all transit times are reduced. At high altitudes, the partial pressure of the ambient O_2 that drives O_2 into the blood is reduced. This effect is shown as a dotted line in Fig. 6.4. Clearly, exercise at high altitudes is the worst of all combinations, except for disease states.

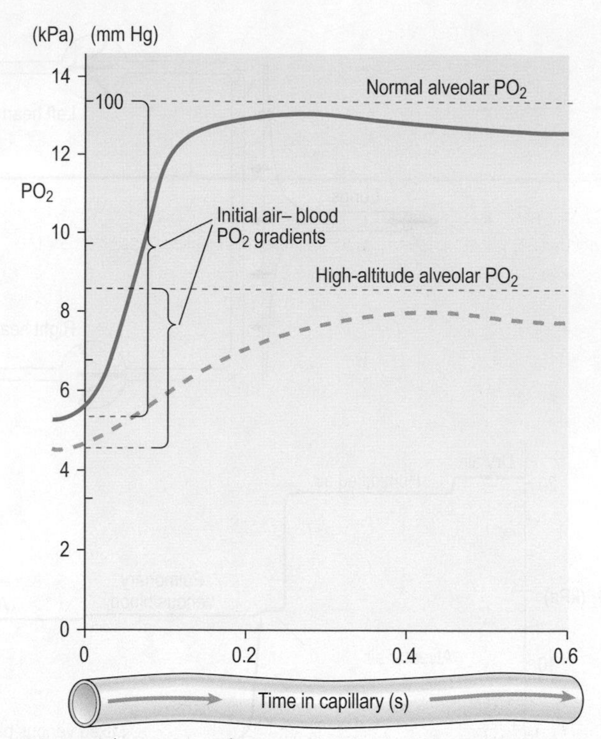

Fig. 6.4 Partial pressures of oxygen, in blood, during its transit through a pulmonary capillary. This example shows the mean transit time for a population which has a high degree of variation. The broken line represents reduced partial pressure of oxygen (as at a high altitude).

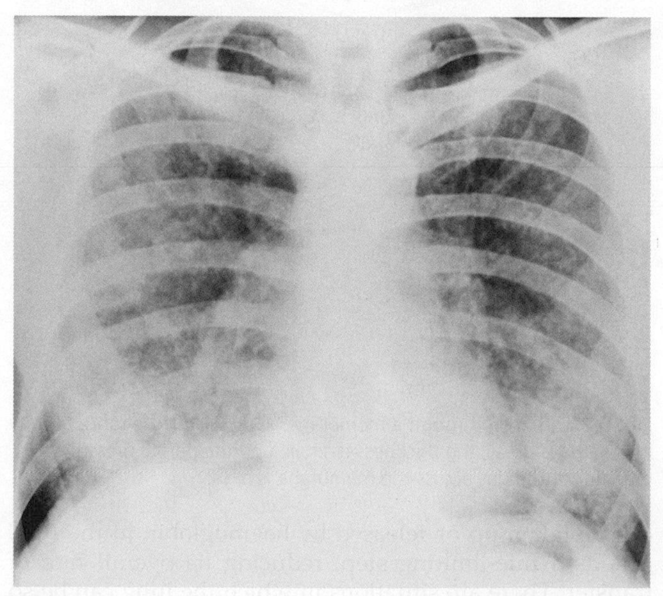

Fig. 6.5 Chest X-ray of a patient with idiopathic pulmonary fibrosis. The image shows fine reticular shadowing, which appears more pronounced towards the outer parts of the lung fields. The shadowing is also more pronounced near the bases of the lungs because there is a reduction in lung volume and it is the bases of the lungs which tend to collapse first.

These combined effects account for many of the challenges of mountaineering achievements.

Crossing the Alveolar Membrane

- The lining epithelia and basement membranes of the alveoli, endothelia, and basement membranes of the pulmonary capillaries are each about 0.2 μm thick on *one side* of the capillary and somewhat thicker on the other, supporting, side (Fig. 6.3); the total thickness of the tissue barrier is around 0.5 μm. The capillaries occupy most of the alveolar wall, generally being less than one capillary diameter apart and with each capillary passing through up to three alveoli.
- It might be expected that diseases such as pulmonary fibrosis, sarcoidosis, asbestosis, and pulmonary oedema, which affect the alveolar/capillary membrane, would interfere with diffusion. Remarkably, however, these problems seem to affect diffusion less than might be expected because they are usually found on the inactive, supporting, side of the pulmonary capillary, leaving the functional side relatively spared. Their major effects are to reduce the surface area available for diffusion by gross destruction of tissue and increased ventilation/perfusion mismatching.
- Chronic heart failure and pulmonary oedema can create barriers to diffusion across the membrane. This may be due to congestion of the pulmonary capillaries, which increases the depth of plasma for O_2 to diffuse across inside the vessels and prior to reaching the RBCs or to a thickened membrane to negotiate, which may be due to interstitial oedema or raised capillary pressure, provoking the proliferation of type II alveolar cells.

Diffusion in blood plasma and the reaction with haemoglobin

- RBCs are approximately the same diameter as pulmonary capillaries, both having diameters of around 7 μm. The RBCs have to be distorted to squeeze through many capillaries, which means there is very little plasma for gas to diffuse through between the corpuscle and the capillary wall. Also, the 'doughnut' shape of the corpuscles means that most of their haemoglobin is close to the wall, again shortening the distance for diffusion. The 'kneading' of the corpuscles as they squeeze through the capillaries probably causes mass movements of haemoglobin within the corpuscle, which also aids diffusion as it has the effect of 'mixing' the haemoglobin with the O_2.
- As the vast majority of O_2 in the blood is carried by haemoglobin, the rate at which they combine is an important and limiting step in O_2 diffusion into the blood. The transfer of O_2 into the blood is profoundly affected by factors such as the reaction rates with haemoglobin and the transit time through pulmonary capillaries, which have nothing to do with the physical process of diffusion. Whilst 'diffusing capacity' is now the preferred term when evaluating the overall process, it should be noted that it is sometimes considered a misnomer because of the other factors involved.

Factors that adversely influence the diffusing capacity include advancing age, female sex, and, in a dose-dependent manner, smoking. Exercise typically enhances diffusing capacity because of the recruitment of pulmonary capillaries in non-dependent lung zones (see Chapter 7) in response to an increase in cardiac output.

Measuring diffusing capacity

It is important to be able to evaluate diffusing capacity when diagnosing and managing certain lung conditions (see the following text and Chapter 11, 'Measuring Diffusing Capacity). Diffusing capacity is the propensity of a gas to diffuse in response to a partial pressure gradient. We need to know the *rate* at which our chosen gas is taken up and the *pressure* which drives it into the body, according to the equation:

$$\text{Diffusing capacity} = \frac{\text{rate of transfer of the gas from lung to blood}}{\text{partial pressure gradient (alveolus to blood)}}$$

The usual units are mmol min^{-1} kPa^{-1}, or mL min^{-1} mm Hg^{-1}. The diffusing capacity is measured as the diffusing capacity of the lung for carbon monoxide (DL_{CO}).

If the blood in the pulmonary capillaries is very quickly saturated with the gas we are using, it cannot take up more and this stops the movement of the gas into the body. In this case, the rate at which blood flows through the lungs, and not diffusion, determines the rate of transfer, and we are measuring pulmonary *blood flow*, not diffusing capacity. Nitrous oxide behaves in this way and is used to measure pulmonary blood flow, but it is useless for measuring diffusing capacity (Fig. 6.6A). Because we are interested in the transfer of O_2, why not use O_2? We can certainly measure the rate at which O_2 is taken up by a subject, but the problem comes in measuring the partial pressure gradient between air and blood. Blood enters lung capillaries that are already carrying some O_2. Venous blood, which contains variable amounts of O_2 is beginning to be oxygenated in the pulmonary arterioles even before it reaches the capillaries, making it very difficult to know the exact driving pressure, for O_2, between alveolar air and these variable levels in the capillary blood. Also, except at low inhaled partial pressures of O_2, blood is almost totally saturated with O_2 when it leaves the lungs, producing the same difficulties as with nitrous oxide, where uptake is governed by blood flow rather than the diffusing capacity (Fig. 6.6B).

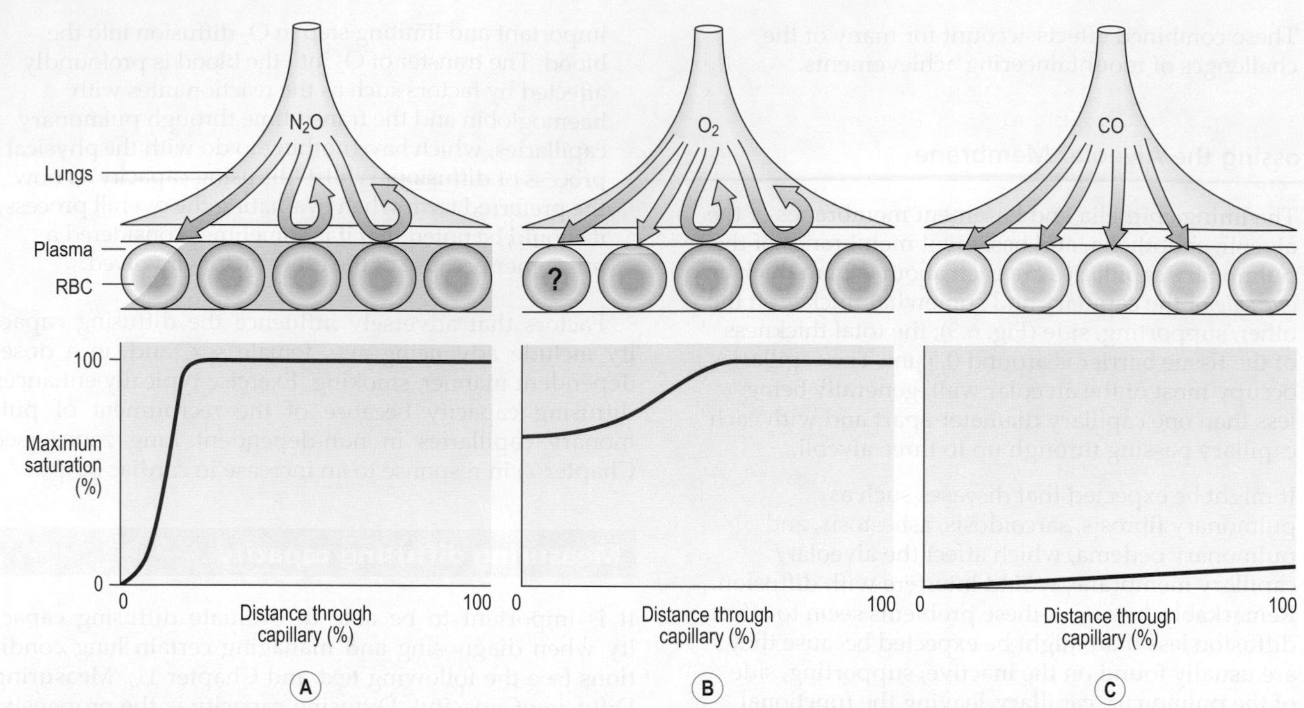

Fig. 6.6 Measuring diffusing capacity. Nitrous oxide (NO) immediately saturates pulmonary capillary blood and prevents any further transfer. Its uptake is therefore limited by pulmonary blood flow, not diffusing capacity. The partial pressure of oxygen (O_2) in the pulmonary capillary is impossible to measure accurately along the capillary, and so the driving pressure into the blood cannot be calculated. Carbon monoxide (CO) is so tightly bound to haemoglobin in the blood that it exerts no partial pressure there. The driving partial pressure is the partial pressure in the inhaled air.

The gas that is most suitable for measuring diffusing capacity is carbon monoxide (CO), using a method first described by the Danish physiologists August and Marie Krogh, in 1915. CO is poisonous because it competes with O_2 for binding sites on haemoglobin; furthermore, it binds haemoglobin 250 times more strongly than O_2 to form carboxyhaemoglobin and thereby denying O_2 access to the haemoglobin; therefore, a patient with CO poisoning dies of a lack of O_2. For this reason, only very low concentrations of CO are used to measure diffusing capacity. Because it binds so strongly, CO is 'locked up' in the haemoglobin and, for all intents and purposes, disappears from the blood. In other words, its partial pressure in the blood is zero. If the rate at which CO disappears from a gas mixture that a subject holds in their lungs for 10 seconds can be determined and the partial pressures of CO in that mixture before and after inhalation are known, the diffusing capacity can be calculated (Fig. 6.6C).

In clinical practice, the measurements of an individual's diffusing capacity are made and then compared with the expected value for someone of the same height, age, and sex, using the following formulae:

$$\text{Males}: \cdot DL_{CO} = 10.9 \times \text{height (m)} - (0.067 \times \text{age (years)}) - 5.89$$

$$\text{Females}: \cdot DL_{CO} = 7.1 \times \text{height (m)} - (0.054 \times \text{age (years)}) - 0.89$$

A healthy 20-year-old male, 1.8-m tall, would have a DL_{CO} of 12.39 mmol·min^{-1}·kPa^{-1}; a healthy female of a similar age and measuring 1.65 m would have a DL_{CO} of 9.75 mmol.min^{-1}·kPa^{-1}. DL_{CO} is considered normal if the value is between 75% and 140% of predicted; mildly impaired if it is between 60% and 75% of predicted; moderately impaired if it is between 40% and 60% of predicted; and severely impaired if it is less than 40% of predicted.

The management of inadequate diffusion

Patients suspected of having a pathology that leads to a diffusion problem may actually have a problem with their ventilation or with $\dot{V}/\dot{Q}$ abnormalities. The rational treatment for patients with lung diffusion problems leading to hypoxaemia depends on understanding the properties of the lung membrane, as illustrated in Fig. 6.2. In these patients, diffusion may have been reduced by membrane thickening (pulmonary fibrosis) or the loss of surface area (emphysema). These conditions are usually irreversible; therefore we are left with only the option of increasing the partial pressure driving O_2 into the blood. Fortunately, this is very effective and increasing the inspired fraction of O_2 from the normal 21% in room air to 30% doubles the O_2 flux into the blood. In appropriate cases of progressive lung disease, O_2 supplied via a nasal cannula or mask, via home oxygen equipment, can significantly improve the quality of life for patients who would otherwise be breathless at rest. Supplemental oxygen should only be administered to patients who obtain relief, and then only when needed, and at the minimum effective dose.

Carbon dioxide and other gases

Gases, such as CO, may be administered experimentally, and volatile anaesthetics, such as isoflurane or sevoflurane, are administered therapeutically (e.g. to induce or maintain anaesthesia). The major determinant of how readily these substances diffuse across the lung membrane is their solubility in water. Nitrogen is about half as soluble in water as O_2 and diffuses at half the rate. CO_2 is 24 times more soluble than O_2 and diffuses 20 times more readily. The rate of diffusion depends on the rate of supply of CO_2, which in turn depends on the chemical reactions that release CO_2 from carbamino compounds and bicarbonate in the blood. The only time hypercapnia occurs, other than as a result of hypoventilation, is when the enzyme that accelerates the equilibrium of bicarbonate and CO_2 in the blood (**carbonic anhydrase**; see Chapter 8 'Carbon Dioxide Transport') is inhibited, that is, the rate of CO_2 removal from the body is determined primarily by **alveolar** ventilation. CO_2 diffuses so readily that its arterial partial pressure ($PaCO_2$) is almost entirely the result of a balance between CO_2 production by metabolism and CO_2 removal by ventilation (Fig. 6.7).

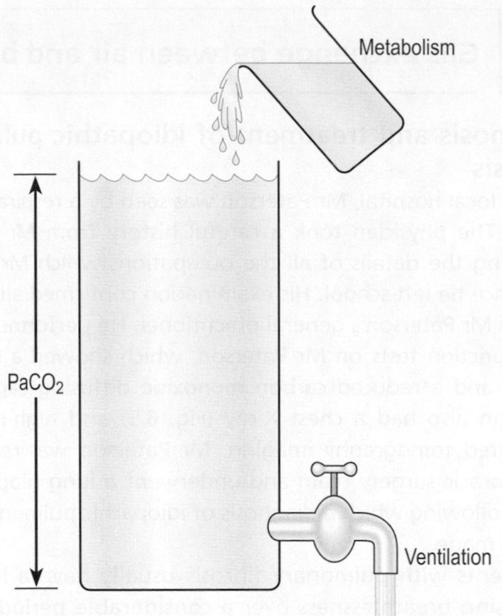

Summary 1

- Diffusion is the result of the random movement of gas molecules which occurs at temperatures above absolute zero.
- The diffusion of gases takes place from a region of high to a region of low partial pressure.
- Fick's law shows that the rate of diffusion of a gas across a membrane is proportional to the concentration gradient, the solubility of the gas in the membrane, and the area of the membrane; it is also inversely proportional to the thickness of the membrane and the square root of the molecular weight of the gas.
- Diffusing capacity (sometimes referred to as 'transfer factor') is a measure of how easily a gas diffuses between the alveoli and pulmonary capillaries. It is usually measured using CO.
- CO_2 is able to diffuse through a membrane around 20 times more readily than O_2.
- Hypercapnia does not result from a reduced diffusing capacity of CO_2 unless the patient is given a carbonic anhydrase-inhibiting drug.

Fig. 6.7 The factors determining the arterial partial pressure of carbon dioxide (PCO_2). In this analogy, the $PaCO_2$ is represented by the height of water in the cylinder which is added to by *metabolism* and removed by *ventilation*.

Case 6.1 Gas exchange between air and blood: 1

Idiopathic pulmonary fibrosis

Mr Paterson is 65 years old. Although he has never smoked, he has become increasingly breathless over the past few months, particularly when he exerts himself. He went to see his doctor, who examined him. He found that Mr Paterson was rather breathless and had clubbing of the fingernails (Fig. 1.4). He found that Mr Paterson's chest expansion was reduced on both sides and, upon auscultation, he heard fine inspiratory crepitations (crackles) all over Mr Paterson's chest, particularly over the bases of his lungs. He decided to refer Mr Paterson to a respiratory physician at the local hospital.

In this overview, we will consider:

1. The clinical features of idiopathic pulmonary fibrosis.
2. The diagnosis and treatment of idiopathic pulmonary fibrosis.

Case 6.1 Gas exchange between air and blood: 2

Diagnosis and treatment of idiopathic pulmonary fibrosis

At the local hospital, Mr Paterson was seen by a respiratory physician. The physician took a careful history from Mr Paterson, including the details of all the occupations which Mr Paterson had since he left school. His examination confirmed all the findings of Mr Paterson's general practitioner. He performed pulmonary function tests on Mr Paterson, which showed a restrictive defect and a reduced carbon monoxide diffusing capacity. Mr Paterson also had a chest X-ray (Fig. 6.5) and high-resolution computed tomography imaging. Mr Paterson was referred to the thoracic surgery team and underwent a lung biopsy procedure, following which a diagnosis of idiopathic pulmonary fibrosis was made.

Patients with pulmonary fibrosis usually have a history of increasing breathlessness over a considerable period of time. A dry cough may be present, but wheeze is unusual. The history may also provide clues as to possible causes of pulmonary fibrosis, such as exposure to metal dust or asbestos. Clues in the history might also point to diseases or drugs that may be complicated by pulmonary fibrosis.

Upon examination, finger clubbing is present in the majority of patients. Fine crepitations at the end of inspiration are present throughout the lungs. In advanced cases, central cyanosis may be present.

Investigations include pulmonary function testing, which may reveal a restrictive defect, and a chest X-ray may demonstrate fine shadowing at the periphery of the lung fields (Fig. 6.5). A computed tomography scan may provide more information than a chest X-ray for diagnosing the disease. Bronchoalveolar lavage, in which fluid is introduced into the airways through a bronchoscope and then recovered for histological analysis, is sometimes used for diagnosis; a lung biopsy provides a definitive diagnosis of the condition.

Case 6.1 Gas exchange between air and blood: 3

Clinical features of idiopathic pulmonary fibrosis

Idiopathic pulmonary fibrosis is a rare condition that affects 10 per 100,000 people, per year, and is more common amongst middle-aged and elderly patients. It encompasses all cases of pulmonary fibrosis in which no cause can be identified. It has been suggested that it may be linked to the Epstein-Barr virus and is more common in smokers. Other causes of pulmonary fibrosis include exposure to inorganic (e.g. asbestos) and organic dusts, infections such as viral pneumonia and HIV, and systemic diseases (e.g. rheumatoid arthritis or sarcoidosis). Pulmonary fibrosis associated with hypersensitivity to dusts involves exposure to very fine dusts containing particles with diameters of 0.5–5 μm. Dusts containing particles with larger diameters would be deposited higher in the respiratory system and would not reach the alveoli. The dust may be associated with a particular occupation, which has led to specific names for particular types of the disease. Hence, there is farmer's lung, bird fancier's lung, mushroom worker's lung, wood worker's lung, and even a sewerage worker's lung and a maple bark stripper's lung! In these cases, the dust may include microorganism spores, animal proteins, or chemicals.

In its early stages, the disease is characterised by thickening of the alveolar walls. There is an increase in type II pneumocytes in the alveolar wall, at the expense of type I pneumocytes. Type II cells have much more cytoplasm than the very thin type I cells and therefore represent more of a barrier to gaseous diffusion. Furthermore, the alveolar walls become infiltrated with cells of the immune system, including neutrophils and lymphocytes, and with time, fibrin is laid down there. Because it is the tissue between the alveoli that is initially affected, pulmonary fibrosis is sometimes known as interstitial pneumonia, to distinguish it from inflammation involving the airways and the alveoli themselves.

The effect of fibrosis on gaseous diffusion is only part of the reason for the hypoxia that accompanies pulmonary fibrosis. Probably equally important is the effect that fibrosis has on the ventilation–perfusion matching of the lungs; in other words, it causes a mismatch of gas flow and blood flow between different areas of the lungs. A recent joint statement on the recommendations for the diagnosis and management of idiopathic pulmonary fibrosis is included in the suggestions for further reading.

References and further reading

Cotes, J.E., Chinn, D.J., Miller, M.R., 2006. Lung Function. Physiology, Measurement, and Application in Medicine. Blackwell.

Hughes, J.M.B., Borland, C.D.R., 2015. Centenary (2015) of the transfer factor for carbon monoxide (TLCO): Marie Krogh's legacy. Thorax 70, 391–394.

Lumb, A.B., Thomas, C.R., 2020. Diffusion of respiratory gases. In: Lumb, A.B., Thomas, C.R. (Eds.), Nunn Applied Respiratory Physiology. Elsevier, pp. 111–121.

Milledge, J.S., 1985. The high level of oxygen secretion is controversial. Lancet 326, 1408–1411.

Raghu, G., Collard, H.R., Egan, J.J., et al., 2011. An official ATS/ERS/JRS/ALAT statement: Idiopathic pulmonary fibrosis: evidence-based guidelines for diagnosis and management. Am. J. Respir. Crit. Care. Med. 183, 788–824.

Stevens, A., Lowe, J.S., Young, B., 2002. Wheater's Basic Histopathology. Churchill Livingstone.

Tedjasaputra, V., Bouwsema, M., Stickland, M.K., 2016. Effect of aerobic fitness on capillary blood volume and diffusing membrane capacity in response to exercise. J Physiol 594, 4359–4370.

7

THE PULMONARY CIRCULATION

Chapter objectives

After studying this chapter, you should be able to:

1. Differentiate the bronchial circulation from the pulmonary circulation.
2. Describe the anatomy of the pulmonary circulation and compare its structure and function with that of the systemic circulation.
3. Describe the relative pressures within the pulmonary and systemic circulations.
4. Describe the mechanisms affecting the distribution of blood within the lungs.
5. Describe ventilation/perfusion matching and discuss how this is achieved.
6. Discuss mechanisms by which lung disease may affect the pulmonary circulation, including shunting.

The bronchial circulation

There are two distinct circulations supplying the lungs:

1. The bronchial circulation.

This is part of the systemic circulation, and its function is to deliver oxygenated blood to meet the metabolic requirements of the airways and lung parenchyma.

2. The pulmonary circulation.

This is not part of the systemic circulation. The pulmonary circulation carries deoxygenated blood from the heart to the lungs, where gas exchange can occur, and then carries oxygenated blood back to the heart, ready to be pumped around the body in the systemic circulation.

The bronchial circulation (Fig. 7.1) receives only 1% of the cardiac output. The bronchial arteries arise from the aorta and supply oxygenated blood, at systemic pressure, to the lower trachea, bronchi, and smaller airways, including the respiratory bronchioles. Blood flowing through the bronchial circulation does not pass through the alveolar capillaries, and therefore does not take part in gas exchange.

Deoxygenated blood from the proximal part of the bronchial circulation around the bronchi drains, via the pleurohilar bronchial veins, into the azygous vein and into the superior vena cava. This blood is effectively part of the systemic circulation, in that it flows from the aorta to the vena cava. However, the deoxygenated blood from the more distal parts of the bronchial circulation drains via the deep bronchial veins into the pulmonary veins. In the pulmonary veins, this deoxygenated blood from the bronchial circulation mixes with oxygenated blood returning from the alveolar capillaries. This reduces (or 'dilutes') the oxygen content of the pulmonary venous blood and constitutes a **shunt**. The significance of this is discussed later in this chapter.

Interestingly, the bronchial circulation is not essential for survival; during a lung transplant, it is severed without any serious ill effects.

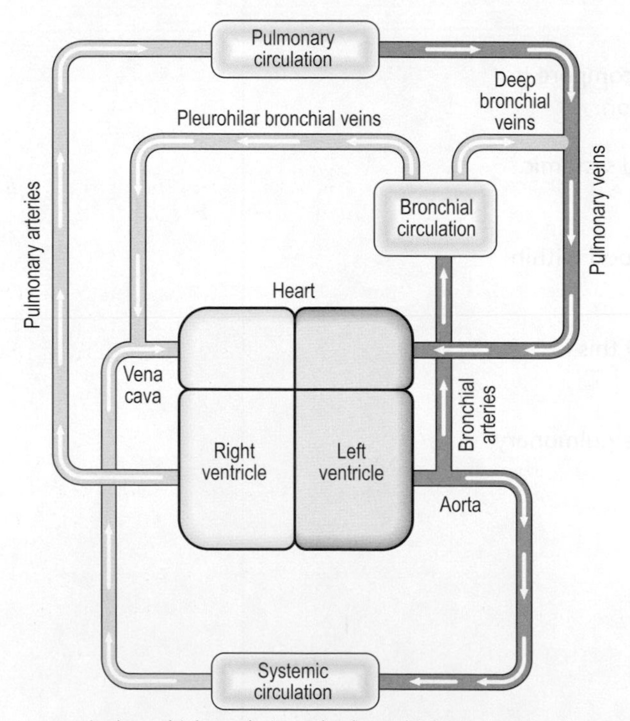

Fig. 7.1 The bronchial circulation. The *bronchial arteries* arise from the *aorta* and therefore carry oxygenated blood. The blood in the *bronchial circulation* supplies tissues within the lung but does not take part in gas exchange; the blood in the *bronchial veins* is therefore deoxygenated. Some of the blood from the bronchial circulation drains via the pleurohilar bronchial veins into the azygous vein or the *vena cava*, whereas blood draining the deep bronchial veins drains into *the pulmonary veins*.

The pulmonary circulation

The main function of the pulmonary circulation is to facilitate oxygenation of blood. This is more complex than simple carriage of blood from the heart to the lungs and back. The pulmonary circulation must deliver the full cardiac output to the lungs with each cardiac cycle, yet not damage the delicate gas exchange barrier in the alveoli. In addition, **ventilation** (gas flow) and **perfusion** (blood flow) to a given area of the lung need to be matched to allow gas exchange to occur efficiently. It is ineffectual to direct air to areas of the lung that have little blood flow, or to direct blood to areas of lung with little or no ventilation. Matching of ventilation and perfusion is vital to maintaining adequate oxygenation and carbon dioxide removal from the blood.

In this chapter, we will consider the anatomy and physiology of the pulmonary circulation and compare it with the systemic circulation. We will then consider the factors that influence the flow of blood to different regions of the lungs. Finally, we will consider the important concepts of ventilation/perfusion matching and shunts and how these can be altered in disease states.

The pulmonary circulation – structure and function

In humans, the circulation behaves as if it consists of two parts. In the **systemic circulation**, the left ventricle pumps oxygenated blood through the organs and tissues of the body, where oxygen is removed, and carbon dioxide is added before the blood returns to the right atrium. In the **pulmonary circulation**, the right ventricle pumps deoxygenated blood through the lungs, where oxygen is added and carbon dioxide is removed (Fig. 7.2). The two parts of the circulation work in parallel to form a single circuit of blood, but there are a number of differences between the pulmonary and systemic circulations which reflect their different functions.

First, virtually the entire cardiac output is directed through the pulmonary circulation. This means that, at any one time, there is as much blood flowing through the lungs as through all the other organs and tissues in the body, put together.

Second, the purpose of the pulmonary circulation is to bring blood and air into very close contact in order to allow gas exchange to take place. This requires a very thin, separating membrane. To avoid damaging this interface, the pressure in the pulmonary circulation needs to be very low compared with that in the systemic circulation. If the pressure in the pulmonary circulation were higher, it would cause fluid to leak from the pulmonary capillaries into the alveoli. In fact, the pressure in the pulmonary artery is about 25/10 mm Hg, compared to 120/80 mm Hg in the systemic circulation. The pulmonary circulation is therefore a *low-pressure, high-flow system,* which implies it has a *low resistance.* The components of the pulmonary circulation differ from their systemic counterparts in a way that reflects this.

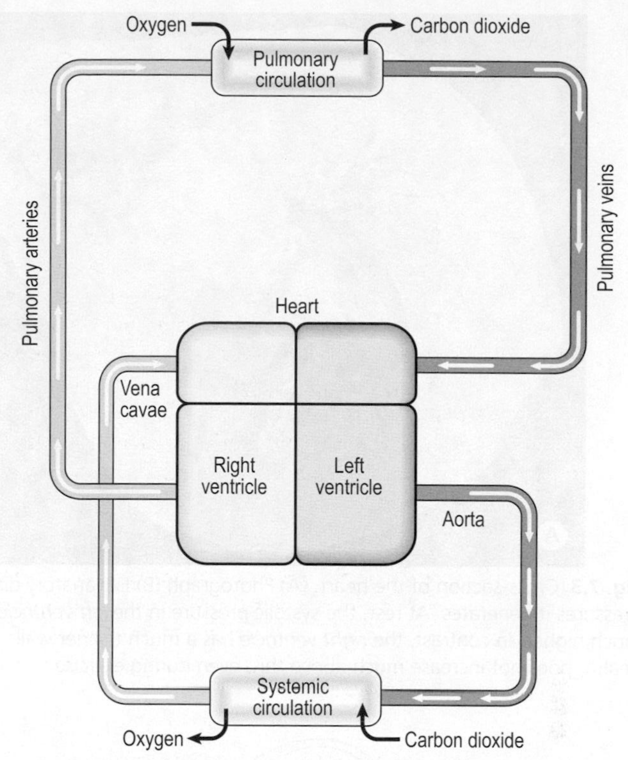

Fig. 7.2 Diagrammatic representation of the circulation. In humans, the circulation behaves as if it consisted of two parts, the *systemic circulation* and the *pulmonary circulation*. The blood flow through the two parts is the same. In both circulations, *arteries* carry blood away from the heart and *veins* carry blood to the heart. For this reason, the *pulmonary artery* carries *deoxygenated* blood, and the pulmonary vein carries *oxygenated* blood.

Gross structure

The pulmonary circulation starts in the right ventricle, where deoxygenated blood is pumped through the pulmonary valve, via a short pulmonary trunk, into the two pulmonary arteries which supply both lungs. The arteries form a branching structure of arterioles leading to capillaries, which are closely adherent to the alveoli and where gas exchange occurs. Oxygenated blood is then carried, via venules, into the four pulmonary veins which empty into the left atrium.

The right ventricle

Every minute, the same volume of blood – about 5 L, at rest – flows through both the right and left ventricles. However, the two ventricles look very different (Fig. 7.3). The left ventricle has a thick, muscular wall that takes up most of the cross-section of the heart. The right ventricle has a much thinner wall, about one-third the thickness of the left. To accommodate the muscle of the left ventricle, the right ventricle almost seems to be 'wrapped around' the left.

The reason for the increased muscularity of the left ventricle is that it pumps blood into the systemic circulation, which has a high resistance and which operates at a relatively high pressure. If cardiac output increases, for example during exercise, this pressure can increase even more, which means that the left ventricle needs a thick, muscular wall to produce these high pressures. On the other hand, the right ventricle pumps blood into the pulmonary circulation, which has a very low resistance, and which operates at a low pressure, always less than that in the systemic circulation. When cardiac output increases, the pulmonary artery pressure does not increase very much. For this reason, the right ventricle needs only a relatively thin, muscular wall compared with the left.

Pulmonary blood vessels

The pulmonary and systemic blood vessels are very different. Pulmonary blood vessels have much thinner walls, reflecting the lower blood pressure they need to withstand; for example, the thickness of the pulmonary artery wall is only about one-third that of the aorta.

In addition to having thinner walls, the pulmonary vessels are much more distensible than systemic arteries, which is important in keeping pulmonary blood pressure low during systole and accommodating increases in cardiac output. In circumstances such as exercise, cardiac output can increase from its normal 5 L/min to as much as 25 L/min. In order to keep pulmonary blood pressure low, the pulmonary circulation is able to reduce its resistance to even lower values than normal and accommodate the increased blood volume by its high capacitance. It does so by two mechanisms, illustrated in Figure 7.4.

1. ***Distension.*** Pulmonary blood vessels are able to dilate or *distend.* A small increase in the diameter of a vessel decreases the resistance of that vessel substantially (see Poiseuille's law, Chapter 4).

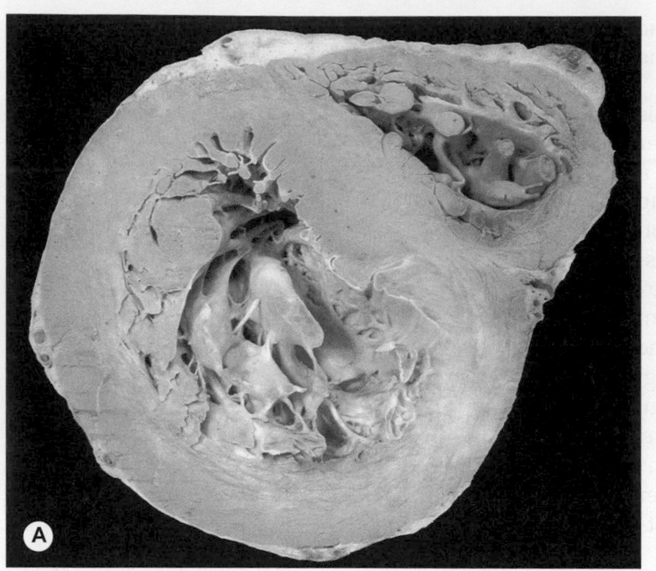

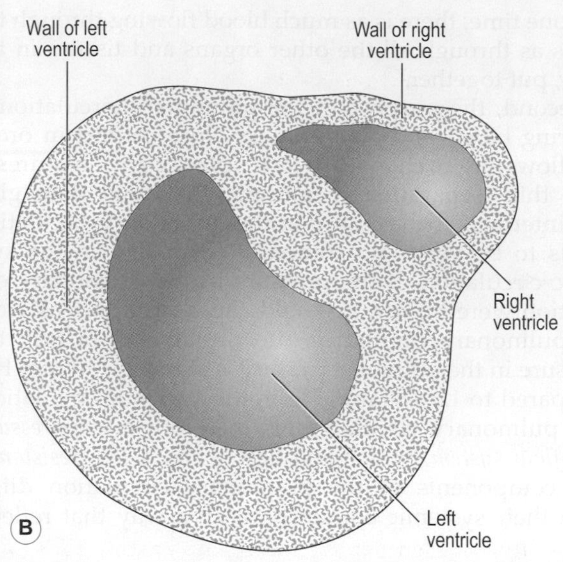

Fig. 7.3 Cross-section of the heart. (A) Photograph (B) Explanatory diagram. Note that the *left ventricle* has a thick wall, reflecting the high pressures it generates. At rest, the systolic pressure in the *left ventricle* is about 120 mm Hg, but during exercise, for example, the pressure can be much higher. In contrast, the *right ventricle* has a much thinner wall. The systolic pressure in the right ventricle is only about 25 mm Hg, and, in health, does not increase much above this, even during exercise.

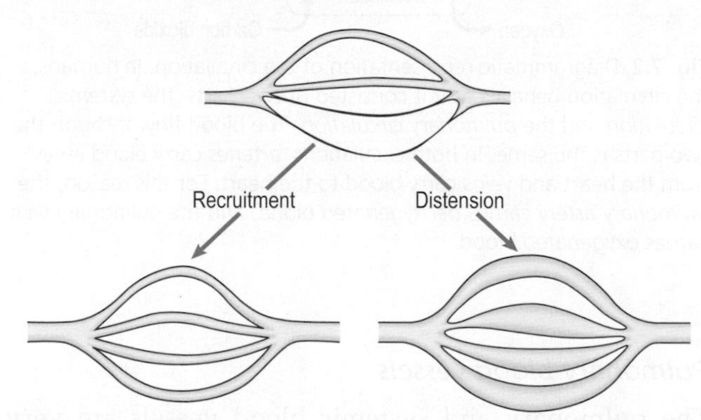

Fig. 7.4 Recruitment and distension of pulmonary blood vessels. If cardiac output increases, the resistance of the pulmonary circulation decreases, meaning that the *pulmonary artery* pressure remains relatively low. This occurs because some pulmonary vessels increase in diameter (distension, lower right of diagram) and because some vessels which were virtually closed begin to open, allowing blood to flow through them (recruitment, lower left of diagram).

2. ***Recruitment.*** During normal conditions, some blood vessels in the lungs are closed. During periods of high cardiac output, these vessels open up and blood is able to flow through them. The increase in the number of blood vessels able to carry blood is called *recruitment*. However, very few vessels are likely to be completely collapsed under normal conditions, and distension is probably much more important than recruitment in reducing vascular resistance.

The anatomical position of the capillaries and their function in gas exchange mean that they differ from their systemic counterparts. The density of the capillary network in the alveolar walls is extremely high so that efficient gas exchange can take place. In fact, there are so few cells between the capillaries in the alveolar walls that the alveolar circulation behaves almost like a film of blood flowing around the alveoli. At rest, blood flows through an alveolar capillary in about 0.8 seconds, which is about three times longer than the time needed for oxygenation of **mixed venous blood**.

There is also very little space between the blood in the pulmonary capillaries and the air in the alveoli. In fact, for the most part, the only cells separating the blood from the air are the endothelial cells of the pulmonary capillary and the epithelial type I cells of the alveolar wall (Fig. 2.9). This is crucial in allowing efficient transfer of gases between the alveoli and the blood (see Chapter 6).

However, because the pulmonary capillaries are very thin-walled and lie within the alveolar walls, they can be readily influenced by changes in the gas pressure within the alveoli. Increased alveolar gas pressure can compress the capillaries, with a consequent increase in capillary resistance and reduction in blood flow which can affect the *distribution* of blood flow within the lungs (see below). This differs from the conditions affecting systemic capillaries, which are better supported by surrounding tissues.

The pressure in the pulmonary *veins* exerts a considerable influence over the pressure in the pulmonary arteries. This is a consequence of the low pressures in the pulmonary circulation and is not the case in the systemic circulation. The difference in pressure between the arterial and venous ends of a capillary bed is called the ***driving pressure,*** and flow is dependent on this. In the systemic circulation, the pressure at the precapillary sphincters (which regulate the blood flow through the capillary beds) is about 90 mm Hg, very much higher than the pressure at the venous ends of the capillary beds. Because the venous pressure in the systemic circulation is so much less than the arterial pressure, changes in systemic venous pressure do not cause large changes in the driving pressure. However, in the pulmonary circulation, the difference between the pulmonary arterial and venous pressures is much less, and a relatively small increase in venous pressure can significantly reduce the driving pressure. To maintain a constant driving pressure, the pulmonary *artery* pressure must increase. In certain pathological situations, this can eventually lead to failure of the right ventricle (**cor pulmonale** – right heart failure due to respiratory disease and pulmonary arterial hypertension; see below).

Summary 1

- The lungs receive their own arterial blood supply: the bronchial circulation.
- The main function of the pulmonary circulation is to deliver deoxygenated blood to the lungs and oxygenated blood to the left heart.
- The pulmonary circulation receives the entire cardiac output.
- Blood vessel recruitment and distension make the pulmonary circulation a high capacitance system so that it can accommodate large blood volumes while maintaining low pressure.
- The low pressure protects the delicate gas exchange barrier.
- The right ventricle and pulmonary arteries are much thinner than the left ventricle and aorta, reflecting the lower pressures in the pulmonary circulation compared with the systemic circulation.

Matching ventilation and perfusion

For gas exchange to occur, the alveoli must be both ventilated and perfused. For maximal efficiency, ventilation should be exactly matched by perfusion, but even in health this is not the case.

In an ideal pair of lungs, all the alveoli would be supplied with equal volumes of air with a uniform gas composition during inspiration and all the alveoli would be supplied with the same flow of mixed venous blood. The ventilation and perfusion of all parts of these ideal lungs would therefore be optimally matched, and gas exchange between the blood and the alveoli would be efficient.

However, in real lungs, this is not the case. Per unit of lung volume, ventilation and perfusion both tend to be greater at the bases of the lungs than at the apices. For most of the lung tissue, the two tend to be fairly well matched. This means that the ratio of ventilation to blood flow, the **ventilation/perfusion ratio**, or $\dot{V}/\dot{Q}$ **ratio**, is close to 1 and varies by a relatively small amount throughout the lungs.

In order to see how ventilation/perfusion matching takes place, we will first look at the way in which the blood flow is distributed throughout the lungs, then we will see how this is matched with ventilation before looking at how regional variations in the $\dot{V}/\dot{Q}$ ratio, in the lungs, affect arterial blood gases.

Distribution of blood flow through the lungs

The distribution of blood to different regions of the lungs is not uniform.

In the systemic circulation, blood flow through organs is almost entirely determined by high-resistance arterioles that regulate the flow through capillary beds. The arterioles in the pulmonary circulation do not have a high resistance and play only a small role in determining the blood flow to different parts of the lungs. The distribution of blood flow through the lungs is influenced, instead, by a number of different factors, including ***gravity***, **alveolar gas pressure**, **hypoxic pulmonary vasoconstriction**, and, to a lesser extent, the ***nervous control*** of blood vessel resistance.

Gravity

Gravity tends to direct blood toward the lung bases.

The diastolic blood pressure in the systemic circulation is about 80 mm Hg, which is enough pressure to raise a column of water by a height of over a metre (80 mm Hg = 109 cm H_2O). In other words, there is more than enough pressure to carry blood from the heart up to the head in the standing adult. However, in the pulmonary circulation, the diastolic blood pressure is only a sixth of this (about 12 mm Hg) or enough pressure to raise a column of water about 16 cm. In other words, there is only just enough pressure to pump blood from the right ventricle up to the lung apices. On the other hand, at the lung bases the blood pressure in the pulmonary circulation is equal to the pressure generated by the right ventricle *plus* the hydrostatic pressure of a column of blood extending up to the height of the heart. Because the pressure generated by the right ventricle is not very high, this extra hydrostatic pressure makes a very significant difference. Thus there is a considerable increase in arterial blood pressure from the apices to the bases of the lungs owing to gravity. In other words, gravity tends to direct blood towards the lung bases.

The regional flow of blood within the lungs can be demonstrated by dissolving a radioactive gas, usually Xenon-133, in saline and injecting this into the right side of the heart via an intravenous catheter. During the injection, the subject holds their breath, and some of the radioactive xenon leaves the blood and enters the alveoli. By measuring the level of radioactivity from outside the body, it is possible to estimate the blood flow to different regions of the lungs.

Gravity is not as important a factor in determining regional differences in blood flow as was once thought. The difference in blood flow per unit lung volume, between the bases and apices of the lungs, is relatively modest and persists in subjects in the supine position. At any given height from the lung base, there is a wide variation in blood flow to different lung regions. It is likely that this variation is due to the fact that when a blood vessel divides, the two vessels formed are not necessarily the same size, leading to an uneven distribution of blood flow between lung regions at the same height. This effect is probably at least as important as gravity in producing variation in regional perfusion of the lungs.

Alveolar gas pressure

Blood flow through the lungs also depends on the alveolar gas pressure. The pulmonary capillaries are thin walled and lie closely adherent to the alveoli, such that raised pressure in the alveoli can compress the capillaries, limiting the blood flow through them. The pressure in the alveoli remains close to atmospheric during quiet breathing but may become significantly positive (and therefore affect blood flow distribution) during exertion or artificial ventilation.

Three zones are described for blood pressure at the beginning (P_a) and end (P_v) of a capillary and the gas pressure (P_A) within the adjacent alveoli (Fig. 7.5):

• *Zone 1.* Apical – little or no blood flow.

$P_A > P_a > P_v$

In this zone, the pressure in the alveoli is greater than the pressure in the capillaries. This means that in Zone 1 there is no blood flow. It is unlikely that such a zone exists in healthy individuals, but if it does, it occupies a very small volume in the apices of the lungs where the pulmonary blood pressure is lowest. Areas of the lung which are ventilated but not perfused are called **dead space.**

• *Zone 2.* Central – increasing blood flow from upper to lower part of zone.

$P_a > P_A > P_v$

In this zone, the alveolar gas pressure is greater than the blood pressure at the venous end of the capillary but less than the blood pressure at the arterial end of the capillary. In Zone 2, the flow through the capillaries is related to the pressure difference between the arterial end of the capillary and the alveolus. If alveolar gas pressure increases, then flow through the capillaries will be reduced.

• *Zone 3.* Basal – unimpeded blood flow

$P_a > P_v > P_A$

In Zone 3, the blood pressure throughout the capillaries, from the arterial end through to the venous end, is greater than the gas pressure in the surrounding alveoli. Therefore, in this zone, flow through the capillaries is influenced only by the difference in blood pressure along the capillary (the 'driving pressure') and is not influenced by changes in alveolar pressure. It is likely that in healthy humans, the *majority* of the volume of the lungs lies within Zone 3, making blood flow independent of alveolar gas pressure.

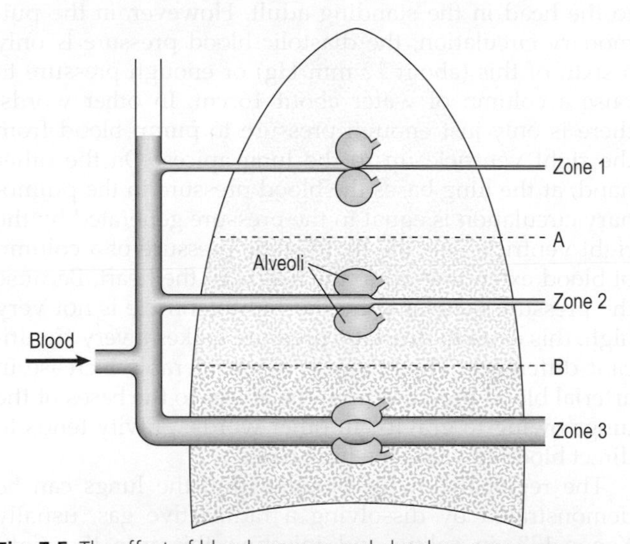

Fig. 7.5 The effect of blood pressure and alveolar pressure on regional blood flow through the lungs. In *Zone 1*, the air pressure in the alveoli is greater than the pressure within the alveolar capillaries and therefore no blood flow takes place. If such a zone exists in healthy individuals, it is very small and situated at the apices of the lungs. In *Zone 2*, the average alveolar gas pressure is lower than the pressure of blood entering the alveolar capillaries but higher than the pressure of blood leaving the capillaries. In *Zone 2*, blood flow varies with changes in alveolar gas pressure. In *Zone 3*, the blood pressure throughout the alveolar capillaries is higher than the alveolar gas pressure, and blood flow through the pulmonary capillaries is independent of alveolar gas pressure. In healthy individuals it is likely that most of the alveoli lie within *Zone 3*.

Hypoxic pulmonary vasoconstriction

Arterioles in the lungs differ considerably from their systemic counterparts in their response to hypoxia. Systemic arterioles **vasodilate** in response to hypoxia. This increases the blood flow to hypoxic tissues and therefore tends to increase oxygen delivery to areas where it is required.

However, arterioles in the lungs **vasoconstrict** in response to alveolar (not arteriolar) hypoxia: this effect is called **hypoxic pulmonary vasoconstriction (HPV).** HPV is important in maintaining ventilation/perfusion matching as it tends to direct blood *away* from underventilated parts of the lungs (which have a low alveolar oxygen concentration) towards better-ventilated parts of the lungs where there is a higher oxygen concentration. In other words, HPV tends to improve the $\dot{V}/\dot{Q}$ ratio for the lungs as a whole by increasing the ratio in areas of the lungs where it is lower than normal. This vasoconstrictor response of blood vessels to low oxygen concentrations is analogous to the bronchodilator response of bronchi to high levels of carbon dioxide (see Chapter 4).

HPV also plays an important role in limiting blood flow through the nonventilated and therefore hypoxic lungs of the foetus. After the baby is delivered and takes its first breath, the oxygen concentration in its lungs increases, the hypoxic pulmonary vasoconstriction reduces, and blood flow to the lungs increases.

The molecular mechanism of HPV is not fully understood. Hypoxia causes membrane depolarisation and therefore contraction of the smooth muscle cells in the pulmonary blood vessel walls (Fig. 7.6). It is thought that the depolarisation of the smooth muscle cells is mediated, at least in part, by a membrane potassium channel called the Kv channel, although there is less certainty regarding whether the channel itself is sensitive to hypoxia or whether it responds to another detector of hypoxia. Membrane depolarisation opens voltage-sensitive calcium channels that allow calcium to enter the cell. A rise in the intracellular calcium concentration triggers smooth muscle contraction, resulting in vasoconstriction. Mediators, such as endothelin (a vasoconstrictor) and nitric oxide (NO, a vasodilator), released from the overlying endothelial cells also influence hypoxic pulmonary vasoconstriction, although they are not necessary for it to take place.

Although HPV is usually beneficial in maintaining ventilation/perfusion matching, it can cause problems in patients with lung conditions, such as chronic obstructive pulmonary disease, that result in long-term hypoxia. This chronic hypoxia affects all parts of the lungs and results in widespread HPV. This means that the resistance of the pulmonary circulation, as a whole, is much higher than normal, and the pulmonary blood pressure increases (**pulmonary hypertension** is defined as a mean pulmonary arterial pressure >20 mm Hg, at rest). The right ventricle is not well suited to producing a high blood pressure and, under these circumstances, can start to fail. The patient may become increasingly breathless upon exertion, as fluid tends to seep into the alveoli as cardiac output increases. Failure of the right ventricle means that the pressure in the systemic veins increases and patients may notice oedema around their ankles. This sort of heart failure that is due to lung disease is called **cor pulmonale**.

Pulmonary vasodilator drugs (e.g. intravenous prostacyclin) can be used to treat pulmonary hypertension but, by causing indiscriminate vasodilation, these drugs cause systemic vasodilation (and a drop in blood pressure) and abolish HPV. This worsens the degree of ventilation-perfusion mismatching seen in lung disease, exacerbates the hypoxaemia, and offsets any benefit achieved in reducing pulmonary arterial pressures. One solution to this is to give inhaled pulmonary vasodilators so that the blood flow is only increased to ventilated lung units. Examples of such drugs include inhaled NO and inhaled prostacyclin.

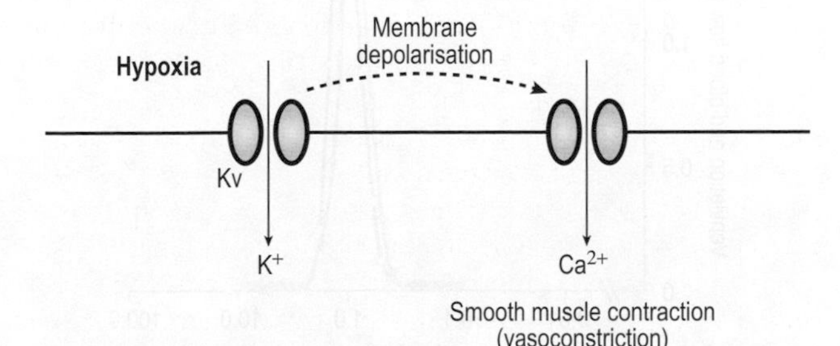

Fig. 7.6 Hypoxic pulmonary vasoconstriction. Pulmonary blood vessels constrict in response to *hypoxia*. The potassium channel K_v, which lies in the vascular smooth muscle membrane, opens in response to *hypoxia*, leading to membrane depolarisation. This results in the opening of a calcium channel which allows extracellular calcium to enter the cell. This, in turn, triggers *muscle contraction*.

Innervation of the pulmonary vessels

Nervous control of the pulmonary vessels may also affect the distribution of blood flow through the lungs but does not seem to be very important in maintaining ventilation/perfusion matching in humans; severing the nerves during lung transplantation does not cause significant postoperative problems. Fibres of the sympathetic and parasympathetic nervous system innervate the pulmonary vessels and may cause vasoconstriction or vasodilatation (Fig. 7.7).

Sympathetic fibres release noradrenaline (norepinephrine), which acts predominantly on α_1 adrenoceptors on the smooth muscle of arteries and arterioles to produce vasoconstriction. Noradrenaline may also act on α_2 receptors to produce vasodilatation, but it is generally accepted that the overall effect of the sympathetic nervous system on the pulmonary vessels is vasoconstriction.

The parasympathetic nervous system produces most of its effects on the pulmonary blood vessels by the release of acetylcholine. Acetylcholine is thought to act on muscarinic M_3 receptors on the *endothelium* of the blood vessels, rather than on the smooth muscle cells themselves. Stimulation of the M_3 receptors results in the release of NO from the vascular endothelial cells. NO is a small, gaseous molecule that is very rapidly broken down and is a very important mediator in many organ systems. NO causes pulmonary vascular smooth muscle cells to relax, and therefore produces vasodilatation.

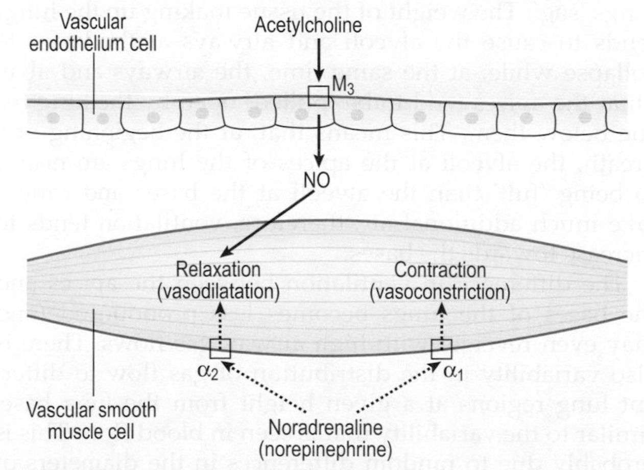

Fig. 7.7 Action of the sympathetic and parasympathetic nervous systems on pulmonary vessels. *Noradrenaline (norepinephrine)* released from sympathetic nerve fibres acts on smooth muscle α_1 receptors to produce *vasoconstriction* and on α_2 receptors to cause *vasodilatation*. Overall, the effect of the sympathetic nervous system is to cause *vasoconstriction*. *Acetylcholine* acts on the *vascular endothelium*, causing the release of *nitric oxide (NO)* that causes *vasodilatation* of the underlying *vascular smooth muscle*.

Like the bronchial smooth muscle, the pulmonary vascular smooth muscle also has a nonadrenergic, noncholinergic parasympathetic innervation. There are many possible neurotransmitters in this system. It seems to produce vasodilatation, and may well act via NO. However, its importance in humans is not fully understood.

Summary 2

- Ventilation should be matched to perfusion for efficient gas exchange.
- The degree of matching for any given lung region is measured as the ventilation/perfusion ratio.
- Areas of the lung which are ventilated but not perfused are called dead space.
- Blood flow (perfusion) in the pulmonary circulation is unevenly distributed.
- Gravity directs blood flow towards the lung bases.
- Uneven division of pulmonary blood vessels contributes to regional differences in perfusion.
- In lung zones where alveolar pressure exceeds pulmonary capillary pressure, blood flow is restricted.
- Pulmonary arterioles vasoconstrict in response to alveolar hypoxia.
- Sympathetic and parasympathetic innervation is not essential for normal functioning of the lung.

Regional differences in ventilation in the lungs

As we have seen, blood flow to different regions of the lung is not uniform but tends to increase toward the lung bases. Fortunately, alveolar ventilation, the volume of air entering the alveoli per minute, is also directed more towards the bases. Essentially, this happens because the lungs 'sag'. The weight of the tissue making up the lungs tends to cause the alveoli and airways at the bases to collapse while, at the same time, the airways and alveoli at the apices tend to be 'pulled' open by the lung tissue below them. This means that, at the beginning of a breath, the alveoli at the apices of the lungs are nearer to being 'full' than the alveoli at the bases and cannot take much additional air; therefore, ventilation tends to increase towards the bases.

The difference in ventilation between the apices and the bases of the lungs becomes less pronounced (and may even reverse) with high airway gas flows. There is also variability in the distribution of gas flow to different lung regions at a given height from the lung base, similar to the variability that is seen in blood flow. This is probably due to random differences in the diameters of bronchi formed at the bifurcation of the airways, comparable to the variation in blood vessel sizes contributing to regional perfusion differences.

Although ventilation and perfusion (per unit volume of lung tissue) both increase towards the bases of the lungs, the *rate* of increase in perfusion is greater than the rate of increase in ventilation, meaning that there is a decrease in the $\dot{V}/\dot{Q}$ ratio from the apices to the bases of the lungs (Fig. 7.8). The *range* of $\dot{V}/\dot{Q}$ ratios found in the healthy lung is relatively narrow at around 0.6–3.3 (Fig. 7.9), with a ratio of 1 around the height of the third rib.

How ventilation and perfusion are so closely matched is not fully understood. Matching is partly due to HPV and the fact that both ventilation and perfusion increase toward the lung bases. It also appears that compliant regions of the lung that are relatively well ventilated seem to have lower vascular resistances and are therefore better perfused.

In contrast to the narrow range of $\dot{V}/\dot{Q}$ ratios found in normal lungs, diseased lungs display a far wider variations, and this affects gas exchange.

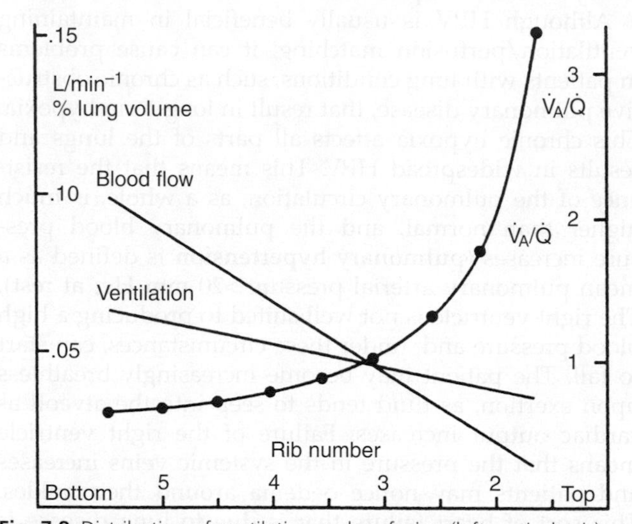

Fig. 7.8 Distribution of ventilation and perfusion (left vertical axis) and the ventilation/perfusion ratio (right vertical axis) in the normal upright lung. Both ventilation and perfusion are expressed in litres per minute per percent alveolar volume. The closed circles mark the ventilation/perfusion ratios of horizontal lung slices. $\dot{V}_A/\dot{Q}$, alveolar ventilation/perfusion ratio (From West JB. Respiratory Physiology. 2nd ed. 1970).

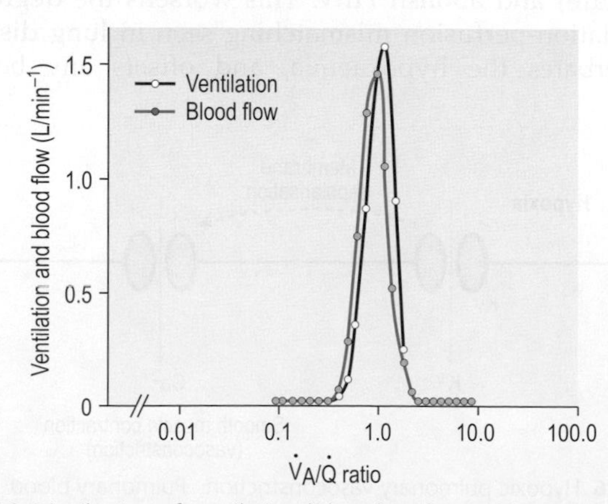

Fig. 7.9 Distribution of ventilation (O) and perfusion (•). Ventilation and perfusion are both plotted against the $\dot{V}/\dot{Q}$ ratio, on a logarithmic scale. Most ventilation and perfusion take place in lung regions having a relatively narrow range of $\dot{V}/\dot{Q}$ ratio.

Ventilation/perfusion matching and its effect on blood oxygen and carbon dioxide content

Oxygen (O_2) and carbon dioxide (CO_2) **tensions** in the alveoli and blood depend on the rate of ventilation of the alveoli, the blood flow rate (perfusion), and the *ratio* of ventilation to perfusion. Where there is a ventilation/perfusion mismatch, there is an impairment of both O_2 and CO_2 transfer.

If the transfer of O_2 and CO_2 were based on a simple mixing effect, it would be straightforward to calculate the composition of gas in an alveolus. In essence, this would be similar to the way we calculate the composition of a beaker of saline (i.e. blood) to which various known amounts of water (i.e. alveolar gas) are added. Adding a small amount of water to the saline would result in a mixture with a composition close to that of the saline. Adding a large volume of water to the saline would result in a mixture with a composition similar to that of water. Figure 7.10 shows how the composition of the saline/water mixture varies with their proportions. If saline represents the composition of mixed venous blood ($\bar{v}$) and water represents the composition of air (I), there would be a straight line joining point $\bar{v}$ (zero $\dot{V}/\dot{Q}$ ratio, shunt) and I (infinite $\dot{V}/\dot{Q}$ ratio, dead space). This straight line would represent the gas tensions at different parts of the lungs with ratios that lie between these two extremes.

However, gas exchange in the lungs is not a simple exchange of one molecule of CO_2 for one molecule of O_2, and the line joining the two extremes of the $\dot{V}/\dot{Q}$ ratio is, in fact, curved (Fig. 7.11), mainly because the oxygen–haemoglobin dissociation curve (see Chapter 8) is sigmoidal in shape. In a region of lung with a high $\dot{V}/\dot{Q}$ ratio, more CO_2 is removed from the blood, but the blood does not take up much more O_2. This is because at the higher PaO_2 that is found here, the haemoglobin is already 97% saturated and can therefore carry very little extra O_2. Similarly, in an area of lung with a low $\dot{V}/\dot{Q}$ ratio, relatively more O_2 is taken up by the blood because at the lower PaO_2, haemoglobin is at the middle, steep part of the oxygen–haemoglobin dissociation curve. However, relatively little extra CO_2 is released from the blood because the CO_2 dissociation curve is straighter than the oxygen–haemoglobin dissociation curve.

In other words, the ratio of CO_2 output to O_2 uptake (usually called the **respiratory exchange ratio, R**) varies throughout the lungs. The value of R for the lungs, as a whole, is about 0.8, varying according to what food is being metabolised. In regions near the lung apices, with high $\dot{V}/\dot{Q}$ ratios, the value of R is as high as 2.0, whereas in regions near the bases, with low $\dot{V}/\dot{Q}$ ratios, the value of R is as low as 0.5.

Figure 7.11 is an ***oxygen-carbon dioxide diagram,*** or O_2-CO_2 diagram. As in Figure 7.10, point $\bar{v}$ represents a $\dot{V}/\dot{Q}$ ratio of zero, meaning there is perfusion but no ventilation (e.g. mucus blockage of a lobar bronchus causing a shunt). As there is no ventilation, the O_2 and CO_2 contents

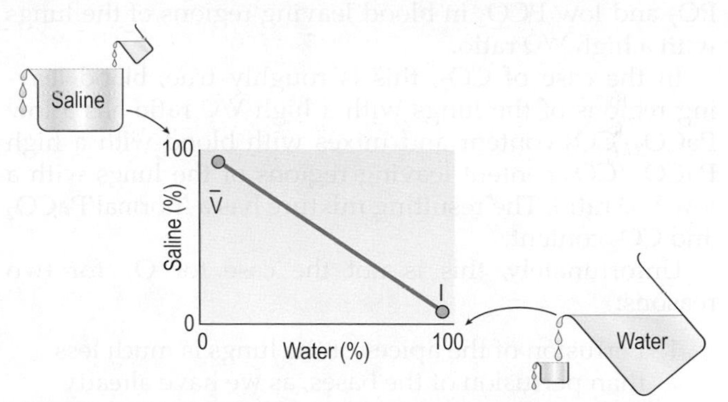

Fig. 7.10 An analogy of under- and overventilated regions of the lung. The exchange of gases is simplified as the displacement of saline by water. Saline represents mixed venous blood and pure water represents alveolar air. The upper represents the composition of blood in poorly ventilated regions of the lung (not enough water being added to wash the salt away). Point I represents regions with ventilation in excess (nearly all the salt is washed away and the composition of I approaches that of pure water).

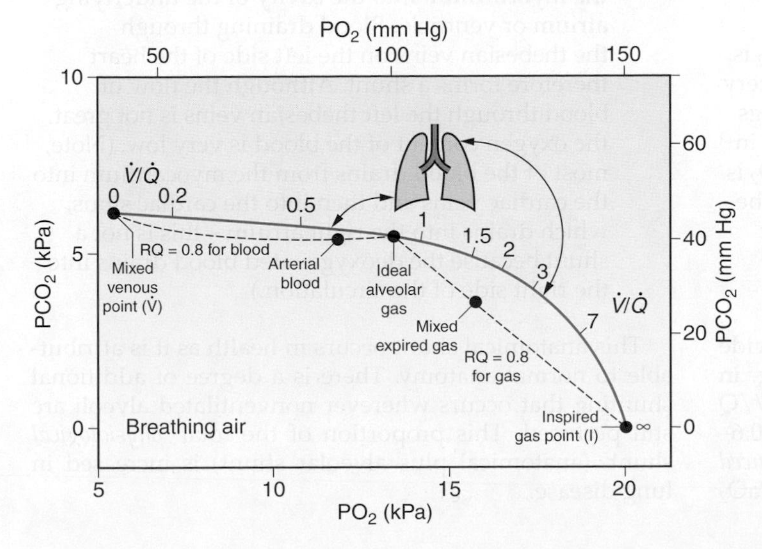

Fig. 7.11 The relationship between PO_2 and PCO_2 in regions of the lungs with different $\dot{V}/\dot{Q}$ ratios. Where the $\dot{V}/\dot{Q}$ ratio is high, as at the lung apices, alveolar gas and end-capillary blood have relatively high PO_2, and relatively low PCO_2. Where the $\dot{V}/\dot{Q}$ ratio is low, as at the lung bases, the mixture has a relatively low PO_2 and a relatively high PCO_2. (From Lumb and Thomas. Nunn and Lumb's Applied Respiratory Physiology. 2021)

in the capillaries remain unchanged from mixed venous blood. Point I represents a $\dot{V}/\dot{Q}$ ratio of infinity. There is ventilation but no perfusion (e.g. an obstructing pulmonary embolism producing **dead space**). Here, the alveolar gas concentrations are the same as in the inspired air.

The different regions of the lungs sit at points between $\bar{v}$ and I. At the base of the lungs, the $\dot{V}/\dot{Q}$ ratio is lower, and the alveolar PO_2 is relatively low while the PCO_2 is high. As the $\dot{V}/\dot{Q}$ ratio increases towards the apices, the PO_2 of the alveoli increases and the PCO_2 decreases. The heterogenous environment of the lungs has clinical implications. For example, the higher ventilation perfusion ratios at the lung apices explain why inhalation of toxic substances primarily damages the upper lobes of the lungs.

Does it matter that the alveoli at the apices of the lungs have a higher PaO_2 and a lower $PaCO_2$ than those at the bases? After all, the blood from different regions of the lungs is mixed together in the left atrium. Surely the low PO_2 and high PCO_2 in blood leaving regions of the lung with a low $\dot{V}/\dot{Q}$ ratio will be 'balanced' by the high PO_2 and low PCO_2 in blood leaving regions of the lungs with a high $\dot{V}/\dot{Q}$ ratio.

In the case of CO_2, this is roughly true; blood leaving regions of the lungs with a high $\dot{V}/\dot{Q}$ ratio has a low $PaCO_2/CO_2$ content and mixes with blood with a high $PaCO_2/CO_2$ content leaving regions of the lungs with a low $\dot{V}/\dot{Q}$ ratio. The resulting mixture has a 'normal'$PaCO_2$ and CO_2 content.

Unfortunately, this is not the case for O_2, for two reasons:

1. Perfusion of the apices of the lungs is much less than perfusion of the bases, as we have already seen. Although blood leaving the apices has higher PaO_2, there is a much less blood flow, here, than at the bases, that is, only a small *volume* of blood with a high PaO_2 is produced.
2. The higher PaO_2 in blood from the apices does not translate into a higher blood O_2 *content*. O_2 is carried in the blood primarily bound to haemoglobin, and only in small quantities as dissolved O_2 (see Chapter 8). The haemoglobin leaving the regions of the lungs with higher PO_2 is 97% saturated with O_2 and can therefore carry very little extra O_2, compared with regions of the lungs with normal PO_2. In other words, the O_2 *content* in blood leaving regions of the lungs with high PO_2 is very similar to that of blood leaving regions of the lungs with 'normal' PO_2. Clearly, then, it cannot 'compensate' for the low O_2 content of blood leaving regions of the lungs with low PO_2.

To summarise these two points: if there is a wide range of $\dot{V}/\dot{Q}$ ratios, as found in diseased lungs (e.g. in chronic obstructive pulmonary disease, the range of V/Q ratios can be as large as 0.03–10 instead of the usual 0.6–3.3), blood in the left atrium will tend to have a *reduced* PaO_2 (because the volume of blood with a low PaO_2 from the bases of the lungs is greater than the volume of blood with high PaO_2 from the apices) and *reduced* O_2 *content* (because the oxygen–haemoglobin dissociation curve indicates that the haemoglobin is already nearly saturated at normal PO_2). Therefore, a narrow range of $\dot{V}/\dot{Q}$ ratios is very important for maximising arterial O_2 content.

In healthy individuals, the degree of ventilation/perfusion matching is so good that arterial blood carries only 2% less O_2 than blood leaving a theoretical 'ideal' set of lungs with perfect ventilation/perfusion matching. This 2% reduction in O_2 content is caused by the small degree of ventilation/perfusion mismatching seen in health, and also by a **shunt**.

Shunt

A *true shunt* refers to a situation where the $\dot{V}/\dot{Q}$ ratio is 0, that is, an area of lung that is perfused but not ventilated at all. For example, if there is total obstruction of a lobar bronchus by mucus or blood, there will be no air flowing into that lung lobe; therefore, there is no ventilation. There will be reduced blood flow due to HPV, but any remaining blood passing through this lobe represents a true shunt. It is important to note that giving a patient 100% oxygen to breathe will not abolish hypoxaemia caused by a shunt as the shunted blood is not exposed to any ventilated alveoli and therefore remains deoxygenated (although the oxygen content of the nonshunted blood will increase somewhat due to the higher P_AO_2).

Anatomical shunt refers to deoxygenated blood which drains into the left side of the heart, thereby reducing the overall PO_2 of the blood which is delivered to the systemic circulation. This comes from two main sources:

1. Blood draining the *bronchial circulation* via the deep bronchial veins (see Bronchial Circulation, above).
2. The *thebesian veins* in the myocardium. These are small vessels that drain deoxygenated blood from the myocardium into the cavity of the underlying atrium or ventricle. Blood draining through the thebesian veins on the left side of the heart therefore forms a shunt. Although the flow of blood through the left thebesian veins is not great, the oxygen content of the blood is very low. (Note, most of the blood drains from the myocardium into the cardiac veins and then into the cardiac sinus, which drains into the right atrium – this is not a shunt because the deoxygenated blood drains into the right side of the circulation.)

This anatomical shunt occurs in health as it is attributable to normal anatomy. There is a degree of additional shunting that occurs wherever nonventilated alveoli are still perfused. This proportion of the total *'physiological* shunt' (anatomical plus alveolar shunt) is increased in lung disease.

The amount of shunting and ventilation/perfusion mismatching may be expressed in a number of ways. One way is to calculate the **alveolar-arterial PO_2 gradient**, which is the drop in PO_2 seen between the alveoli and arteries (A-a difference = $P_AO_2 - PaO_2$). The oxygen tension in the alveoli (P_AO_2) is calculated using the alveolar gas equation (Chapter 5) and the oxygen tension in the systemic arteries (PaO_2) is measured directly from an arterial blood gas sample. In health, the difference is typically 0.5–1 kPa (5 mm Hg) but can be much higher in patients with respiratory disease.

Another way of expressing the amount of shunting and ventilation/perfusion mismatching that is taking place is to calculate the **venous admixture**. This is defined as the amount of mixed venous blood that would need to be added to blood leaving a well-perfused and well-ventilated area of lung in order to produce the arterial O_2 concentration that is actually seen in the systemic arteries. The venous admixture is usually expressed as a proportion of the total cardiac output (**shunt fraction**). The venous admixture is a theoretical volume of blood, as the blood that actually flows through the physiological shunts has an O_2 content that may be higher (deep bronchial veins) or lower (thebesian veins) than that of mixed venous blood. The venous admixture may nevertheless be estimated using the **shunt equation** (Fig. 7.12):

$$\frac{\dot{Q}s}{\dot{Q}t} = \frac{(Cc'O_2 - CaO_2)}{(Cc'O_2 - C\bar{v}O_2)}$$

where $\dot{Q}_s$ is the venous admixture flow, $\dot{Q}_t$ is the total blood flow, Cao_2 is the O_2 content of arterial blood, CvO_2 is the O_2 content of mixed venous blood and $Cc'o_2$ is the O_2 content of the capillary blood draining an alveolus with an ideal ventilation/perfusion ratio.

The O_2 content of blood can be calculated by knowing the partial pressure of O_2, the haemoglobin concentration, and using the O_2 dissociation curve. Mixed venous blood needs to be obtained from a catheter placed in the pulmonary artery. The O_2 content of capillary blood draining an 'ideal' alveolus cannot be measured but it can be inferred by calculating the PaO_2, using the alveolar gas equation (see above) and then calculating the O_2 content of blood at equilibrium within such an alveolus.

The shunt fraction in normal individuals is usually less than 5% of the total cardiac output, and is mostly due to ventilation/perfusion mismatching, with only a small portion attributable to shunting of blood from the deep bronchial and thebesian veins.

Disease processes can increase the extent of $\dot{V}/\dot{Q}$ mismatching or shunting, and therefore increase the alveolar-arterial PO_2 gradient and shunt fraction.

A salutary tale

A student illicitly eating peanuts in the library is surprised by the approach of the librarian. He inhales a nut, which completely blocks his *right* main bronchus. Leaping about in an attempt to expel the offending fruit,

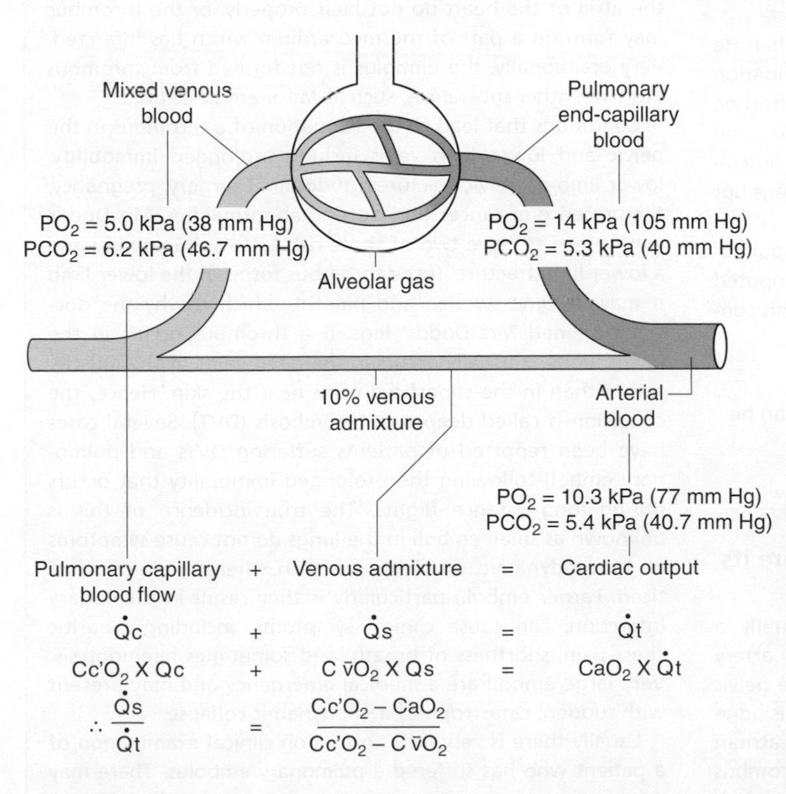

Fig 7.12 Calculation of shunt fraction. The oxygen carried in the *arterial blood* equals the sum of the oxygen carried in the *capillary blood* plus that in the shunted blood. It makes the assumption that all the *arterial blood* has come either from alveoli with normal ventilation/perfusion ratios or from a shunt carrying only *mixed venous blood*. This is never true, but it forms a convenient method for quantifying *venous admixtures* from whatever cause. The amount of oxygen in 1 minute's flow of blood equals the product of blood flow rate and the oxygen content of the blood. Qt, total cardiac output; Qs, blood flow through shunt; CaO_2, oxygen content of arterial blood; $Cc'O_2$, oxygen content of pulmonary end-capillary blood; CvO_2 oxygen content of mixed venous blood (From Lumb and Thomas. Nunn and Lumb's Applied Respiratory Physiology. 2021).

our hero merely succeeds in dislodging a large clot which has formed in a leg vein due to the hours of immobility he has spent at his studies. If the clot obstructs his *right* pulmonary artery, all will probably be well; although his right lung will be functionally non-existent, his left lung will be normal and sufficient for him to survive. If the clot lodges in the *left* pulmonary artery, the consequences of this extreme case of ventilation/perfusion mismatch will be grave. Despite the fact that his *total* lung ventilation and *total* lung perfusion may be sufficient for survival, both lungs will be functionally useless, each for a different reason. The right lung will have no ventilation and will be a shunt and the left lung will have no perfusion and will be dead space. This story may help you understand the importance of matching ventilation and perfusion and maintaining a law-abiding lifestyle.

Summary 3

- Ventilation increases from the lung apices to the bases, but not as much as perfusion increases from the apices to the bases.
- $\dot{V}/\dot{Q}$ ratios decrease from the lung apices to the bases.
- The relatively small range of ventilation–perfusion ratios in the healthy lung is increased during disease.
- Regions of the lung which are perfused but not ventilated constitute shunts ($\dot{V}/\dot{Q}$ ratio zero).
- Administering 100% oxygen does not reverse hypoxaemia arising from shunt.
- Regions of the lung which are ventilated but not perfused are called dead space ($\dot{V}/\dot{Q}$ ratio infinity).
- Ventilation/perfusion mismatching can cause depression of arterial PO_2 and reduction in arterial O_2 content but has less effect on $PaCO_2$.

Case 7.1 The pulmonary circulation

Pulmonary embolus

Mrs Dodds is an 80-year-old woman who tripped and fell at home, fracturing her right hip. She was taken to hospital and, the next day, she went to the operating theatre where her hip was fixed surgically. Postoperatively, she was initially doing well, although she was quite slow to mobilise. However, on the third day after her operation, she developed left-sided chest pain. The pain was pleuritic (sharp in nature and made worse with breathing) and was associated with breathlessness.

The doctor who came to see Mrs Dodds examined her. He thought she looked a little cyanosed, but the examination of her chest did not reveal anything remarkable. Her trachea was not deviated, the expansion of her chest was normal, and there was no abnormality evident upon percussion or auscultation of her chest. The doctor examined Mrs Dodds' legs but found no abnormality.

The doctor felt that the most likely diagnosis was a pulmonary embolus and he sent Mrs Dodds to undergo a computed tomography (CT) pulmonary angiogram (Fig. 7.13A). This confirmed the diagnosis of a pulmonary embolus.

In this case, we will consider:

1. The causes of a pulmonary embolus and how it can be diagnosed.
2. How a pulmonary embolus can be treated.
3. Massive pulmonary embolus.

What causes a pulmonary embolus? What are its symptoms and how can it be diagnosed?

A pulmonary embolus occurs when something, usually a thrombus (blood clot), occludes part of the pulmonary artery tree. Generally, the thrombus forms in the veins of the pelvis or lower limbs, and part or all of that thrombus may dislodge and pass through the vena cava, through the right atrium and ventricle, and into the pulmonary artery. The thrombus finally lodges in a branch of the pulmonary artery, occluding it. The segment of lung tissue supplied by the obstructed artery has a reduced blood supply (although it often receives some blood – remember the bronchial circulation) and may, ultimately, infarct.

In a small number of cases (probably less than 10% of the total number of pulmonary emboli) the thrombus originates from the upper extremity deep veins or in the right side of the heart, itself. This may be a result of atrial fibrillation, in which the atria of the heart do not beat properly, or the thrombus may form on a part of the myocardium which has infarcted. Very occasionally, the embolus is not formed from thrombus but from other substances, such as fat or amniotic fluid.

Conditions that lead to the formation of a thrombus in the pelvic and lower limb veins include prolonged immobility, lower limb or pelvic fractures, abdominal surgery, pregnancy, the presence of cancer, and clotting abnormalities. Mrs Dodds was known to have two of these risk factors: immobility and a lower limb fracture. If the thrombus forms in the lower limb it may become swollen and painful, which is why the doctor examined Mrs Dodds' legs. If a thrombus occurs in the lower limbs, it usually occurs in the deep veins of the muscle, rather than in the superficial veins near the skin. Hence, the condition is called deep vein thrombosis (DVT). Several cases have been reported of patients suffering DVTs and pulmonary emboli following the prolonged immobility that occurs during long-distance flights. The true incidence of this is unknown as small emboli in the lungs do not cause symptoms or haemodynamic problems and can, therefore, go unnoticed. Larger emboli, particularly if they result in pulmonary infarction, can cause clinical symptoms, including pleuritic chest pain, shortness of breath, and sometimes haemoptysis. Very large emboli are a medical emergency and may present with sudden, catastrophic haemodynamic collapse.

Usually there is very little to find on clinical examination of a patient who has suffered a pulmonary embolus. There may be a few crackles upon auscultation and occasionally a pleural

Case 7.1

The pulmonary circulation – cont'd

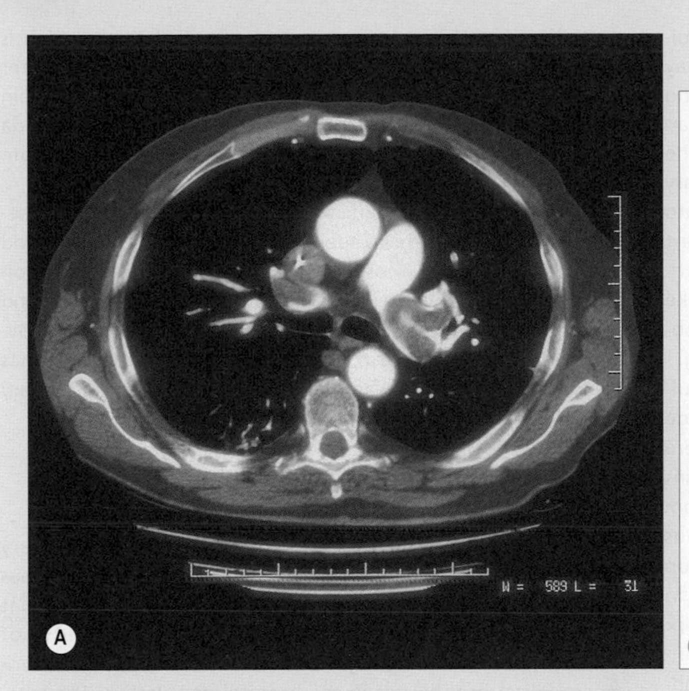

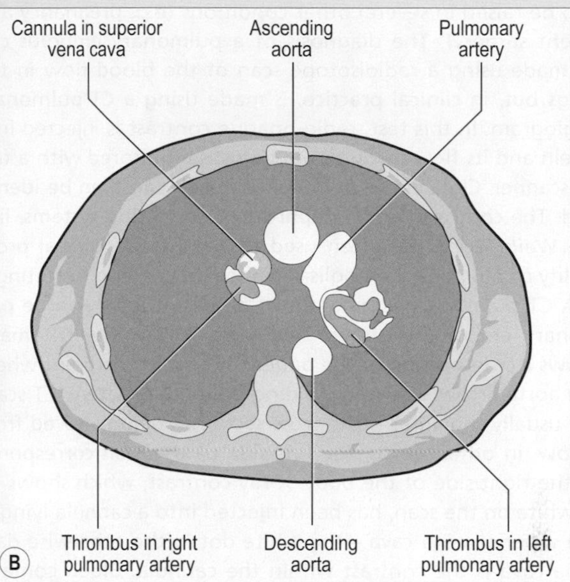

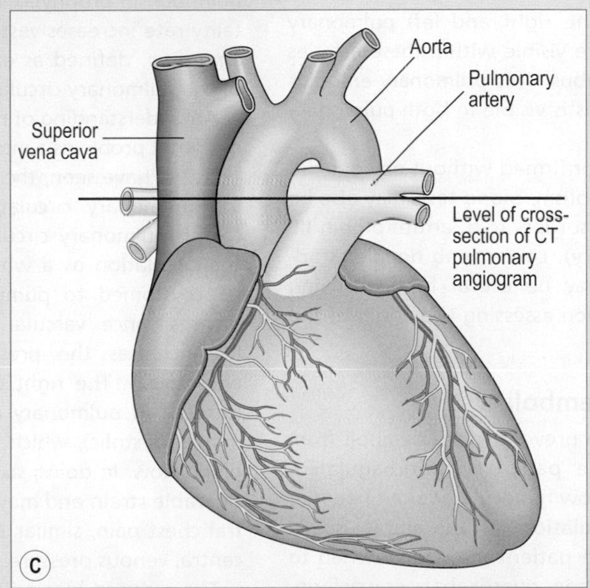

Fig. 7.13 Computed tomography pulmonary angiogram (CTPA) of a patient with a large pulmonary embolus (A). The relevant structures seen on the CT image are labelled in (B). The CT images depict a cross-section at about the level shown in (C). The clot is clearly visible in both pulmonary arteries as dark areas against the white of the X-ray contrast medium. Courtesy of Dr J. T. Murchison, Royal Infirmary, Edinburgh.

rub may be heard over an area of infarcted lung. A plain chest X-ray is not generally very helpful in diagnosing a pulmonary embolus; if there is quite a large embolus, it is said that the affected lung fields can appear 'oligaemic' (i.e. they contain less blood so appear darker on the chest X-ray). This is not always easy to see, however. Larger pulmonary emboli increase the amount of work that the right ventricle has to do, as it has to pump blood into the partially obstructed pulmonary circulation. This can result in changes in the electrocardiogram. Classically, these changes consist of S waves in lead I, and Q waves and inverted T waves in lead III (hence, the mnemonic: 'S1 Q3 T3'), but these changes are rarely seen in practice.

Continued

Case 7.1 The pulmonary circulation – cont'd

D-dimer levels are usually increased in patients with pulmonary emboli, but this test is non-specific as the levels may also be raised in several other conditions (e.g. pregnancy and recent surgery). The diagnosis of a pulmonary embolus can be made using a radioisotope scan of the blood flow in the lungs but, in clinical practice, is made using a CT pulmonary angiogram. In this test, radio-opaque contrast is injected into a vein and its flow through the lungs is monitored with a fast CT scanner. Clots in the pulmonary vessels can then be identified. The contrast can be nephrotoxic so scoring systems, like the *Wells Score*, are often used to stratify the clinical probability of pulmonary embolism before proceeding to testing.

A CT pulmonary angiogram of a patient with a large pulmonary embolus is shown in Figure 7.13A. The CT image shows a cross-section of the patient's chest at the point where the aorta arches over the dividing pulmonary artery. CT scans are usually shown as if the cross-section is being viewed from *below*, in other words, the left side of the scan corresponds to the right side of the body. X-ray contrast, which shows up as white on the scan, has been injected into a cannula lying in the superior vena cava – the white dot in the otherwise dark vena cava is the contrast within the cannula. Blood containing contrast is clearly visible in the ascending and descending aorta. There is blood in the right and left pulmonary arteries; however, dark areas are visible within these arteries which correspond to the thrombus. This pulmonary embolus is a large one, and the thrombus is visible in both pulmonary arteries.

If a pulmonary embolism is confirmed without obvious risk factors for venous thromboembolism, blood tests may also be sent to look for coagulation disorders (e.g. antithrombin III, protein C or protein S deficiency). Lower limb doppler studies and an echocardiogram may be useful for identifying thrombi in the legs or heart when assessing the origin of the pulmonary embolism.

Treatment of pulmonary emboli

The mainstay of treatment is to prevent further emboli from occurring. For this reason, the patient is anticoagulated. Initially, this is achieved with a low molecular weight heparin, a drug which inhibits the coagulation cascade and is usually given subcutaneously. Later, the patient may be switched to an oral anticoagulant like apixaban, rivaroxaban, or warfarin, which are often taken for several months following a pulmonary embolism. This combination of treatment is used for the type of pulmonary embolism suffered by Mrs Dodds.

Following a very large pulmonary embolism, an attempt may be made to break down the thrombus that is in the lungs. Drugs, such as streptokinase, may be used to activate the fibrinolytic pathway, resulting in the breakdown of the clot. In extreme circumstances, after a very major pulmonary embolus, a surgical operation may be carried out to remove the clot, particularly if it lies in the proximal pulmonary artery. If warfarin does not prevent further pulmonary emboli, it may be necessary to insert a caval filter, which is a small filter that fits into the inferior vena cava. The filter is inserted, folded, through a puncture in the femoral vein before being opened up and wedged into the inferior vena cava, under X-ray guidance. The filter 'catches' emboli from the lower limb veins and prevents them reaching the lungs.

Pulmonary emboli can sometimes have serious consequences and, as we have seen, are promoted by surgery and immobility. For this reason, all patients admitted to hospital are assessed for their venous thromboembolism risk and given prophylactic, small, daily, subcutaneous doses of low molecular weight heparin, if appropriate. This treatment has been shown to significantly reduce the risk of pulmonary emboli in these patients.

Massive pulmonary embolism – a rare medical emergency

The mortality rate for patients presenting with pulmonary emboli is quoted as being between 1 and 15% and increases with age and comorbidity. Postmortem studies suggest that pulmonary emboli are implicated in approximately 10% of all hospital deaths, highlighting the need for venous thromboembolism prophylaxis in the hospital population. The mortality rate increases vastly in the case of a *massive pulmonary embolism*, defined as embolism obstructing more than 50% of the pulmonary circulation.

An understanding of respiratory physiology allows us to predict what problems a massive pulmonary emoblism will cause.

As we have seen, the entire cardiac output passes through the pulmonary circulation, therefore a major obstruction to the pulmonary circulation means a major obstruction to the circulation as a whole. Furthermore, the right ventricle is accustomed to pumping blood through a low-pressure, low-resistance vascular bed. A massive pulmonary embolus increases the pressure in the pulmonary circulation enormously. The right ventricle can produce only a modest increase in pulmonary artery blood pressure (say, up to 60 mm Hg systolic), which is insufficient to sustain an adequate blood flow. In doing so, the right ventricle is put under considerable strain and may start to fail, leading to crushing central chest pain, similar to that of angina, as well as a raised central venous pressure.

The reduced blood flow to the lungs leads to a large mismatch in ventilation and perfusion, and leads to arterial hypoxia. The reduced blood flow through the lungs also means that the filling of the left ventricle starts to diminish, and the circulation as a whole therefore begins to fail. The patient may become pale and shocked and may lose consciousness. In severe cases, death follows quickly.

The treatment of a massive pulmonary embolism is initially supportive, with the administration of oxygen and fluids. Anticoagulation, thrombolysis, acute surgery, or heart bypass may be necessary. However, the result of a massive pulmonary embolus is often death.

References and Further reading

Hensley, M.K., Levine, A., Gladwin, M.T., et al., 2018. Emerging therapeutics in pulmonary hypertension. Am. J. Physiol. Lung. Cell. Mol. Physiol. 314, L769–L781.

Hughes, J.M.B., 1997. Distribution of pulmonary blood flow. In: Crystal, R.G., West, J.B., Barnes, P.J., Weibel, E.R. (Eds.), The Lung: Scientific Foundations, second ed. Raven Press.

Lumb A. and Thomas C., 2021. Nunn and Lumb's Applied Respiratory Physiology, ninth ed. Elsevier, Oxford.

Tapson, V.F., 2008. Acute pulmonary embolism. N. Eng. J. Med. 358 (10), 1037–1052.

Venous thromboembolic diseases: diagnosis, management and thrombophilia testing. NICE guideline [NG158] Published date: 26 March 2020.

Weir, E.K., Reeves, J.T. (Eds.), 1989. Pulmonary Vascular Physiology and Pathophysiology. Marcel Dekker.

West JB. Respiratory Physiology. 2nd ed. Baltimore: Williams & Wilkins; 1970.

West, J.B., 2005. Ventilation-Perfusion relationships. In: West, J.B. (Ed.), Respiratory Physiology: The Essentials, seventh ed. Lippincott Williams and Wilkins, 55–73.

CARRIAGE OF GASES BY THE BLOOD AND ACID/BASE BALANCE

8

Chapter objectives

After studying this chapter, you should be able to:

1. Define the oxygen content of blood, and explain how this changes in anaemia
2. Discuss the properties of red cells
3. Discuss abnormal haemoglobins
4. Describe factors affecting the oxyhaemoglobin dissociation curve
5. Describe carbon monoxide poisoning
6. List the ways carbon dioxide is transported in the blood
7. List the major buffers in blood
8. Describe common acid–base abnormalities resulting from disease, and how physiological compensation may occur

Introduction – why do we need to transport gases in the blood?

Cell survival requires the expenditure of energy. This energy is obtained by the oxidation of food, mainly in the form of glucose:

$$C_6H_{12}O_6 + 6O_2 \rightarrow 6CO_2 + 6H_2O + \text{Energy}$$

This equation represents the reaction that occurs when glucose is oxidised, producing energy as a burst of heat. This does not happen as a crude, single step, in vivo; rather, the reaction takes place as a series of small steps within the mitochondria of cells. Oxygen is the terminal electron acceptor in the electron transport chain in the mitochondrial inner membrane. Most of the energy released is immediately stored as **adenosine triphosphate** (ATP), a high-energy coenzyme molecule which is made by combining adenosine diphosphate (ADP) with inorganic phosphate:

$$\text{ADP} + \text{Phosphate} + \text{Energy} \leftrightarrow \text{ATP}$$

This simplistic representation explains why oxidative metabolism in our mitochondria requires oxygen (O_2) and produces carbon dioxide (CO_2) and water, as well as the energy crucial to our survival. This chapter will consider how O_2 is supplied to the cells and how CO_2 is removed.

O_2 moves into and CO_2 moves out of our cells by the passive process of **diffusion**. There must be a difference in the concentrations of the diffusing substance for diffusion to take place (see Chapter 6). O_2 diffuses down its concentration gradient from the high partial pressure found in the alveoli to the lower O_2 tension found in deoxygenated blood in the pulmonary capillaries. O_2 then reaches the various tissues of the body by bulk transport in the blood. The energy for this active process comes from the pumping of the heart. At the tissues, O_2 again diffuses passively down its concentration gradient, this time from oxygenated blood in the systemic capillaries to the metabolically active tissues. CO_2 moves in the opposite direction, from tissues to the lungs, resulting in the differences in composition between venous and arterial blood shown in Table 8.1.

Blood is a liquid tissue (plasma) containing formed elements (cells). The red blood corpuscles (RBCs, **erythrocytes**) play an important part in the transport of O_2 to and CO_2 away from the tissues. RBCs are strictly called corpuscles because they do not contain a nucleus, but the term *cell* is often used. Although RBCs play an important role in the carriage and exchange of gases (carrying the majority of O_2 and processing CO_2 at both the lungs and tissues), the gases must first enter into simple solution, in the plasma, before being carried or processed by the RBCs.

O_2 in the blood is mainly carried in loose combination with haemoglobin (Hb) within the RBC. CO_2 is carried partly in solution, partly in combination with proteins (particularly Hb), but mainly as bicarbonate in the plasma. The carrier mechanisms in blood have evolved such that the uptake or loss of O_2 promotes the loss or uptake of CO_2, and vice versa.

Table 8.1 Some values for normal blood

	Systemic arterial blood	*Mixed venous blood*
Oxygen		
Tension (kPa)	13.3	5.3
Blood content (mL L^{-1})	200	150
Saturation (%)	98	75
Carbon dioxide		
Tension (kPa)	5.3	6.1
Blood content (mL L^{-1})	490	530
Plasma content (mL L^{-1})	600	640
Acidity		
Plasma [H^+] (nM)	40	43
Plasma pH	7.40	7.37

The addition of CO_2 to the blood at the tissues would cause a dangerously large change in acidity if the blood did not contain efficient buffering systems, in particular proteins, bicarbonate, and phosphate, which take up hydrogen ions added to the blood and release them when the blood becomes more alkaline, thereby **buffering** (resisting) changes in acidity.

Oxygen transport

Because we are large and complicated animals, most of the cells of our bodies are far removed from the atmosphere. O_2 has, therefore, to be carried from the lungs to these cells via the blood. All gases dissolve in water to a greater or lesser extent, but O_2 dissolves only to 3 mL L^{-1} in the plasma leaving the lungs. While exercising vigorously, we may need up to 3 L of O_2 per minute. This implies that if O_2 was only carried to the tissues dissolved in simple solution, we would need a blood flow of 1000 L min^{-1} to supply our bodies with O_2. Normal cardiac output is 5–6 L min^{-1}, at rest. Olympic athletes can increase the output of their hearts to about 30 L min^{-1} which, you can see, is still far short of the blood flow required to supply the tissues with O_2. The answer to this problem is that, like all other vertebrates, we have evolved a carrier molecule in the blood which picks up and then releases a great deal of O_2. In us, this molecule is **Hb**, and it is contained within RBCs.

Hb vastly increases the O_2-carrying capacity of blood. We have seen that normal arterial blood contains only 3 mL of *dissolved* O_2 per litre (due to the low solubility of oxygen in plasma), but a further 200 mL of oxygen can be carried when attached to Hb (about 180 mL in women, because they have less Hb). So, about 60 times as much O_2 is carried by Hb as is in solution.

Henry's law tells us that the amount dissolved is proportional to the pressure of O_2 (its partial pressure in a mixture, such as air). So, the amount of dissolved O_2 can be increased by increasing the pressure (unlike the amount attached to Hb, which reaches a maximum at atmospheric pressure). If a subject breathes pure O_2, the alveolar and arterial PO_2 increase more than sixfold, and the amount of O_2 in solution rises from 3 to 20 mL per litre of blood. Furthermore, if a subject breathes pure O_2 at 3 atmospheres pressure (e.g. in a hyperbaric chamber) he can theoretically obtain sufficient O_2 to meet metabolic requirements from that dissolved in plasma, and Hb is not necessary as an O_2 transporter.

Table 8.1 illustrates the important point that we do not extract all the O_2 present in arterial blood. Mixed venous blood is still 75% saturated with O_2, and there is an arteriovenous content difference of 50 mL O_2/L blood.

Haemoglobin

Hb has remarkable O_2-carrying properties which are related to its molecular structure (Fig. 8.1). Each Hb molecule consists of a protein (globin) and haem (protoporphyrin and ferrous iron). The globin is made up of four polypeptide chains, each carrying a haem group, which means there are *four sites, each capable of carrying one O_2* on each Hb molecule. It is conceptually useful to consider each Hb molecule as having four 'hooks'. On each hook can hang one O_2. This structure explains many of the properties of Hb, as we will see below.

Each of the four polypeptide chains can vary in a way which will alter the O_2-carrying properties of the blood. The chains are named according to their structure. Adult Hb consists of two α and two β chains, with 141 and 146 amino acid residues per chain, respectively. Thus each Hb molecule has 574 amino acids and four haems, which gives the molecule a weight of about 64 500 Da. The various other forms of normal and abnormal Hb comprise other combinations of polypeptide chain structures. These are discussed under 'Haemoglobin variants', below. Men have about 150 g L^{-1} Hb in their blood, women about 130 g L^{-1}.

Oxygen combination with haemoglobin

This reversible reaction can be summarised as follows:

$$Hb + O_2 \leftrightarrow HbO_2$$

which will be driven to the right (to oxyhaemoglobin, HbO_2) by increased PO_2 and to the left (to deoxyhaemoglobin, Hb) by low PO_2.

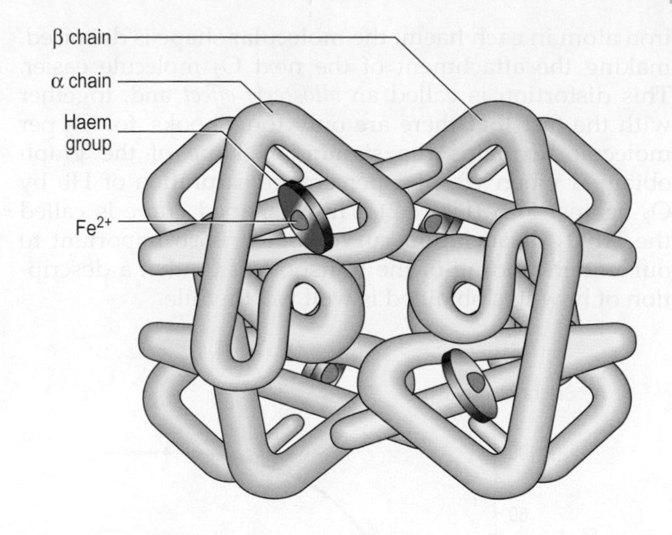

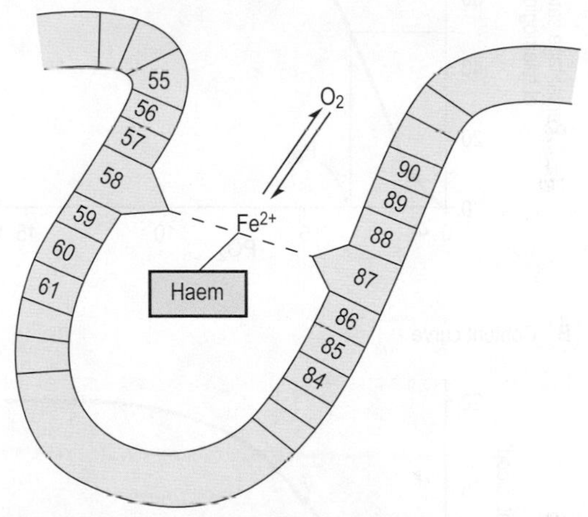

Fig. 8.1 The structure of haemoglobin. Each of the four globin chains (two α chains and two β chains) is made up of a spiral of just over 100 amino acids. Each chain is attached to an iron (Fe^{2+})-containing *haem group*. Each *haem group* can carry a molecule of oxygen (O_2), so each haemoglobin molecule has four 'hooks', each of which can carry one O_2.

As each of the four haem groups of the Hb molecule represents a site for combination with O_2; it might be more correct to consider each Hb molecule as Hb_4, with which association or dissociation with O_2 takes place in four steps. Thus the previous equation should be written:

$$Hb_4 + O_2 \leftrightarrow Hb_4O_2$$
$$Hb_4O_2 + O_2 \leftrightarrow Hb_4O_4$$
$$Hb_4O_4 + O_2 \leftrightarrow Hb_4O_6$$

and finally,

$$Hb_4O_6 + O_2 \leftrightarrow Hb_4O_8$$

The haem and the globin of each molecule are held in a fixed relationship to each other by links (salt bridges) between the polypeptide chains. In each of the steps in the above equation, when a molecule of O_2 binds to the iron atom in each haem, the molecular shape is distorted, making the attachment of the next O_2 molecule easier. This distortion is called an *allosteric effect* and, together with the fact that there are only four 'hooks' for O_2 per molecule, explains the sigmoidal shape of the graph obtained when we plot percentage saturation of Hb by O_2 against PO_2 (Fig. 8.2). This S-shaped curve is called the **HbO_2 dissociation curve**, and it is so important to our understanding of the transport of O_2 that a description of how it is obtained is well worthwhile.

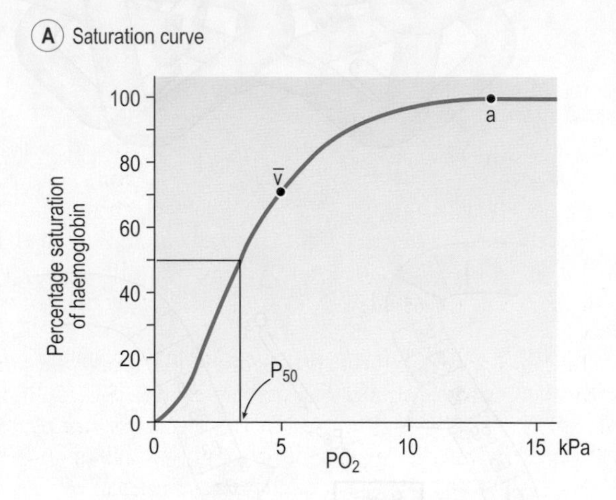

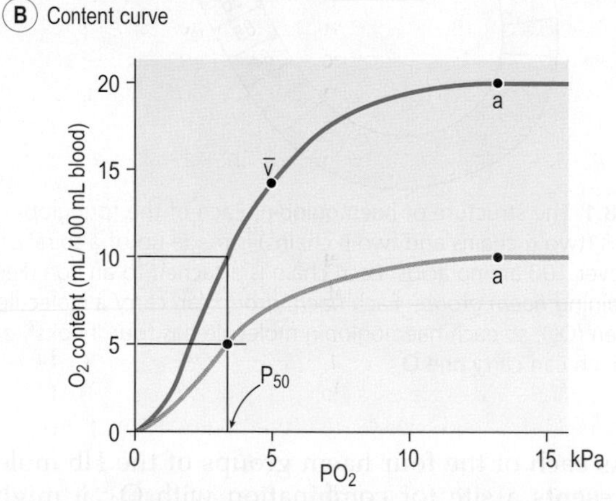

Fig. 8.2 The oxyhaemoglobin dissociation curve. This curve is obtained by exposing blood to a number of partial pressures of O_2 and measuring how much of its total O_2-carrying capacity is occupied. This can be expressed in two ways. The *saturation curve* (A) represents the percentage of the total number of 'hooks' for O_2 that are occupied (the 50% occupancy, P_{50}, is shown). This curve gives us no idea of the amount of O_2 being carried, which depends on the amount of Hb present and is shown by the content curve (B). The lower curve represents anaemic blood, demonstrating that content is dependent on Hb concentration. Both this and the normal curve are equally saturated at different PO_2, as shown by their identical P_{50} values, but the amount they are carrying is very different. Because temperature and pH affect the properties of Hb, we must state that these curves were obtained at pH 7.4 and 37°C. The important loading and unloading conditions for blood are from arterial blood at (a) and into mixed venous blood at ($\bar{v}$). Note that the slopes of the curve are very different at these two points.

Obtaining an oxyhaemoglobin dissociation curve

If you take, say, five test tubes of blood and expose each of them to a different partial pressure of O_2 (say, 0, 2, 4, 8, and 16 kPa O_2), each tube will contain a different percentage of Hb that has been converted to HbO_2, depending on the partial pressure it has been exposed to. Each sample will also have a different colour because HbO_2 is brighter red than Hb (arterial blood is red; venous blood is dark red). An instrument called a spectrophotometer can use this colour variation to measure the percentage of Hb that has been converted to HbO_2, allowing us to plot a graph of the percentage saturation (percentage of the O_2-carrying 'hooks' occupied) against the PO_2 to which that particular sample of blood was exposed (Fig. 8.2A). We have seen that each Hb molecule has four hooks, each of which can carry one O_2 molecule. This might suggest that blood can only be 25% (one hook), 50% (two hooks), 75% (three hooks), or 100% (four hooks) saturated with O_2. This is true for each individual molecule, but ignores the fact that even a drop of blood contains millions of Hb molecules, any one of which can be carrying from zero to four O_2 molecules.

Properties of the oxyhaemoglobin dissociation curve

When 100% saturated (all 'hooks' occupied), 1 g of Hb carries about 2 mg – 1.34 mL – of O_2, at normal body temperature. Therefore, 1 L of your blood, containing 150 g of Hb, can transport 200 mL (150 × 1.34) of O_2 as HbO_2. Comparing this with the 3 mL carried in simple solution gives some idea of the advantage of having Hb in our blood.

The carriage of O_2 in our blood is not quite as simple as hanging O_2 molecules on hooks, like coats on a stand; evolution has refined this already efficient process even further. To understand these refinements requires the definition of four terms:

1. *Oxygen tension (PO_2; kPa).* Oxygen **tension** is sometimes called the **partial pressure** of O_2 in solution. The difference in PO_2 between two sites determines the rate and direction of diffusion of O_2. This is because the partial pressures correspond to the concentrations in solution (Henry's law). Thus, dissolved O_2 will diffuse down its concentration (partial pressure) gradient. The PO_2 of active skeletal muscle may be as low as 1 kPa. Arterial blood supplying that muscle has a PO_2 of about 13 kPa, and this large pressure difference 'pushes' O_2 strongly into the tissues.

2. *Hb content (Hb, g L^{-1}).* It is Hb that has the haem 'hooks' that carry the O_2. The number of 'hooks' determines the maximum O_2-carrying capacity per mL of blood. If blood has only 50% (say) of the normal amount of Hb (it is anaemic), it will only have 50% of the normal number of 'hooks', and

even when fully saturated with O_2 will only be able to carry 100 mL, rather than 200 mL, of O_2.

3. *Hb saturation (%)*. This is the percentage of the total number of 'hooks' that are in fact occupied. It has nothing to do with the *number* of 'hooks' present. The number present may be normal, increased (polycythaemia), or reduced (anaemia). The measurement of Hb saturation is technically simple using a spectrophotometer, as described above, and gives useful information for clinical assessment (e.g. 100% saturation of arterial blood implies that the lungs are doing a good job of gas exchange). However, other measurements, particularly PO_2 and Hb content, are necessary to provide a complete picture. Students sometimes find it helpful to think of saturation as the 'appetite' Hb has for O_2. If Hb finds itself in a PO_2 where its saturation should be high (say, 10 kPa, in Fig. 8.2), it is 'hungry' and will readily accept O_2 until it is appropriately saturated or 'full'. At low PO_2 (say, 2 kPa, in Fig. 8.2), it is not so 'hungry', and does not readily accept oxygen.
4. *O_2 content* ($mL\ L^{-1}$). This refers to the amount of O_2 in a litre of arterial blood, which is the sum of the O_2 combined with Hb plus that O_2 dissolved in plasma. It is dependent on the Hb concentration, the Hb saturation, and the arterial O_2 tension (which in turn is dependent on the PO_2 of the air in the lungs driving O_2 into the blood). The O_2 content of arterial blood (CaO_2) is the volume of O_2 carried in each 100 mL of blood. It is calculated by:

(O_2 carried by Hb) + (O_2 in solution)

$$= (1.34 \times Hb \times SpO_2 \times 0.01) + (0.023 \times PaO_2).$$

Where:

1.34 = *Hüfner's constant*. Each gram of Hb can carry a maximum of 1.34 mL of O_2.

Hb = Hb concentration in grams per 100 mL of blood

SO_2 = percentage saturation of Hb with O_2

PaO_2 = O_2 tension of arterial blood

(0.023 = mL of O_2 dissolved per 100 mL of plasma per kPa, or 0.003 mL/mm Hg)

For a normal adult male, with an Hb level of 15 g dL^{-1} (from a full blood count), SpO_2 of 100% (from plethysmography), and a PaO_2 of 13.3 kPa (from an arterial blood gas sample), the oxygen content of arterial blood is:

CaO_2 = 20.1 +0.3 = 20.4 mL O_2 per 100 mL of blood

The difference between 'saturation' and 'content' is very important to understand. If everything else is normal, the O_2 content in blood depends on the amount of Hb present *and the* PO_2 whereas the O_2 saturation (percentage Hb saturation with O_2) depends only on PO_2.

Cyanosis

Clinicians are often alerted to reduced blood O_2 content by **cyanosis**, a bluish tinge to the skin. This arises because the colour of blood depends on the Hb content, and the proportions of Hb that are in the oxygenated (bright red) or deoxygenated (dark red) state. In normal blood, the appearance of cyanosis corresponds to about 70% saturation and a PO_2 of 5 kPa; this means the blood contains 50 g L^{-1} deoxygenated Hb, which gives cyanosed skin its blue colour. If the patient is anaemic, there is not sufficient Hb to produce this effect, and anaemic patients can be severely hypoxic without cyanosis. On the other hand, polycythaemic patients, with excess Hb, may be cyanosed with little hypoxia.

The shape of the oxyhaemoglobin dissociation curve

The HbO_2 dissociation curve (Fig. 8.2A) demonstrates the relationship between PO_2 and saturation, which is independent of blood Hb content. The O_2 content curve (Fig. 8.2B) shows the relationship between PO_2 and O_2 content (this does depend on Hb level), with the curve displaced downwards in anaemia (where the Hb content is low).

Whether expressing the relationship between PO_2 and saturation or content, the curves in Figure 8.2 have the same characteristic shape, which has an important influence on function. The major function of Hb is to *load* with O_2 in the lungs and *unload* at the tissues. Although red cells are of great importance (see 'Why is Hb kept in cells?', below), the only way O_2 can get from the lungs to the red cells, or from the red cells to the tissues, is by going into solution in plasma and tissue fluid. Hence, loading and unloading of O_2 occur solely due to differences in *partial pressure,* which provides the gradient for oxygen diffusion. These functions are carried out in the flat *loading region* at the top of the curve and in the steep *unloading region* (Fig. 8.2). The difference in the slopes of the curve at these two points has the following consequences:

- *Loading region (a; used in the lungs)*. Above about 10 kPa, Hb cannot take up much more O_2; it is 100% saturated because the molecules of Hb are carrying their full complement of four O_2 molecules each, and this number cannot be exceeded, regardless of how high the PO_2 level becomes. Alveolar ventilation can decrease by up to 25% or increase indefinitely without affecting O_2 *content* significantly. O_2 *tension* varies, however. The evolutionary advantage of this is that normal activities, such as talking, sighing, coughing, etc., do not greatly alter the amount of O_2 per litre of blood leaving the lungs for the tissues.
- *Unloading region (v; used at the tissues)*. Blood in the capillaries of active tissues is in an environment of low PO_2. O_2diffuses from blood to tissues, and even a small decline in blood PO_2 causes a large unloading of O_2 (i.e. the blood is working on the steep part of the HbO_2 dissociation curve). If it stays in the tissue long enough, the blood PO_2

will equilibrate with the tissue PO_2. If the blood is anaemic (low Hb content), however, removal of even a small amount of O_2 causes a large fall in PO_2 because there is little O_2 in the blood to begin with. A situation is quickly reached where there is little possibility of further supply to the tissues, along with a reduced PO_2 to drive it in. Thus anaemia can cause tissue hypoxia even though the arterial blood has a normal PO_2 and Hb *saturation* – it is the overall oxygen *content* that is low.

To identify the position of the steep part of the HbO_2 dissociation curve (usually to see if it is being oxygenated properly), the PO_2 at which 50% of the Hb is saturated is measured: this is called the P_{50} and is about 3.2 kPa for normal adult human arterial blood.

Displacement of the oxyhaemoglobin dissociation curve (Fig. 8.3)

We have seen (Fig. 8.2) that abnormal amounts of Hb in the blood will displace the O_2 content curve vertically (but will not affect the *saturation* curve). Various factors displace, or shift, the curve horizontally along the x-axis, making Hb an even more efficient oxygen carrier. Each circuit of the blood between the lungs and the tissue and between the tissue and the lungs results in cyclical changes in the properties of Hb, which favour oxygen unloading at the tissues. We will now look at factors that displace the curve horizontally and the way in which this improves the supply of O_2 to the tissues, specifically the effects of hydrogen ions, CO_2, temperature, and 2,3-diphosphoglycerate (DPG).

1. *Hydrogen ion concentration ([H+]).* In metabolising tissues, the release of acids or CO_2 (which increases $[H^+]$) shifts the HbO_2 dissociation curve to the *right* (Fig. 8.3). This **Bohr shift** is due to H^+ acting on the Hb molecule to decrease its affinity for O_2. This does not affect the loading region of the curve because it is horizontal, and so movement to left or right does not produce a change in saturation. The steep unloading region of the curve is a different matter. The rightward shift has two major consequences:
   - Take a vertical line at some PO_2 on the steep part of the curve, say 4 kPa in Figure 8.3. If the curve moves to the right, the saturation corresponding to that PO_2 will fall. The Hb has less 'appetite' for O_2 and it releases the excess. This is clearly an advantage, liberating O_2 to diffuse down the concentration gradient to the actively metabolising tissues.
   - What is not so immediately obvious, but equally important, is revealed if you take a *horizontal* line at, say, 50% saturation. When the curve moves to the right, the PO_2 corresponding to that saturation *increases.* This increases the partial pressure gradient driving O_2 into the tissues.

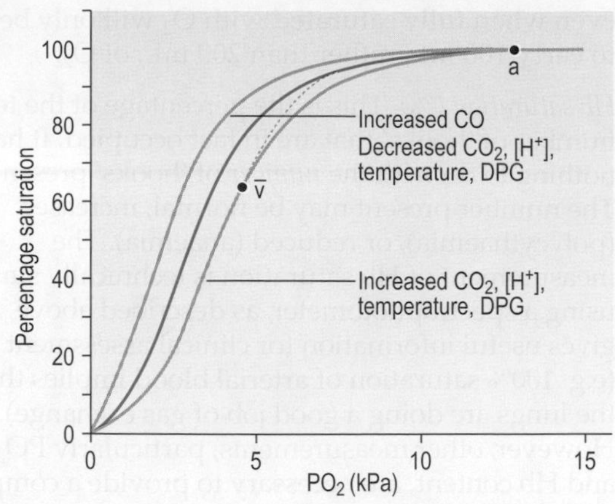

Fig. 8.3 Shifts of the dissociation curve. Conditions in terms of $[H_+]$, CO_2, temperature, and 2,3-diphosphoglycerate are very different at the sites of loading (the lungs) and unloading (the tissues) of haemoglobin with O_2. These differences shift the dissociation curve and improve its carrying properties. For example, the effect of increased $[H_+]$ and CO_2 in the tissues is to shift the curve to the right (this is called the Bohr shift), and this steepens the functional dissociation curve to that shown as a dotted line.

These effects of acidity are so powerful that a decrease of 0.2 pH units can increase the O_2 release by 25%, at low PO_2.

2. *CO_2.* In addition to its acid properties, which are dealt with above, CO_2 reacts with Hb to form **carbamino Hb.** This also moves the curve to the right. If hypercapnia (increased PCO_2) persists for several hours, with chronic acidosis, the levels of an RBC metabolite, ***2,3-diphosphoglycerate*** (DPG, see below), is decreased, shifting the curve back to the left.
3. *Temperature.* A decrease in temperature shifts the curve to the left. Blood therefore gives up its O_2 less readily in cold tissues, and blood leaving them may still be well oxygenated because of this effect. Also, cold will reduce the metabolic demand for O_2. For this reason, children playing in the snow have pink ears and noses when their vasoconstricted skin might have been expected to turn blue. This effect is not very important in the lungs because the air in them is so well warmed. It is important, however, in patients made hypothermic during open heart surgery. In these patients, even if arterial PO_2 is low, the Hb is relatively well saturated, and the patient does not look hypoxic.
4. *(DPG).* In most cells, under anaerobic conditions, 1,3-diphosphoglycerate (1,3-DPG) is converted to 3-phosphoglycerate, with the release of energy which is stored in the form of ATP. In red cells, however, 1,3-DPG is converted to 2,3-DPG, without the release of energy (Fig. 8.4). This 2,3-DPG reacts with HbO_2, causing a release of O_2 by shifting the dissociation curve to the right, suggesting that DPG is relevant:
   - in chronic hypoxia, caused by disease or residence at high altitude, when DPG levels are increased, O_2 is released into the hypoxic tissues

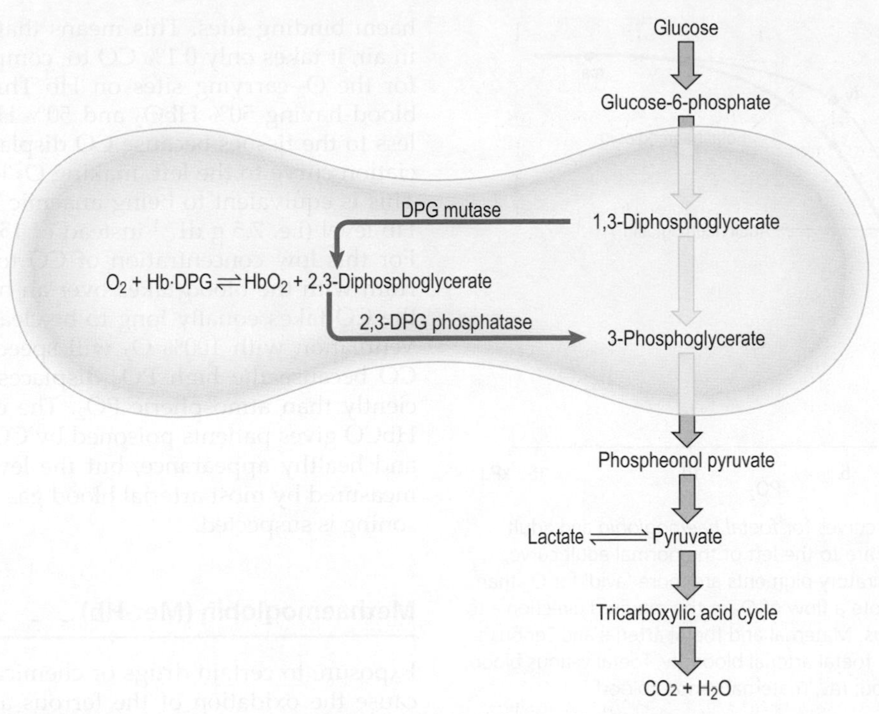

Fig. 8.4 The 2,3-diphosphoglycerate (2,3-DPG) shunt. The glycolytic pathway of red corpuscles has an extra 'shunt' which produces 2,3-DPG. This substance shifts the oxyhaemoglobin curve to the right, but this effect is of little functional importance.

- during prolonged exercise, the DPG concentration increases
- when blood is stored, as in blood banks, the DPG level decreases. This blood will not give up its oxygen so easily, a disadvantage for patients receiving transfusions
- in red cells containing abnormal Hbs, as in sickle cell anaemia or patients with enzyme abnormalities, abnormal levels of DPG may exist.

Why is haemoglobin kept in red cells?

Having Hb isolated from the plasma and packaged into red cells has a number of advantages:

- If the 15 g dL^{-1} Hb were free in the plasma, it would raise the viscosity to dangerous levels, especially in capillaries which would be at risk of being blocked, and colloid oncotic pressure would also increase considerably.
- Hb molecules are just small enough to be filtered out of the blood at the renal glomeruli and would therefore be lost in the urine if not contained within erythrocytes.
- Crucial enzyme systems are restricted to within RBCs (e.g. *carbonic anhydrase* which has a crucial role in CO_2 transport, and *methaemoglobin reductase* (met-Hb) which converts met-Hb back into Hb (see 'Haemoglobin variants' next)).
- The presence of 2,3-DPG in RBCs displaces the HbO_2 dissociation curve to the right and aids the unloading of O_2 at the tissues.

Haemoglobin variants

There are a number of normal and abnormal Hb variants, some of which reduce the O_2- carrying capacity of the blood.

Myoglobin

Myoglobin is a molecule normally found in muscle and, in part, gives muscle its red colour. Unlike Hb, with its four chains carrying oxygen, myoglobin consists of only one molecule of haem and one polypeptide chain. Its dissociation curve is to the left of that of Hb (Fig. 8.5), so it readily takes up O_2 from Hb in capillary blood. Myoglobin may act as a small store of O_2 that is available during anaerobic conditions. This is useful during muscle, particularly heart muscle, contraction because contraction cuts off blood flow. This effect is very limited in the case of sustained contractions of skeletal muscle because the O_2 stored in myoglobin is depleted within a few seconds.

Foetal haemoglobin (HbF)

HbF is a normal variant. It has a higher affinity for O_2 than adult Hb (Fig. 8.5) and this facilitates transfer from mother

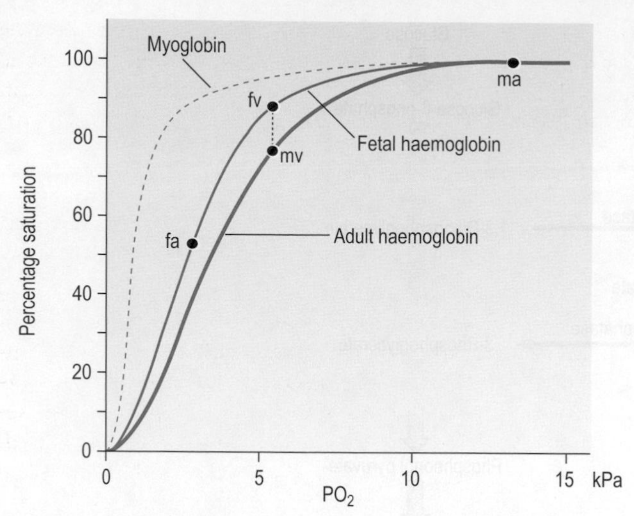

Fig. 8.5 The dissociation curves for *foetal haemoglobin* and adult *myoglobin*. These curves are to the left of the normal adult curve, indicating that these respiratory pigments are more 'avid' for O_2 than the adult form and promote a flow of O_2 in the required direction—to the muscles or to the fetus. Maternal and foetal arterial and venous saturations are shown fa, foetal arterial blood; fv, foetal venous blood; ma, maternal arterial blood; mv, maternal venous blood.

to foetus. HbF has two γ-polypeptide chains in place of the β chains of adult Hb. Foetal blood in the placental circulation takes up O_2 mainly because its PO_2 is lower than that of the maternal uterine arterial blood. In addition, inspection of Figure 8.5 will show that, because its dissociation curve is to the left of the maternal one, at most PO_2 levels foetal blood is more saturated and therefore 'hungry' for O_2. The transfer of O_2 from mother to foetus is aided by another mechanism produced by the unloading of CO_2 in the other direction, from foetus to mother. We have seen, above ('Displacement of the oxyhaemoglobin curve'), that the acidic effects of CO_2 cause the release of O_2 from HbO_2. The effect of the transfer of CO_2 from foetus to mother first moves the foetal dissociation curve to the left (CO_2 is leaving this blood), and then the same CO_2 moves the mother's dissociation curve to the right (CO_2 is being added to this blood). The overall effect of this **double Bohr shift** is to widen the gap between the two dissociation curves, enhancing the transfer of O_2 to the foetus. The mechanisms that make HbF so efficient at obtaining O_2 from the mother also make it less efficient at releasing it to the foetal tissues. This results in a degree of hypoxia, which the foetal tissues are better able to withstand than those of the adult. Furthermore, because HbF is more acidic than adult Hb, it is less able to carry CO_2, and so the foetus tends towards acidosis. The level of HbF gradually decreases and reaches adult levels (less than 1% of total Hb) within the first year of life, as adult Hb is produced.

Carboxyhaemoglobin (HbCO)

Carbon monoxide (CO) binds to Hb 250 times more strongly than does O_2 and competes with it for the haem binding sites. This means that as there is 21% O_2 in air, it takes only 0.1% CO to 'compete' on equal terms for the O_2-carrying sites on Hb This results in arterial blood having 50% HbO_2 and 50% HbCO, which is useless to the tissues because CO displaces the HbO_2 dissociation curve to the left, making O_2 less readily released. This is equivalent to being anaemic to half your normal Hb level (i.e. 7.5 g dL^{-1} instead of 15 g dL^{-1}, for a male). For this low concentration of CO to come into equilibrium with the blood takes over an hour, but once there, the CO takes equally long to be cleared from the blood. Ventilation with 100% O_2 will speed the elimination of CO because the high PO_2 displaces the CO more efficiently than atmospheric PO_2. The cherry-red colour of HbCO gives patients poisoned by CO a deceptively pink and healthy appearance, but the level of HbCO can be measured by most arterial blood gas analysers if CO poisoning is suspected.

Methaemoglobin (Met-Hb)

Exposure to certain drugs or chemicals (e.g. nitrites) can cause the oxidation of the ferrous atom of Hb into the ferric form. The resulting 'Met-Hb' cannot combine with O_2. Therefore, like carboxyhaemoglobinaemia, this can cause life-threatening tissue hypoxia. Met-Hb can also be formed because of a congenital defect. The *methaemoglobin reductase* enzyme found in RBCs slowly converts Met-Hb back into Hb.

Sickle cell disease (HbS)

More than 100 different types of human Hb have been discovered. Most variations consist of the substitution of a single amino acid in the globin chain, with the haem group being normal. These differences are usually identified by electrophoresis and only a few result in clinical manifestations. Some of these Hbs have abnormal dissociation curves because the Hb itself is changed, or because the changes lead to alterations of the RBC, such as abnormal DPG content. Hb abnormalities may also change the shape of the RBC and make it more fragile, as in sickle cell disease.

In the genetically determined sickle cell disease, deoxygenation of the abnormal Hb (HbS) causes it to polymerise and distort the RBC into the shape of a sickle. Heterozygotes for this disease are said to carry the trait for sickle cell disease; about 40%–50% of their total Hb is HbS and they are asymptomatic, except under hypoxic conditions. Homozygotes always manifest the disease, which may be fatal during childhood. The disease is found in regions where falciparum malaria is endemic, and people who carry the sickle cell gene are protected against malaria.

Clinical symptoms develop at about 6 months of age. They include bone pain and painful vaso-occlusive crises caused by sickled erythrocytes blocking small blood vessels. Leg ulceration is common, and splenic infarction results in splenic atrophy. HbF reduces the risk of sickling, which explains why symptoms do not develop before the age of 6 months, by which time HbF has been almost completely replaced by adult Hb.

No specific therapy has been found to prevent sickling. The steady state of anaemia in this condition frequently requires no treatment. Acute attacks require intravenous fluids, O_2, and antibiotics, if necessary. Transfusions are only given if there is severe anaemia. Genetic counselling should be given to prospective parents who carry the trait.

Thalassaemia

Thalassaemias are a group of inherited disorders resulting in reduced production of the α (causing α-thalassaemia) or β (causing β-thalassaemia) polypeptide chains of Hb. It is more common in Mediterranean, African, and Asian populations. The severity of the anaemia varies depending on the pattern of inheritance; management includes repeated blood transfusions and genetic counselling.

Summary 1

- O_2 is carried in the blood, mostly bound to Hb, with a small amount dissolved in the plasma.
- Blood O_2 content refers to the amount of O_2 being carried by a litre of blood. It depends on the Hb concentration and PO_2.
- Saturation refers to the percentage of sites on the Hb which are occupied by O_2. It is independent of Hb concentration.
- Each molecule of Hb has four binding sites for O_2.
- Allosteric binding of O_2 produces the sigmoid shape of the O_2 dissociation curve.
- The shape of the curve facilitates O_2 loading in the lungs and unloading at the tissues.
- $[H^+]$, PCO_2, temperature, and 2,3-DPG all shift the O_2 dissociation curve.
- There are a number of normal and abnormal Hb variants.
- HbF has a greater affinity for O_2 than adult Hb.

Carbon dioxide transport

Almost all the CO_2 in the blood comes from tissue metabolism. The amount produced depends on the rate of metabolism and the food source metabolised. Approximately 200 mL min^{-1} is produced at rest when eating a mixed diet. Just like O_2 moving in the opposite direction, CO_2 diffuses down its concentration gradient in the tissues, from the cell interior to the extracellular fluid, to plasma, and into the RBC. CO_2 in the blood is found both in the RBCs and in the plasma. It is transported in three main forms: dissolved in plasma (approximately 5%), in the form of HCO_3^- (85%), or combined with the amino groups of proteins like Hb (10%). Very small amounts of carbonic acid (H_2CO_3) and carbonate ion (CO_3^{2-}) are also present. In the lungs, the whole process is reversed, releasing CO_2 into the alveolar air.

Dissolved carbon dioxide

CO_2 is 20 times more soluble in blood than O_2 is. The amount dissolved is proportional to the partial pressure of CO_2 (PCO_2) (Henry's law), and solubility increases as temperature falls. At 37ºC, approximately 0.5 mL kPa^{-1} CO_2 is dissolved in every 100 mL of blood. So, in 100 mL of arterial blood with a PCO_2 of 5.3 kPa, there is about 2.6 mL of dissolved CO_2, and in 100 mL of venous blood with a PCO_2 of 6.1 kPa, there is about 3 mL of dissolved CO_2.

Carbon dioxide in the form of bicarbonate

Plasma water reacts with CO_2 to form carbonic acid, which dissociates into HCO_3^- and H^+.

$$CO_2 + H_2O \leftrightarrow H_2CO_3 \leftrightarrow HCO_3^- + H^+ \quad \text{Equation (i)}$$

Like any chain reaction, the overall speed of this reaction is determined by its slowest step. In plasma, the first stage of this reaction ($CO_2 + H_2O \leftrightarrow H_2CO_3$) is slow, taking 100 seconds to reach 90% equilibrium, at body temperature. Adding even small quantities of CO_2 to whole blood will therefore increase the plasma PCO_2 appreciably, and as this occurs in the tissues, a gradient for CO_2 forms to allow diffusion into the RBCs (Fig. 8.6). Unlike the plasma, RBCs contain an enzyme called **carbonic anhydrase**, which accelerates the normally slow formation of H_2CO_3 from CO_2 and H_2O. Thus, in the RBC, the reaction (Equation i) proceeds quickly to the right, increasing the concentrations of H^+ and HCO_3^-. These ions are rapidly removed, allowing the reaction to continue moving to the right. H^+ is mopped up by Hb and HCO_3^- diffuses out of the cell into the plasma, down its concentration gradient. The HCO_3^- ions carry a negative charge out of the cell and, to maintain electrical neutrality in the cell, chloride ions (Cl^-) move in. This exchange of ions is called the **chloride shift**. If this did not occur, HCO_3^- would be held in the RBC by its negative charge, Equation (i) would be blocked by the build-up of HCO_3^-, and less CO_2 could be converted to HCO_3^-.

Carbon dioxide combined with proteins

The amino groups of plasma proteins (albumin, globulins, and fibrinogen) carry CO_2 in the form of carbamino compounds:

$$\text{Protein-}NH_2 + CO_2 \leftrightarrow \text{Protein-}NHCOO^- + H^+ \quad \text{Equation (ii)}$$

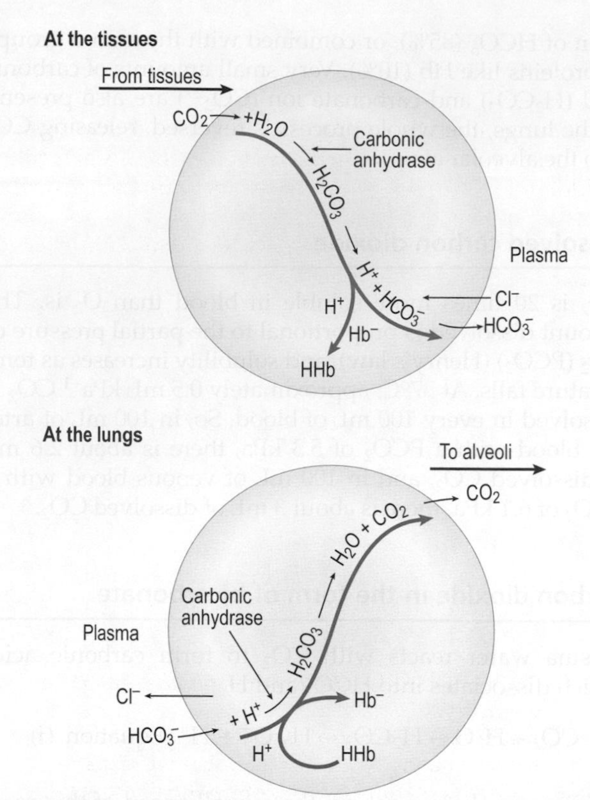

Fig. 8.6 Bicarbonate formation. The erythrocytes, because of the haemoglobin (Hb) and *carbonic anhydrase* they contain, are essential for the rapid loading and unloading of the plasma with CO_2 in the form of HCO_3^-.

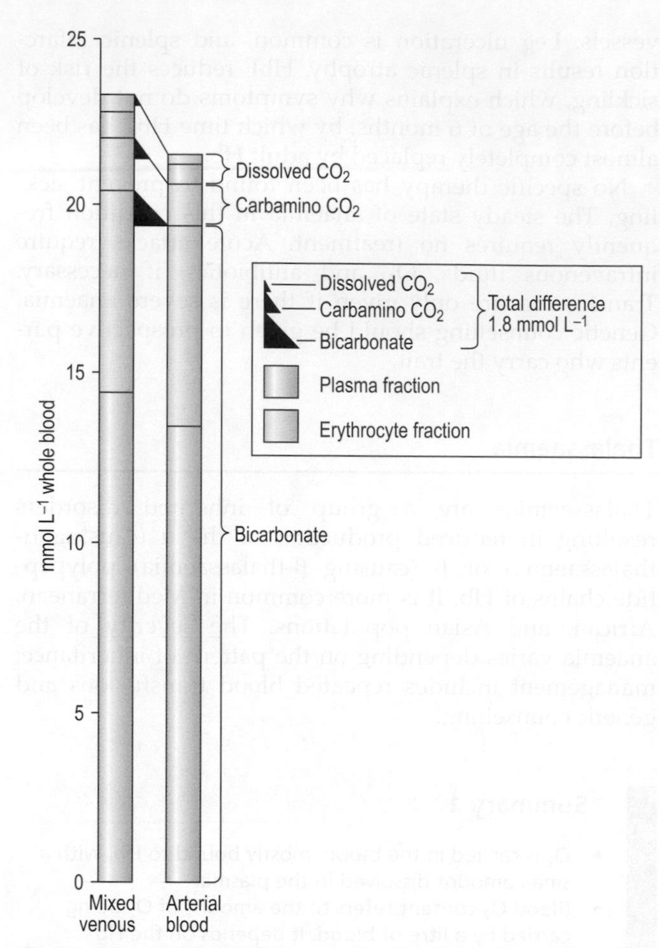

Fig. 8.7 The quantities of CO_2 carried in the blood. The amounts lost in the lungs are shown; note that different proportions are lost from different sources.

Compared to the plasma proteins, Hb in the RBCs has a threefold greater affinity for CO_2 and is present at four times the concentration. Therefore Hb is the most important carrier molecule for CO_2 in the blood. CO_2 combines with Hb to form **carbaminohaemoglobin**. This is a special case of the reaction represented by Equation (ii):

$$Hb\text{-}NH_2 + CO_2 \leftrightarrow Hb\text{-}NHCOO^- + H^+ \quad \text{Equation (iii)}$$

It releases CO_2 very readily in the lungs, and the first 30% of the total CO_2 released in the lungs is from this source (Fig. 8.7).

The H^+ produced in Equations (i), (ii), and (iii) has to be **buffered** to prevent unacceptable increases in acidity. A chemical buffer is a substance that accepts or releases protons (H^+) and so minimises changes in pH. The H^+ formed in the RBCs is buffered by Hb. Deoxygenated Hb is a weaker acid than HbO_2, so it has more sites available to accept protons. It, therefore, absorbs more H^+ and Equation (iii) shifts to the right. In other words, the release of O_2 from HbO_2 into metabolically active tissues allows the Hb to take up and carry more CO_2 at the same PCO_2. This effect of deoxygenation increasing the ability of blood to carry CO_2 is called the **Haldane effect** and, like the Bohr effect, it demonstrates the interaction between O_2 and CO_2 carriage in creating an efficient system of gas transport.

Gas exchange in the lungs

In the lungs, the processes taking place at the tissues are reversed (Fig. 8.6). As CO_2 is blown off, Equations (i), (ii), and (ii) move to the left and the chloride shift is reversed. The oxygenation of Hb in the lungs aids the release of CO_2 from the RBCs into the plasma and alveoli. It should be remembered that before CO_2 can move from the RBC to the air, it must enter into solution in the plasma (as with O_2 moving from the air to the RBC).

The quantities of transported carbon dioxide

The quantities of the forms of CO_2 carried in venous blood are shown in Figure 8.7 and Table 8.1. Although the total *amount* of CO_2 carried in the RBCs is much less than that carried in the plasma, the chemical reactions of CO_2 in the RBCs and the buffering of the H^+ produced are much greater than in the plasma. The RBCs act like factories, processing CO_2 and producing HCO_3^- to be stored in the plasma. Thus the *exchange* of CO_2 in lungs and tissues depends more on the processing power of the RBCs than on

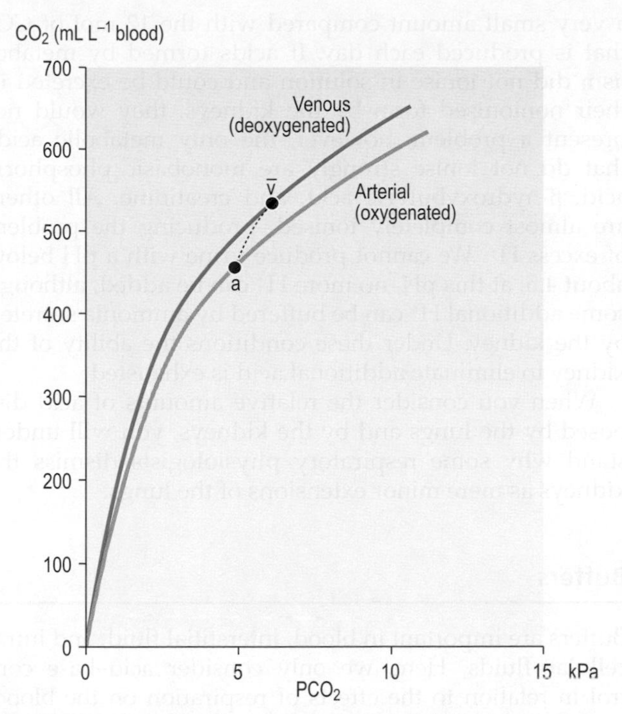

Fig. 8.8 The CO_2 dissociation curve. Oxygenated blood carries less CO_2 at the same PCO_2 than does deoxygenated blood. This means that the 'true' dissociation curve, as occurs in the body, is steeper than might be expected (the broken line) because this Haldane effect results in PCO_2 being about 0.5 kPa lower than if the blood were oxygenated, which helps the unloading of CO_2 from the tissues.

the plasma content. This is clearly demonstrated by inhibiting carbonic anhydrase in the RBCs using a suitable drug. CO_2 entering the blood is then only slowly converted to HCO_3^-, and the amounts of CO_2 in solution and as plasma carbamino compounds build up, causing acidosis.

Carbonic anhydrase does not exist solely in the RBCs. It is also found in other tissues, including the gastric mucosa, renal tubules, eyes, and pancreatic cells. Some carbonic anhydrase inhibitor drugs are used clinically; for example, acetazolamide is a mild diuretic used in the prevention/treatment of altitude sickness, and brinzolamide is used in the treatment of glaucoma.

The dissociation curve for carbon dioxide

The relationship between PCO_2 and the concentration of CO_2 in whole blood is shown in Figure 8.8. This plot is similar to that for O_2 (Fig. 8.2), except that for CO_2 we cannot plot *saturation* against *partial pressure* because, in the case of CO_2, there is no carrier molecule (Hb in the case of O_2) to be saturated.

The relationship between PCO_2 and total CO_2 in the blood is approximately linear over the physiological range of CO_2 partial pressures, from mixed venous (6.1 kPa) to arterial (5.3 kPa) blood. We have already seen that HbO_2 has a weaker affinity for CO_2 than deoxygenated Hb. This means that oxygenation of blood causes the curve to be displaced to the right (the Haldane shift). Also, HbO_2 is a stronger acid than deoxygenated Hb and releases H^+, which drives Equations (i), (ii), and (iii) to the left with the formation of free CO_2. The Haldane shift results in the 'functional' CO_2 dissociation curve (the normal range of blood PCO_2 over which we function) being steeper than would be expected because it joins points a and $\bar{v}$ on Figure 8.8. We have seen, for O_2, that a steep curve improves unloading and, as a result of the Haldane shift, at any PCO_2 blood loads and unloads extra CO_2 when it is unloading or loading O_2. Because the quantity of Hb in a sample of blood is fixed, the O_2 capacity of that blood is also fixed. Because the CO_2 dissociation curve cannot be saturated, the CO_2 content of our blood is much more variable, even in health, than its O_2 content.

Summary 3

- CO_2 is an acid product of metabolism which must be removed; it is a major determinant of blood pH.
- In solution, CO_2 forms H_2CO_3 which dissociates into H^+ and HCO_3^-.
- CO_2 is mainly transported in the plasma as HCO_3^-, which is first formed in the RBCs.
- Just as the change in levels of CO_2 in the blood between lungs and tissues improves the carriage of O_2, the changes in levels of O_2 also improve the carriage of CO_2.
- The dissociation curve for CO_2 from the blood is almost a straight line, quite different from the S-shape for O_2.

Acid–base balance

A little chemistry

Our metabolism is largely aerobic (i.e. it uses O_2). The word O_2 means 'acid producer', in Greek, and acids are continually being produced in our bodies. Oxidation of proteins and nucleic acids produces sulphuric and phosphoric acids, CO_2 is hydrated to carbonic acid, and, in the absence of O_2, lactic and other acids are released during the anaerobic metabolism of fats and carbohydrates (e.g. during heavy exercise). These acids dissociate (ionise) to increase the $[H^+]$ (proton concentration) of the blood. H^+ is a proton, and acids, by definition, are proton *donors*. When an acid releases a proton, it forms a **base** which, as an anion, is a proton *acceptor*.

$$HB \leftrightarrow H^+ + B^-$$

In aqueous solution, acids increase $[H^+]$ and the H^+ combines with H_2O to form H_3O^-, but it is conventional, and more convenient, to speak of hydrogen ions, H^+.

Because the $[H^+]$ in a solution involves very small numbers, chemists sometimes express it in terms of pH, which makes the numbers manageable and understandable:

$$pH = -\log[H^+]$$

Logs are used to compress the scale, thus log(10) = 1, log(1,000,000) = 6, etc., and negative log numbers are used when the raw numbers are less than 1, which is awkward, so we use the mathematical trick of:

$$-\times- = +$$

In this system, pH 7.0 represents neutrality, higher pHs represent alkalinity and lower pHs represent acidity. Thus, when $[H^+]$ rises (i.e. the solution gets more acidic) the pH reduces. This does not lead to an intuitive grasp of what is happening when changes take place.

Also, because there is not a linear relationship between pH and $[H^+]$, increases or decreases of equal amounts of pH are brought about by different changes in $[H^+]$. A solution containing 40 nmol L^{-1} $[H^+]$ has a pH of 7.4. To raise the pH 4 points (to 7.8), we must remove 24 nmol L^{-1} of H^+; to lower the pH 4 points (to 7.0), we need to add 60 nmol L^{-1} of H^+.

Life is only possible within a blood pH range of 7.0 to 7.8, which represents only a sixfold range in $[H^+]$, from 10.0×10^{-8} to 1.6×10^{-8}.

The most immediate and serious effect of a build-up of $[H^+]$ in the body is interference with enzyme activity. This has far-reaching implications, given the many essential roles of enzymes across body systems. Changes in $[H^+]$ in the body are resisted by chemicals known as **buffers**. Buffers are chemicals, or combinations of chemicals, which 'mop up' or release H^+ when acids or bases are added to them, thereby resisting changes in $[H^+]$. Buffers within the cells and buffers in the blood neutralise H^+, but their ability is limited and only give respite against the constant stream of acid produced by metabolism. Over the long term, the body must get rid of as much acid as it produces. Buffers are a kind of 'overdraft' that enables the body to keep going, but eventually the acid 'debt' has to be removed.

Metabolic acids can be categorised as **volatile acids** (removed in gaseous form; the only one of interest to us is carbonic acid, which is removed as CO_2 by the lungs) and ***fixed*** or ***nonvolatile acids*** (removed by the kidneys, in particular, as sulphate and phosphoric acid). As the normal pH of urine is about 6.0 (acidic), the body is producing an excess of acid beyond that removed by respiration, despite the acid load being removed by the lungs being about fourold greater than that removed by the kidneys. The lungs do not, of course, 'excrete' acid: they excrete CO_2, which as you can see from Equation (i) is in equilibrium with H^+ in the plasma. The $[H^+]$ determines pH, and it does not matter where the H^+ comes from or in what form it is removed. When acids, such as lactic acid, are added to the blood they add H^+, which displaces Equation (i) to the left, forming CO_2 and water. Water is harmless and diffuses away; the removal of CO_2 by the lungs allows Equation (i) to continue moving to the left, removing H^+ and limiting acidosis.

More than 50 mmol of nonvolatile acids are produced, each day, by a normal healthy man. It is essential that these acids be disposed of; in quantitative terms, this is a very small amount compared with the 12 mol of CO_2 that is produced each day. If acids formed by metabolism did not ionise in solution and could be excreted in their nonionised form by the kidneys, they would not present a problem; however, the only metabolic acids that do not ionise strongly are monobasic phosphoric acid, β-hydroxybutyric acid, and creatinine. All others are almost completely ionised, producing the problem of excess H^+. We cannot produce urine with a pH below about 4.5; at this pH, no more H^+ can be added, although some additional H^+ can be buffered by ammonia secreted by the kidney. Under these conditions the ability of the kidney to eliminate additional acid is exhausted.

When you consider the relative amounts of acid disposed by the lungs and by the kidneys, you will understand why some respiratory physiologists dismiss the kidneys as mere minor extensions of the lungs.

Buffers

Buffers are important in blood, interstitial fluid, and intracellular fluids. Here, we only consider acid–base control in relation to the effects of respiration on the blood. In terms of *total* CO_2, H^+, and HCO_3^-, blood is the least important buffered compartment. In terms of purely chemical buffering, the cells of our bodies, with their high protein content, are by far the most important chemical buffer. However, as we will see shortly, this system is finite, whereas the mechanisms that have evolved for the respiratory system have an almost infinite capacity. We will see that the cell system is like a nonrechargeable battery: once used, it is finished. However, the system involving respiration is rechargeable and is used over and over again. To explain how this system works we can consider it in isolation, but in clinical situations the interactions between the three buffer compartments (blood, interstitial fluid, intracellular fluid) are of great importance.

Normal plasma hydrogen ion concentration

Normal plasma $[H^+]$ = 40 nmol (pH 7.40). Increases in $[H^+]$ cause **acidaemia** while decreases cause **alkalaemia**. Because the pH scale is logarithmic, a shift of one pH unit represents a 10-fold change in $[H^+]$. The addition to or removal from the blood of H^+ activates compensatory changes in respiratory excretion of CO_2 and in the excretion of H^+ and HCO_3^- by the kidneys.

Blood buffering

A **strong acid** is one that dissociates vigorously and almost completely in solution. Strong in this chemical sense should not be confused with concentrated. Hydrochloric acid, for example, is a strong acid and dissociates vigorously into H^+ and Cl^-, whether it is in a concentrated or dilute solution.

On the other hand, a **weak acid** (such as acetic acid) does not dissociate strongly into ions (N.B., an undissociated molecule of acid does not have acidic properties, it is the H^+ that is acidic.)

We have already noted that buffers are solutions that resist changes in $[H^+]$ when acids or bases are added to them. Buffers consist of a weak acid (H^+B^-) which only weakly dissociates into H^+, anion B^-, and its salt (in this case, a sodium salt NaB, which dissociates more strongly into its ions Na^+ and B^-). In an aqueous solution of the two, the following reaction takes place with the equilibrium well to the left:

$$HB + B^- + Na^+ \leftrightarrow B^- + H^+ + NaB \qquad \text{Equation (iv)}$$

(weak acid) (ions of salt) (ions of acid) (salt)

The addition of a strong acid, such as HCl, will shift the equilibrium further to the left because of the strong affinity of Cl^- for the added H^+. Thus, the potential increase in H^+ is minimised. The added Cl^- associates with Na^+ to form neutral NaCl.

pK of a buffer

The pK of a buffer system is the pH at which the buffer works best to resist changes in *either* direction.

From Equation (iv), you can see that the source of the ions on the left side of the equation is the salt, and on the right side, the acid. For this buffer to work most efficiently at reducing changes of pH in *either* direction, there should be equal amounts of acid or salt. If there is already a lot of acid in the buffer system, it can resist the effects of added base very well but cannot deal with the addition of more acid. If there is a lot of salt, the buffer system can deal with additional acid but not base. So, in the ideal state for resisting changes of pH in either direction, the system should be 'in the middle', with the buffer salt and the acid both half-dissociated; the pH at which a buffer system is in this ideal state is called its **pK**. Normal plasma has a pH of 7.40, and a buffer system with a pK of this value will be at its most powerful in the blood. Figure 8.9 illustrates the performance of the buffer systems for phosphate and bicarbonate. It would seem that the HCO_3^- system, with its pK far from the plasma pH, would be a poor buffer in the body, but it has other attributes that make it perhaps the most important buffer we have; we will consider these a little later. The main buffers in the blood are bicarbonate, proteins (in particular, Hb), and phosphate.

Proteins as buffers

Plasma proteins and Hb constitute the major *chemical* blood buffers for limiting the effects of added acid (we will see shortly that another system which does not rely solely on chemical means is at least as important). Hb is more important than plasma protein because molecule for molecule, it is a more efficient buffer and also because there is more of it (150 g L^{-1} for Hb compared with 40 g L^{-1} for plasma protein). Buffering actions are based on Equation (ii), where the protein can be Hb or another plasma protein.

Phosphates as buffers

The phosphate buffer system, illustrated in Figure 8.9, is made up of the acidic (H_2PO_4) and basic ($NaHPO_4$) forms of ***phosphoric acid*** and its salts. In plasma, phosphate buffers are not very important because the concentrations of the radicals involved are small. In the kidney, however, the system is particularly important in regulating the excretion of H^+. At pH 7.4, urine contains four parts of basic phosphate to one part of acidic phosphate. If more acid is excreted and the pH of the urine is reduced to 5.8, say, the ratio of acidic to basic phosphate becomes 10:1. Phosphates may form a more important buffer system inside cells than in the plasma or interstitial fluid.

Bicarbonate as a buffer

At the beginning of this section on CO_2 transport, we saw that carbonic acid is formed when CO_2 dissolves in water:

$$CO_2 + H_2O \leftrightarrow H_2CO_3$$

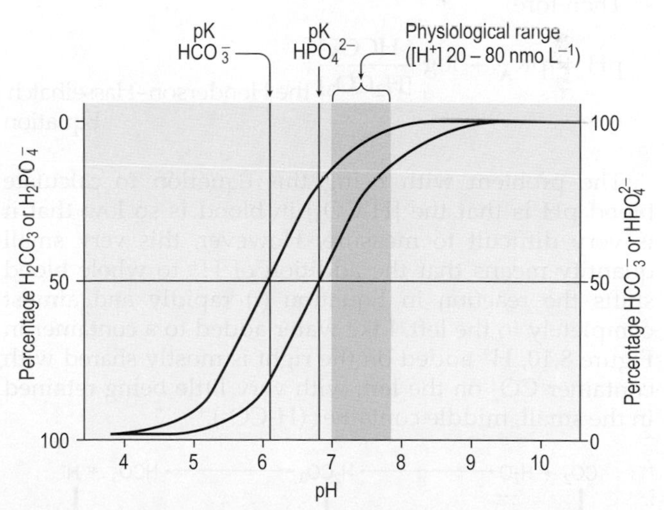

Fig. 8.9 pK. The pK of a buffer is where there are equal amounts of its two components. At this point the curve is at its steepest, so changes in the proportions of the components produce the minimum effect on pH, i.e., the buffer is most efficient at stabilising pH. For reasons explained in this chapter, the bicarbonate buffer system is probably the most important in the blood, even though its pK is not the pH of plasma. The phosphate buffer system has a pK close to the intracellular pH.

Carbonic acid is a weak acid which dissociates:

$$H_2CO_3 \leftrightarrow H^+ + HCO_3^-$$

This is a buffer system: the addition of H^+ will shift the reaction to the left, and because of the formation of undissociated H_2CO_3, the H^+ will be taken up with little change in pH. Removal of H^+ will shift the reaction to the right, producing more H^+ and again minimising the change in pH.

The law of mass action describes the equilibrium of reversible reactions, such as the dissociation of carbonic acid, above, as follows:

$$\frac{[H^+][HCO_3^-]}{[H_2CO_3]} = K_A$$

where K_A is the dissociation constant for H_2CO_3. This equation can be converted to a special equation relating CO_2 and pH in the blood: **the Henderson–Hasselbalch Equation**, as follows:

pH is the negative logarithm of $[H^+]$ so, taking logs of both sides of the above equation and rearranging, we get:

$$\log \frac{[H^+][HCO_3^-]}{[H_2CO_3]} = \log K_A$$

$$\log [H^+] + \log \frac{[HCO_3^-]}{[H_2CO_3]} = \log K_A$$

$$\log [H^+] = \log K_A - \log \frac{[HCO_3^-]}{[H_2CO_3]}$$

pH and pK_A are the negative logarithms of $[H^+]$ and K_A, respectively.

Therefore,

$$pH = pK_A + \log \frac{[HCO_3^-]}{[H_2CO_3]}$$ the Henderson–Hasselbalch Equation

The problem with using this equation to calculate blood pH is that the $[H_2CO_3]$ in blood is so low that it is very difficult to measure. However, this very small quantity means that the addition of H^+ to whole blood shifts the reaction in Equation (i) rapidly and almost completely to the left. Like water added to a container in Figure 8.10, H^+ added on the right is mostly shared with container CO_2 on the left, with very little being retained in the small, middle container (H_2CO_3).

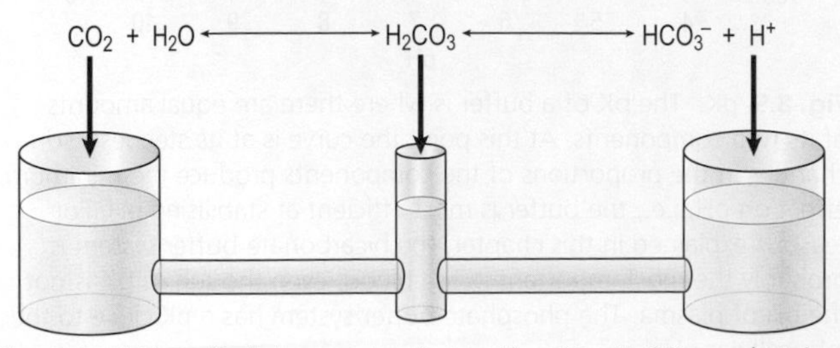

Fig. 8.10 'Water finds its own level', just like CO_2, H_2CO_3, and H^+ in this reaction.

At equilibrium, which is reached very rapidly because of the carbonic anhydrase in RBCs, $[CO_2] = 809[H_2CO_3]$. Thus, the Henderson-Hasselbalch equation can be written as:

$$pH = pK' + \log \frac{[HCO_3^-]}{[CO_2]}$$

Note pK_A has changed to pK' because we have changed from considering $[H_2CO_3]$ to considering $[CO_2]$.

The amount of CO_2 dissolved, the $[CO_2]$, is proportional to the PCO_2 (Henry's law), and the Henderson–Hasselbalch equation is usually written as:

$$pH = pK' + \log \frac{[HCO_3^-]}{[\alpha PCO_2]}$$

where α is the solubility of CO_2 in plasma per kPa PCO_2, at body temperature (0.23 mmol kPa^{-1} L^{-1}). Expressing the equation this way has the advantage that PCO_2 is easy to measure in blood using a *CO_2 electrode*.

Although this system buffers H^+ added to the blood by other acids, it is not a buffer system for CO_2. Remember the reaction:

$$CO_2 + H_2O \leftrightarrow H_2CO_3 \leftrightarrow HCO_3^- + H^+$$

The reaction reaches equilibrium to the right, the $[HCO_3^-]$ being 20-fold higher than the $[CO_2]$. You can see from the equation that every molecule of CO_2 involved forms not only a HCO_3^- but also an H^+, and so this is not buffering of CO_2.

It may seem illogical that CO_2 and therefore H_2CO_3 can cause acidosis because each H^+ (acid) produced is accompanied by the production of a HCO_3^- (base), but the effect of adding one H^+ to a concentration of 40 nmol L^{-1} H^+ is much greater than adding one HCO_3^- to 26 nmol L^{-1} bicarbonate ion.

The ability of the blood to *transport* CO_2 makes up for its weakness as a purely chemical buffer. By carrying CO_2 to the lungs for excretion, the blood achieves the same results as a good buffer: it minimises the acidaemia that results from the addition of CO_2 to the blood. By transporting CO_2 to the lungs, and HCO_3^- to the kidneys, the blood assists in controlling the levels of these substances and hence pH.

The lungs excrete or retain CO_2 and the kidneys eliminate or reabsorb HCO_3^-; together, they work to maintain the $HCO_3^-:CO_2$ ratio at 20:1. Although not a buffer system in the chemical sense of the word, the kidney/lung combination is a more powerful controller of blood pH than excellent chemical buffers, such as Hb. The ability of Hb to deal with excess acid or base is limited by the amount of Hb present. When that is 'used up', its buffering capacity ceases. The kidneys and lungs, on the other hand, can deal with an almost infinite excess of acid or base because they simply expel them from the body. This explains why renal or respiratory failure leads to loss of pH homeostasis, even if blood Hb levels are high: the Hb has a finite buffering capacity.

Calculation and illustration of acid–base status

The Henderson–Hasselbalch equation is important because if any two of the variables (pH, [HCO_3^-] or PCO_2) is known, the third can be calculated. Furthermore, theoretically, it allows the calculation of what would happen if one of the three variables were changed. For example, if CO_2 were added to the blood, pH and/or [HCO_3^-] must change in a clearly defined way. Knowing the values of the three variables, allows an accurate assessment of the acid–base status of the blood. For example, normal arterial blood has a pH of 7.40 and pK of 6.10, which allows the HCO_3^-:CO_2 ratio to be calculated:

$$pH = pK_A + \log \frac{[HCO_3^-]}{[H_2CO_3]}$$

$$7.4 - 6.1 = \log \frac{[HCO_3^-]}{[H_2CO_3]} = \log \frac{20}{1}$$

In patients with acid–base abnormalities, the Henderson–Hasselbalch equation can be applied to discover the source of the abnormality. Many automated systems for analysing arterial blood now carry out these calculations to provide this information. The figures provided by these systems are of little use if their relevance is not understood, and one of the most useful systems for displaying the relationship between pH, CO_2, and [HCO_3^-] is known as the ***Davenport diagram*** (Fig. 8.11). The problem with displaying the Henderson–Hasselbalch relationship graphically on a page is that you have to display three variables on a two-dimensional surface. The Davenport diagram gets round this by displaying PCO_2 as a series of ***isobars*** (lines consisting of points of equal partial pressure) plotted against plasma [HCO_3^-] and pH, laid out along axes as in a conventional graph.

Disturbances in the normal acid–base situation may be manifest as **acidosis** or **alkalosis** and result from:

- *Respiratory* malfunction, where ventilation is too great (respiratory alkalosis) or too little (respiratory acidosis).
- *Metabolic* malfunction, where excess acid is ingested or generated (metabolic acidosis) or acid is lost from the body e.g. by vomiting gastric contents (metabolic alkalosis). The acute changes (1) and the chronic compensatory changes (2) that take place primarily to restore pH to normal are shown in Figure 8.11.

Clinical measurements

In the clinical situation [H^+] and PCO_2 are measured in arterial blood samples in an instrument known as a blood gas analyser, which consists of a series of ion-sensitive electrodes. The blood samples are usually drawn from the radial artery into a syringe containing an anticoagulant (heparin). It is important to exclude air from the sample, as the partial pressures between blood and air will equilibrate. If the sample is to be kept for any length of time before analysis, it should be stored in ice to arrest the metabolism of the white cells.

Modern blood gas analysers measure [H^+] and PCO_2 directly and calculate a multitude of other values. These include:

- *Standard bicarbonate*, which is the [HCO_3^-] expected if the arterial blood sample were equilibrated to a normal PCO_2 of 5.3 kPa, and
- *Base excess*, which is the amount of acid (or base, in the case of a *base deficit*) which has to be added to

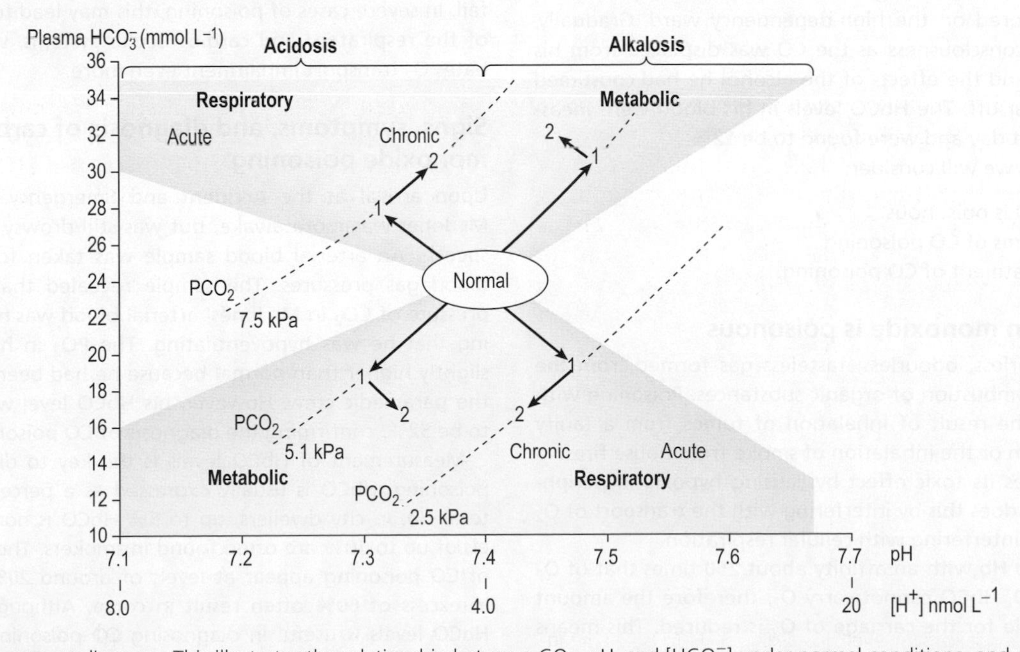

Fig. 8.11 The Davenport diagram. This illustrates the relationship between CO_2, pH, and [HCO_3^-] under normal conditions, and during *acidosis* and *alkalosis*.

the blood (which is first restored to a physiological PCO_2 to remove any respiratory component) to restore the pH to normal. Base excess is, therefore, zero in normal situations, and is represented in the pathological situation by the broken line in Figure 8.11.

When interpreting acid–base results, these biochemical measurements are only a means of quantifying the severity of the disorder. The patient's clinical history is the most important factor in deciding the nature of the disorder, or whether more than one disorder is present.

Summary 4

- O_2 means acid producer. Our oxidative metabolism produces acids.
- There are 'fixed acids' (excreted in solution by the kidneys) or 'volatile acid' (the only one of interest to us being carbonic acid, excreted by the lungs as CO_2).
- A buffer is a substance that resists changes in pH.
- The carbonic acid/bicarbonate system in the blood would not be a powerful buffer in a test-tube. But because it can enlist the aid of the lungs and kidneys, it is arguably the most powerful buffer in the body.
- Acid/base imbalance can result in acidosis or alkalosis.
- These imbalances can be metabolic due to excess acid production/ingestion/loss or respiratory where ventilation of the lungs is excessive/insufficient.

Case 8.1 Carriage of gases by the blood and acid/base balance: 1

Carbon monoxide poisoning – a failure of oxygen transport

Mr Jones is a pensioner who lives alone. One winter's evening, he turned on his gas fireplace and settled down to watch the television. The gas fireplace was very old and had never been serviced, as far as Mr Jones could remember. As the evening wore on, Mr Jones became increasingly drowsy. Eventually, he fell deeply asleep. Later that evening, Mr Jones' daughter called round to see him. She found her father unconscious on the sofa and called an ambulance. Upon his arrival at the Accident and Emergency Department, an arterial blood sample was taken from Mr Jones for analysis of blood gas tensions. The sample revealed that his arterial blood gases were close to normal. However, his HbCO level was measured at 52%, confirming the diagnosis of CO poisoning.

He was treated with high concentrations of O_2 and was closely monitored on the high-dependency ward. Gradually, he regained consciousness as the CO was displaced from his blood by O_2 and the effects of the alcohol he had consumed began to wear off. The HbCO levels in his blood were measured later that day and were found to be 12%.

In this case, we will consider:

1. Why CO is poisonous.
2. Symptoms of CO poisoning.
3. The treatment of CO poisoning.

Why carbon monoxide is poisonous

CO is a colourless, odourless, tasteless gas formed from the incomplete combustion of organic substances. Poisoning with CO may be the result of inhalation of fumes from a faulty heating system or the inhalation of smoke from house fires.

CO produces its toxic effect by causing hypoxia in peripheral tissues. It does this by interfering with the transport of O_2 by Hb and by interfering with cellular respiration.

CO binds to Hb with an affinity about 250 times that of O_2 to form HbCO. HbCO cannot carry O_2; therefore the amount of Hb available for the carriage of O_2 is reduced. This means that even if the PO_2 in arterial blood is normal and, therefore, the *O_2 saturation* of the available Hb is maintained, the *O_2 content* of the blood is reduced because the amount of Hb available to carry O_2 is reduced. Furthermore, in the presence of HbCO the O_2–Hb dissociation curve is distorted and shifted to the left. As a result of this, O_2 tends to remain bound to Hb in the peripheral circulation, rather than being released into the tissues. In other words, less O_2 is carried in the circulation, and of the O_2 that is carried, much remains bound to Hb and is not available for tissue respiration.

In addition to these effects on O_2 carriage by the blood, CO also interferes with electron transport in the mitochondria and with other cellular processes. Overall, then, its effect is to reduce O_2 delivery to peripheral tissues and to reduce the ability of these tissues to use what O_2 they obtain. As a result, cellular ATP levels fall, and vital cellular functions begin to fail. In severe cases of poisoning, this may lead to impairment of the respiratory and cardiovascular systems, which exacerbates O_2 transport impairment even more.

Signs, symptoms, and diagnosis of carbon monoxide poisoning

Upon arrival at the Accident and Emergency Department, Mr Jones was more awake, but was still drowsy, with slurred speech. An arterial blood sample was taken for analysis of blood gas pressures. The sample revealed that the partial pressure of CO_2 in Mr Jones' arterial blood was high, suggesting that he was hypoventilating. The PO_2 in his blood was slightly higher than normal because he had been given O_2 by the paramedic crew. However, his HbCO level was measured to be 52%, confirming the diagnosis of CO poisoning.

Measurement of HbCO levels is the key to diagnosing CO poisoning. HbCO is usually expressed as a percentage of the total Hb. In city dwellers, up to 5% HbCO is normal and levels of up to 10% are often found in smokers. The toxic effects of CO poisoning appear at levels of around 20%, and levels in excess of 60% often result in coma. Although measuring HbCO levels is useful in diagnosing CO poisoning, it is often

Case 8.1 Carriage of gases by the blood and acid/base balance: 1 – cont'd

difficult to relate these measurements to the patient's clinical condition. This is because once the patient is removed from the source of CO, blood levels fall very quickly, and the clinical picture is thought to be more closely related to peak HbCO levels.

The signs and symptoms of CO poisoning are related to the tissue hypoxia that it causes. Many organs, but particularly the brain, heart, and lungs, can be affected. In mild cases of CO poisoning, patients develop a frontal headache that may be associated with drowsiness or agitation and confusion, particularly in the elderly. Often these symptoms are associated with nausea or vomiting. In more severe cases of poisoning, patients may lose consciousness or start to fit. CO may also affect the heart, causing electrocardiogram abnormalities; CO is recognised as a cause of cardiac failure and myocardial infarction. Its effects on the lungs include hyperventilation and pulmonary oedema. It may affect the nervous system, producing hemiplegia or peripheral nerve damage, and recovery from poisoning may be complicated by long-term psychiatric problems, such as personality changes and memory loss, which are thought to be consequences of hypoxic brain damage.

Classically, patients with CO poisoning are said to have pink skin and 'cherry-red' mucosae owing to the presence of HbCO, which has a bright red colour. This is not a reliable sign, and in severe cases of CO poisoning associated with a failing circulation, it may not be apparent.

Treatment of carbon monoxide poisoning

After the diagnosis of CO poisoning had been made, Mr Jones was treated with high concentrations of O_2 (60% inspired oxygen) and was closely monitored on the high-dependency unit. Gradually, he regained consciousness as the CO was displaced from his blood by O_2 and the effects of the alcohol he had consumed began to wear off. The HbCO levels in his blood were measured later that day and were found to be 12%.

O_2 is the treatment for CO poisoning. By administering high concentrations of O_2, CO is dissociated from HbCO, producing Hb, which is then free to combine with O_2. In some centres, CO poisoning is treated with hyperbaric O_2, that is, the patient is placed in a pressurised chamber and breathes 100% O_2. Under these circumstances, the PO_2 is very high because the ambient pressure is high. The high PO_2 leads to an even more rapid removal of CO. It is also possible that an improvement in oxygenation occurs because the administration of a high PO_2 results in an increase in the amount of dissolved O_2 in the blood, possibly to a clinically significant level. The use of hyperbaric O_2 remains controversial, however, and it is only useful if it is quickly available, which is not the case in most centres.

Case 8.2 Interpretation of arterial blood gases

The analysis of blood gas tensions, usually in arterial blood, provides key information about a patient's respiratory system. Generally, a blood gas analyser measures the PO_2 and PCO_2 in the blood, as well as its pH. From these measurements, the machine calculates other values, such as the actual and standard bicarbonate concentrations and the base excess. An example of blood gas results from a patient without respiratory disease is given below, with normal ranges for the measured variables:

		Normal range
pH	7.4	(7.35–7.45)
$[H^+]$	40 nmol L^{-1}	(36–44)
PCO_2	5.3 kPa	(4.4–6.0)
PO_2	12.4 kPa	(12.0–14.0)
$HCO_{3\,act}$	24 mmol L^{-1}	
$HCO_{3\,std}$	24 mmol L^{-1}	(22–26 mmol L^{-1})
Base excess	0.1 mmol L^{-1}.	(-2 to +2)

In this example, pH has been given alongside $[H^+]$; pH is related to $[H^+]$ by the equation:

$$pH = -\log_{10} [H^+]$$

In other words, a change in pH of one unit is equivalent to a 10-fold change in $[H^+]$. For example, a $[H^+]$ of 10 nmol·L^{-1} is equivalent to a pH of 8.0 and a $[H^+]$ of 100 nmol·L^{-1} is equivalent to a pH of 7.0. This makes the pH scale very versatile in fields of chemistry where $[H^+]$ may vary widely. In medicine, blood $[H^+]$ varies comparatively little and, for this reason, a logarithmic scale is not necessary. However, pH is commonly used in medical practice.

Plasma bicarbonate is calculated from pH and PCO_2, using the Henderson–Hasselbalch equation. Two values of bicarbonate are often quoted: the actual bicarbonate ($HCO_{3\,act}$) and the standard bicarbonate ($HCO_{3\,std}$). The $HCO_{3\,act}$ is calculated at the PCO_2 measured in the blood sample and $HCO_{3\,std}$ is calculated using a 'normal' value for PCO_2 (often, 5.3 kPa). In other words, the $HCO_{3\,act}$ is an estimate of the bicarbonate concentration in the sample and the $HCO_{3\,std}$ is what the concentration of bicarbonate would be, *if the* PCO_2 *were normal*. The purpose of calculating these two values is to differentiate between respiratory and metabolic acidaemia and alkalaemia. If a patient has a purely respiratory acidosis, then his *actual* bicarbonate will be *abnormal*, but his $HCO_{3\,std}$ will be *normal* since all the abnormalities in the bicarbonate are due to the abnormal PCO_2. On the other

Continued

Case 8.2 **Interpretation of arterial blood gases – cont'd**

hand, a metabolic acidosis or alkalosis will tend to cause a change to the $HCO_{3\ std}$.

Another way to differentiate between respiratory and metabolic acidaemia and alkalaemia is to calculate the base excess. This is defined as the amount of H^+ that need to be added to a litre of blood to bring the pH back to normal, *at a normal* PCO_2. The key part of this definition is 'at a normal PCO_2', that is, the base excess is a measure only of metabolic abnormalities in acid–base status. If a patient has *acidosis*, then the base excess will be *negative*, since H^+ will have to be *removed* to return the pH to normal.

Armed with this information, you should be able to answer the following questions about a patient by studying their blood gases:

1. Is the patient's oxygenation adequate?
2. Does the patient have acidaemia or alkalaemia?
3. Does the patient have a respiratory acidosis or alkalosis?
4. Does the patient have a metabolic acidosis or alkalosis?

Is the patient's oxygenation adequate?

This question can be answered by knowing the patient's Po_2 and inspired oxygen concentration. Knowing the Po_2, alone, is not enough; a patient with a Po_2 of 11 kPa while breathing room air clearly has better gas exchange than a patient with a Po_2 of 12 kPa breathing 60% oxygen.

Does the patient's blood have a normal pH/[H+]?

If the answer to this question is 'yes', it does not mean that the patient's acid–base balance is normal. Remember, a patient may have respiratory acidosis that is partially compensated by a metabolic alkalosis, leading to a near normal pH. A high $[H^+]$ (or low pH) is acidaemia and a low $[H^+]$ (or a high pH) is alkalaemia.

Does the patient have a respiratory acidosis or alkalosis?

This question is answered by looking at the PCO_2. A raised PCO_2 results in respiratory acidosis, whereas a low PCO_2 results in respiratory alkalosis.

Does the patient have a metabolic acidosis or alkalosis?

This question is answered by looking at either the $HCO_{3\ std}$ level or the base excess. A low $HCO_{3\ std}$ indicates metabolic acidosis, whereas a raised $HCO_{3\ std}$ indicates metabolic alkalosis. Similarly, a large negative base excess indicates metabolic acidosis, and a large positive base excess indicates metabolic alkalosis.

The principles of blood gas interpretation are best illustrated by a few examples:

Arterial blood gas analysis example 1

		Normal range
pH	7.26	(7.35–7.45)
$[H^+]$	55.6 nmol L^{-1}	(36–44)
PCO_2	8.84 kPa	(4.4–6.0)
PO_2	7.66 kPa	(12.0–14.0)
$HCO_{3\ act}$	28.7 mmol L^{-1}	
$HCO_{3\ std}$	24.1 mmol L^{-1}	(22–-26 mmol L^{-1})
Base excess	-0.3 mmol L^{-1}.	(-2 to +2)

This patient suffered from severe chronic obstructive pulmonary disease. She had sustained a fractured leg and had been given a lot of morphine to control her pain. At the time this sample was taken, she was receiving oxygen with an inspired concentration of 35%.

These results show:

1. There is impaired oxygenation: the patient's Po_2 is low, particularly given the fact that she is breathing 35% oxygen.
2. The pH of the patient's plasma is low and the $[H^+]$ is high: she is acidaemic.
3. There is a respiratory acidosis: the PCO_2 is high.
4. There is neither metabolic acidosis or alkalosis: the $HCO_{3\ std}$ and base excess are both normal.

The combination of this patient's respiratory disease and opioid administration resulted in hypoxia and CO_2 retention. The CO_2 retention had led to respiratory acidosis.

These are the results for the same patient, 36 hours later. The patient is still breathing 35% oxygen. However, the patient is no longer receiving opioid drugs and the analgesia is now being provided by a local epidural anaesthetic, which does not cause respiratory depression:

		Normal range
pH	7.4	(7.35–7.45)
$[H^+]$	40 nmol L^{-1}	(36–44)
PCO_2	6.43 kPa	(4.4–6.0)
PO_2	9.5 kPa	(12.0–14.0)
$HCO_{3\ act}$	29.1 mmol L^{-1}	
$HCO_{3\ std}$	27.6 mmol L^{-1}	(22–26 mmol L^{-1})
Base excess	3.5 mmol L^{-1}.	(-2 to +2)

1. The patient's oxygenation has improved, although it is still abnormal.
2. The patient's blood is at a normal pH and $[H^+]$.
3. The patient still has respiratory acidosis (high PCO_2), although this has improved.
4. The patient has metabolic alkalosis (high standard bicarbonate, positive base excess).

The patient is clearly improving; her oxygenation is better since her opioids were stopped and her PCO_2 is returning towards normal. She has developed metabolic alkalosis which, in this case, has compensated fully for her respiratory acidosis. Note that this has taken many hours; metabolic alkalosis develops in response to increased acid excretion by the kidneys and this takes time. It is unusual for a metabolic alkalosis to compensate completely for a respiratory acidosis;

Case 8.2 Interpretation of arterial blood gases – cont'd

in this lady's case, it is likely that her respiratory acidosis was improving anyway.

Arterial blood analysis example 2

These results were obtained from a gentleman who had recently returned to the ward following major emergency surgery for an obstructed bowel. He is receiving 40% inspired oxygen:

		Normal range
pH	7.29	(7.35–7.45)
[H+]	51.8 nmol L^{-1}	(36–44)
PCO_2	6.27 kPa	(4.4–6.0)
PO_2	21.08 kPa	(12.0–14.0)
$HCO_{3\ act}$	21.9 mmol L^{-1}	
$HCO_{3\ std}$	20.6 mmol L^{-1}	(22–26 mmol L^{-1})
Base excess	−4.7 mmol L^{-1}.	(−2 to +2)

These results show:

1. Good oxygenation. The patient's PO_2 is well above normal.
2. A raised [H+] and low pH; the patient is acidotic.
3. The patient has respiratory acidosis; his PCO_2 is abnormally high.
4. The patient has metabolic acidosis; his $HCO_{3\ std}$ is abnormally low and his base excess is abnormally negative.

This patient has both respiratory and metabolic acidosis. The respiratory depression causing his respiratory acidosis may be due to the administration of postoperative opioids or as a result of drowsiness due to the hangover effects of the general anaesthetic. Notice that this degree of respiratory impairment in a man with healthy lungs does not cause a problem with oxygenation, if he is breathing supplemental O_2. Metabolic acidosis is not unusual following major, emergency surgery. It is likely that the patient was relatively dehydrated prior to his surgery and this may have led to poor organ perfusion and oxygenation. This, in turn, often leads to the production of lactic acid.

Arterial blood gas analysis example 3

These blood gases were taken from a lady in intensive care, on a mechanical ventilator, with an inspired O_2 concentration of 40%:

		Normal range
pH	7.04	(7.35–7.45)
[H+]	91.2 nmol L^{-1}	(36–44)
PCO_2	5.9 kPa	(4.4–6.0)
PO_2	18.8 kPa	(12.0–14.0)
$HCO_{3\ act}$	10.8 mmol L^{-1}	
$HCO_{3\ std}$		
Base excess	−18.9 mmol L^{-1}.	(−2 to +2)

These results show:

1. Adequate oxygenation, PO_2 is 18.8.
2. The patient is very severely acidaemic, a very high [H+]/ low pH.
3. The patient does not have respiratory acidosis/alkalosis.
4. The patient has severe metabolic acidosis (base excess, −18.9).

This patient is very ill and has very severe metabolic acidosis, which was thought to be due to renal and liver disease. If this patient was able to breathe spontaneously, her tidal volume would probably be very large, and she would produce respiratory alkalosis in an attempt to compensate for her metabolic acidosis. As she is on a mechanical ventilator, this does not happen.

References and Further reading

Arthurs, G.J., Sudhakar, M., 2005. Carbon dioxide transport. BJA Education. CEACCP 5 (6), 207–210.
Collins, J.A., Rudenski, A., O'Driscoll, B.R., 2008. Clinical validation of the severity of oxygen dissociation curve. Thorax 63, A4–A73.
Dunn, J.-O.C., Grocott, M.P., 2016. Physiology of oxygen transport. BJA Education. CEACCP 16 (10), 341–348.
McLellan, S.A., Walsh, T.S., 2004. Oxygen delivery and haemoglobin levels. Continuing Education in Anaesthesia, Critical Care, and Pain 4, 123–126.
NICE Guidance, 2018. Carbon monoxide poisoning. Available at https://cks.nice.org.uk/topics/carbon-monoxide-poisoning/. Accessed on 20 December 2020.
West, J.B., 2005. Gas transport by the blood. In: West, J.B. Respiratory Physiology: The Essentials, seventh ed. Lipincott Williams & Wilkins, 75–92.

9

NERVOUS CONTROL OF BREATHNG

Chapter objectives

After studying this chapter, you should be able to:

1. Identify the major sites in the brainstem which contribute to the control of the pattern of breathing.
2. Explain why 'respiratory centre' is not a precise term.
3. Describe the changes in the pattern of breathing seen in chronic obstructive pulmonary disease.
4. Compare voluntary and automatic control of breathing.
5. Discuss efferent innervation of the respiratory muscles.
6. Discuss neuromuscular disorders of breathing.
7. Define dyspnoea.
8. Outline the major afferent neural influences on the pattern of breathing.
9. Describe three classes of vagal mechanoreceptors in the lungs, together with their effects on breathing.
10. Discuss neurally mediated respiratory reflexes, such as coughing and sneezing.
11. Discuss the effect of coning on breathing.

Introduction

The objective of the respiratory system is to maintain the oxygen and carbon dioxide levels (PO_2 and PCO_2) in arterial blood within a narrow range. Metabolism uses up oxygen and produces carbon dioxide. Oxygen demand and carbon dioxide production can vary widely, depending on metabolic rate. Despite this, the respiratory system maintains the levels of oxygen, carbon dioxide, and hydrogen ions in the blood within a remarkably narrow range by producing a minute ventilation appropriate to the metabolic rate at that time. This is achieved by a series of receptors (in the lungs and peripherally) which feed information via **afferent** nerves to the 'respiratory centres' in the brain (Fig. 9.1). The respiratory centres integrate this information and send outputs along **efferent** nerves, travelling through the spinal cord, to the effectors (respiratory muscles), resulting in a particular rate, depth, and pattern of breathing. The muscles also send information back to the respiratory centres to modify the respiratory pattern (an example of negative feedback).

This fine control of breathing is brought about by chemical and neural mechanisms. In practice, the two occur simultaneously and nerves are involved in the pathways of the chemical control of breathing; however, for ease of understanding, neural and chemical control are considered separately in this chapter and the next.

Minute ventilation ($\dot{V}_E$) is equal to

$$V_T \times f$$

where V_T and f are the tidal volume (volume of each individual breath) and respiratory rate, respectively. This means any given minute ventilation can be achieved by a huge number of combinations of tidal volumes and frequencies; for example, a minute ventilation of 6 L min^{-1} could be achieved by twelve 500-mL breaths per minute or by twenty-four 250-mL breaths per minute. The particular pattern 'chosen' is determined predominantly by the neural mechanisms controlling breathing.

Economy of energy is an evolutionary advantage, and the pattern of breathing chosen by our bodies is aimed at minimising the amount of work we have to do to produce a particular minute ventilation. This work of breathing is directly related to the force exerted by the respiratory muscles. The most energy-efficient respiratory rate to produce a particular minute ventilation is

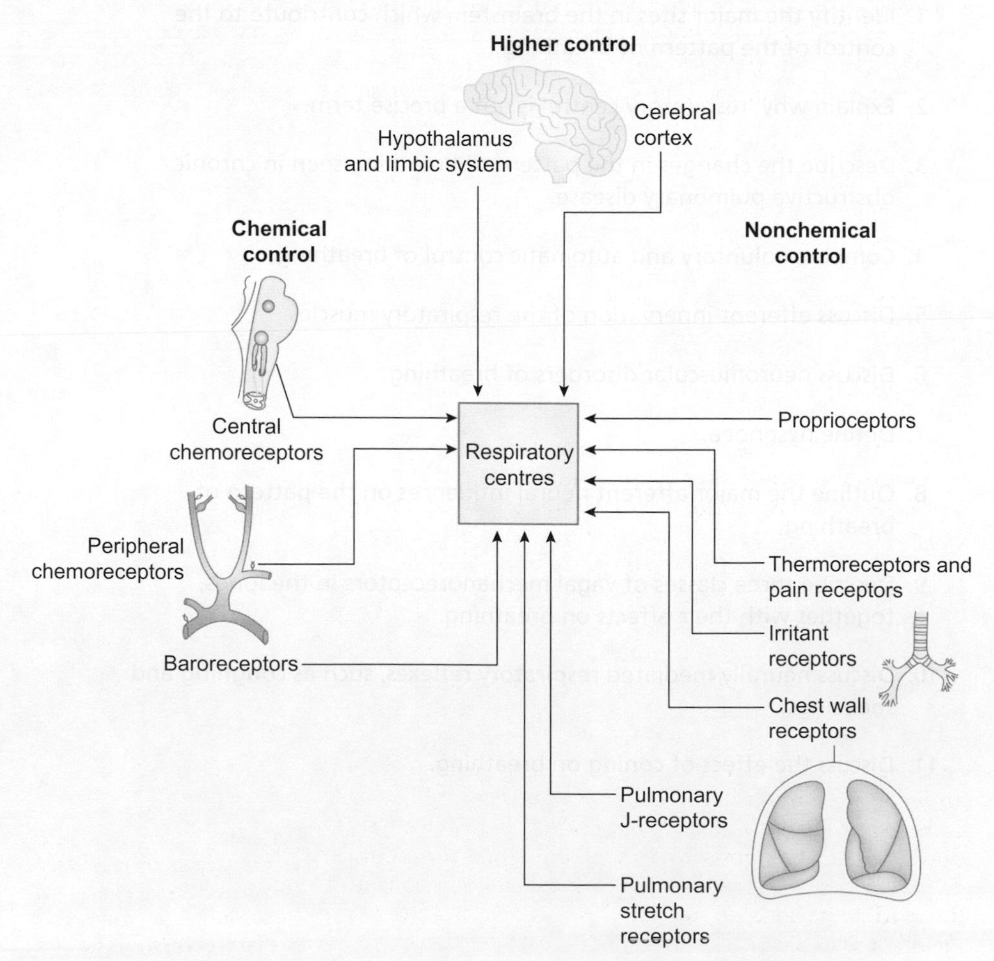

Fig 9.1 Afferent impulses to respiratory centres. There are a number of different receptors involved in sensing change in the respiratory system. These feed information via afferent impulses to the *respiratory centre*, which integrates the information and conveys efferent impulses to the effectors (the respiratory muscles). There are both chemical and nonchemical (neural) mechanisms involved. Higher centres of the brain also send afferents to the *respiratory centre* to adjust breathing (From Khurana I. et al. Textbook of Medical Physiology, 3e. 2020.).

called the resonance frequency, and this depends on the mechanical properties of the lungs (which were dealt with in Chapters 3 and 4). The process of matching the breathing pattern with the physical properties of the lungs can be likened to pushing someone on a swing. If you get the timing right, it requires very little effort to keep the swing going and the timing of the push (respiratory rate) depends on the length of the ropes (mechanical properties of the lungs). The optimal respiratory rate required to minimise the energy expenditure to achieve a given minute ventilation, therefore, varies from person to person, depending on the mechanical properties of their individual lungs.

Central control of breathing

The neural mechanisms that bring about alternating inspiration and expiration are still not completely understood. In quiet breathing, expiration is passive. So, to bring about a pattern of quiet breathing, all that is required is an intermittent signal to the inspiratory muscles. However, there must be some sort of negative feedback loop that stops inspiration, allowing a return to resting muscle tone and passive expiration. Further, active expiration is needed during more forceful breathing (e.g. during exercise). This requires an intermittent signal to the expiratory muscles/accessory muscles of respiration. It has therefore been suggested that there are two groups of neurons that each function in a synchronised manner to produce either inspiration or expiration, and they reciprocally inhibit each other to limit the duration of action of the other group (Fig. 9.2)

The actual control of respiration is far more complicated than this simple model. The rhythmic process of breathing originates in the **central pattern generator (CPG)** in the medulla, which is part of the brainstem (Fig 9.3).

The central pattern generator

There are numerous respiratory 'centres' in the brain. It is important to note that these are not anatomically discrete areas, that is cannot be found macro- or microscopically. Rather, they are areas with a high density of groups of neurons with common function.

Experiments involving transections of the brainstem, at various points, have revealed that breathing remains remarkably normal if the brainstem is transected above the medulla, but breathing ceases if connections between the medulla and spinal cord are severed (this can be the mechanism of death in high spinal cord injuries, e.g. from hanging). This is because breathing originates from an area in the medulla, which is called the pre-Bötzinger complex. This houses the respiratory CPG. The CPG plays a role analogous to that of the sinoatrial node in initiating rhythmic cardiac contractions; however, unlike the cardiac pacemaker, the CPG is actually an ill-defined group of neurons.

The CPG contains glutamatergic neurons which send excitatory nerve impulses to bilateral premotor neurons (upper motor neurons), which activate lower motor neurons (the phrenic and intercostal nerves) and, in turn, cause contraction of the respiratory muscles (mainly the diaphragm and intercostals), resulting in inspiration. Other nerves to accessory muscles (e.g. those innervating the larynx) synchronise their contractions with the phases of breathing. The Bötzinger complex, rostral to the pre-Bötzinger complex, is thought to control switching from inspiration to expiration, possibly by inhibitory neurons to the CPG.

The CPG produces a basic pattern of breathing. This pattern is finetuned by other regions of the brain, for example inputs from the pons, hypothalamus, and limbic system can modify breathing patterns during hyperthermia or emotions like panic, fear, or rage. This occurs by the inputs to the CPG or premotor neurons from these regions of brain, and a number of neurotransmitters and neuron types are involved. For example, adrenergic activity (i.e. the fight-or-flight response to perceived danger) enhances CPG activity via α_1-adrenoceptor activation. Conversely CPG activity is inhibited by α_2-adrenoceptor activation.

The efficiency of the breathing pattern generated by the CPG is also improved by afferent inputs from receptors in other parts of the body, particularly in the lungs and chest (Figs 9.1 and 9.4). This produces a refined respiratory pattern, which is efficient and can respond to changed conditions within seconds.

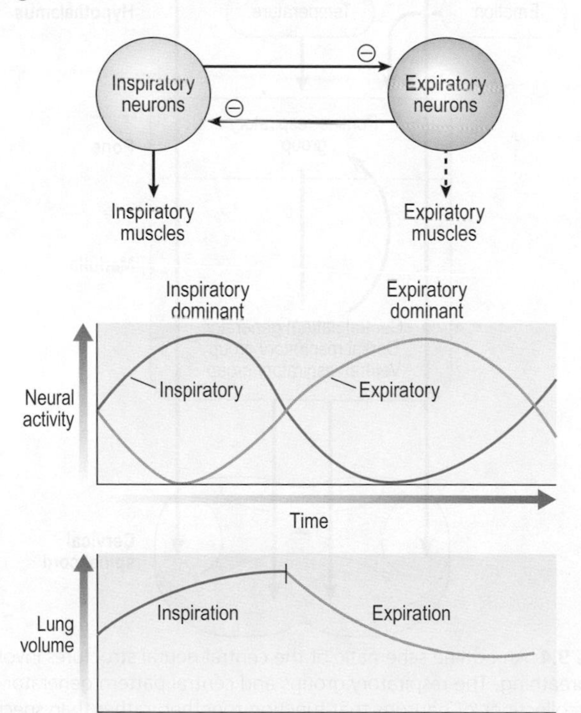

Fig. 9.2 A simple oscillator model of the generation of breathing. Groups of *inspiratory* and *expiratory* neurons alternately become dominant by inhibiting the other group. This model implies there is a 'self-inhibition' within each group that causes it to switch itself off. If that were not so, breathing would 'stick' in inspiration or expiration.

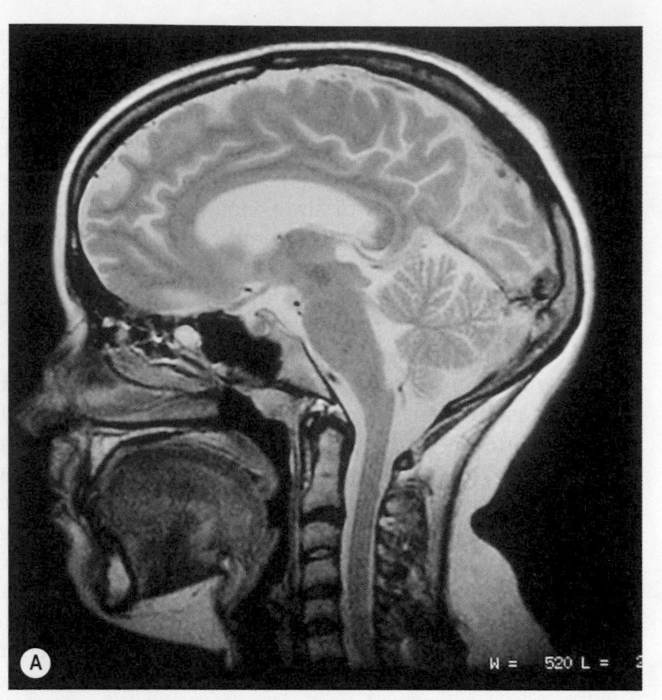

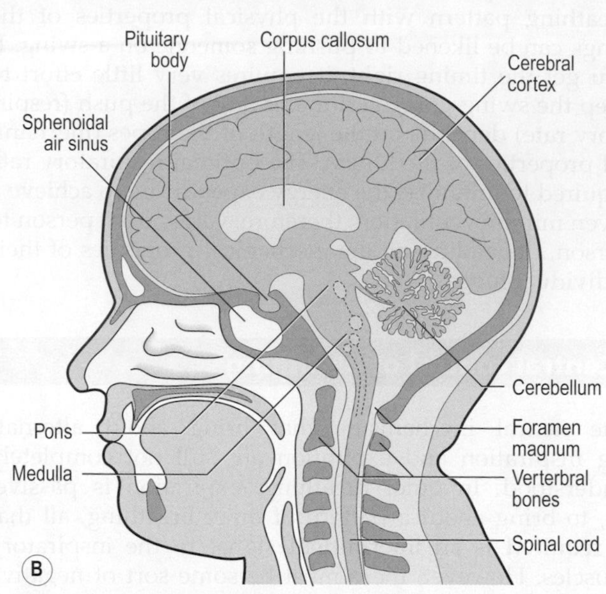

Fig. 9.3 The anatomical origin of breathing rhythm. This MRI scan (A) and corresponding diagram (B) show the areas of the central nervous system (*pons* and *medulla*) from which our basic pattern of breathing originates. These areas are influenced by many afferent inputs.

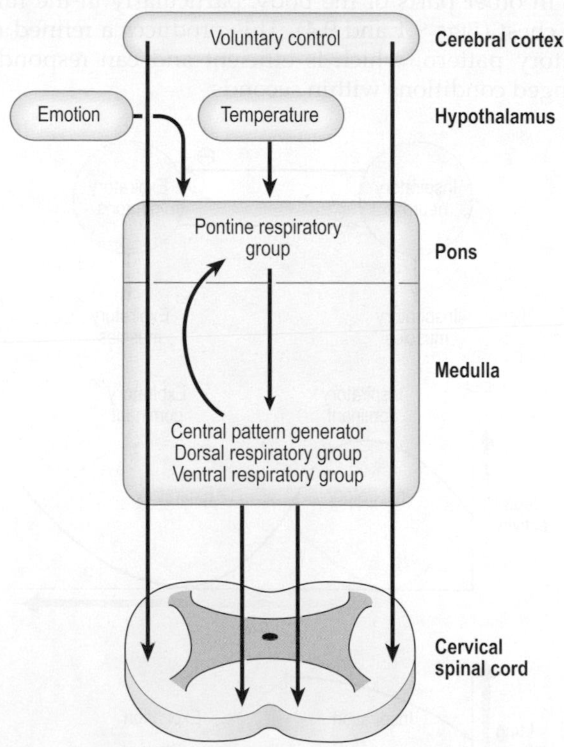

Fig. 9.4 An outline schematic of the central neural structures involved in breathing. The respiratory groups and central pattern generator are collections of neurons that function together, rather than specific anatomical structures.

Medullary respiratory centres

Within the medulla, in the reticular formation beneath the floor of the fourth ventricle, there are two functionally distinct groups of respiratory premotor neurons (Fig. 9.5). These are the descending excitatory (glutamatergic) neurons.

The dorsal respiratory group (DRG)

This is made up of exclusively inspiratory neurons in the region of the *nucleus tractus solitarius* and controls the timing of the respiratory cycle. The DRG neurons integrate information from chemoreceptors and mechanoreceptors related to breathing, for example, by receiving afferent inputs from cranial nerves IX and X (the glossopharyngeal and vagus nerves). The nerve cells of the DRG have a spontaneous rhythm of discharge. This intrinsic periodic firing is thought to be responsible for the basic pattern of breathing. These repetitive bursts of action potentials are transmitted to the respiratory muscles. Following a latent period, action potentials increase in a crescendo pattern, causing a 'ramped' increase in respiratory muscle activity. The action potentials then cease, allowing a return of the muscles to resting tone.

The ventral respiratory group (VRG)

This consists of both inspiratory and expiratory motor neurons (unlike the exclusively inspiratory DRG).

The rostral portion of the VRG is called the *nucleus ambiguus*. This innervates the accessory muscles of respiration on the same side of the body and is involved in dilating the pharynx and larynx.

The caudal part of the VRG contains the *nucleus retroambigualis*, which is predominantly expiratory. This innervates the contralateral diaphragm, abdominal muscles, and expiratory intercostal muscles. The caudal VRG also contains the *nucleus paraambigualis*, which controls the force of contraction of the contralateral inspiratory muscles.

The DRG and VRG, in the medulla, have numerous complex interconnections. For example, inspiratory activity in the DRG excites inspiratory activity in the VRG and inhibits VRG expiratory activity.

The pontine respiratory group (PRG)

The neurons that make up this 'centre' are found in and around the *nucleus parabrachialis medialis* (Fig 9.5). The PRG was previously referred to as the *pneumotaxic centre*. A normal respiratory rhythm can exist without this centre, but it is believed to be important in 'finetuning' the respiratory pattern by switching off inspiration to regulate the V_T and control the respiratory rate.

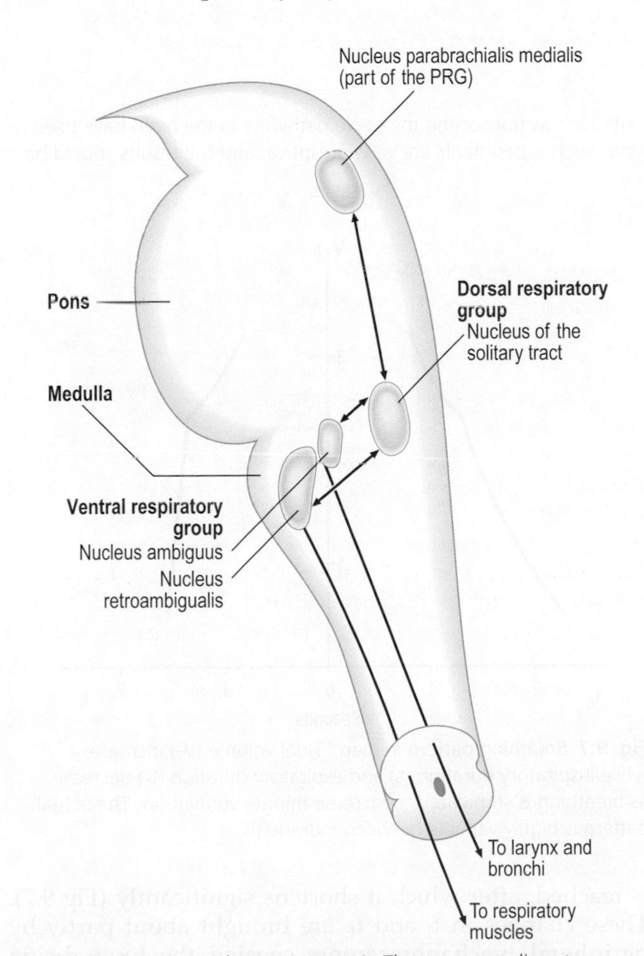

Fig. 9.5 Brainstem respiratory 'centres'. These are not discrete anatomical centres, rather they are areas of the brainstem which have a large percentage of neurons with a common function relating to the automatic control of breathing. PRG, pontine respiratory group.

The PRG receives afferents from the hypothalamus, cortex, and DRG, suggesting it coordinates inputs from a number of areas to optimise the breathing pattern. The PRG may have evolved as a means of mediating the rapid, shallow breathing (panting) initiated for thermal or emotional reasons by higher parts of the brain. It is thought that the inspiratory neurons of the DRG stimulate the PRG, which, after a short delay, sends inhibitory impulses back to the DRG, cutting short inspiratory activity (and hence reducing the action potentials to the inspiratory muscles, for example in the phrenic nerve to the diaphragm). This is an example of a negative feedback arrangement. Shortening one breath, in this way, means that the next breath can start earlier, that is the frequency of breathing is increased and the volume of breaths is reduced.

The vagus nerves (cranial nerves X) can produce the same effect of cutting short inspiration and limiting tidal volume. Experimentally removing the PRG *and* cutting the vagi (Fig 9.6) results in *apneusis* – long, powerful inspiratory efforts interspersed with brief expirations (Greek, *apneusis, without breath*). This led to the suggestion that there was an *apneustic centre* in the lower pons, an idea which is no longer popular. This apneustic pattern of breathing can be seen in individuals with severe brain injuries.

Conscious control of breathing

The control of breathing described, so far, is automatic and independent of the brain above the pons. Normal breathing is involuntary, that is we are not conscious of it. However, we are able to voluntarily change the rate, pattern, or depth of our breathing, for example when blowing, whistling, speaking, performing lung function tests (see Chapter 11), or when locking the ribcage to provide a framework against which the arms can act. This voluntary control is achieved by higher centres in the brain (the cerebral cortex) overriding the automatic pattern.

The voluntary pathways bypass the CPG and brainstem respiratory centres to descend in the pyramidal tracts found laterally in the spinal cord (Fig. 9.4). The involuntary pathways from the brainstem run in the anterior region, near the outlets of the ventral roots. As a result of their separate anatomical locations, the voluntary pathways can be destroyed independently of the involuntary pathways, for example by a stroke. Patients with such a stroke breathe normally, respond to reflex and chemical stimuli, but cannot voluntarily change their pattern of breathing; they will cough if their larynx is stimulated, but cannot cough on command. Very rarely, the opposite situation is seen, where the automatic pathways have been destroyed but the pyramidal tracts are left intact. The patient can breathe deliberately but not automatically, as in sleep. This condition is

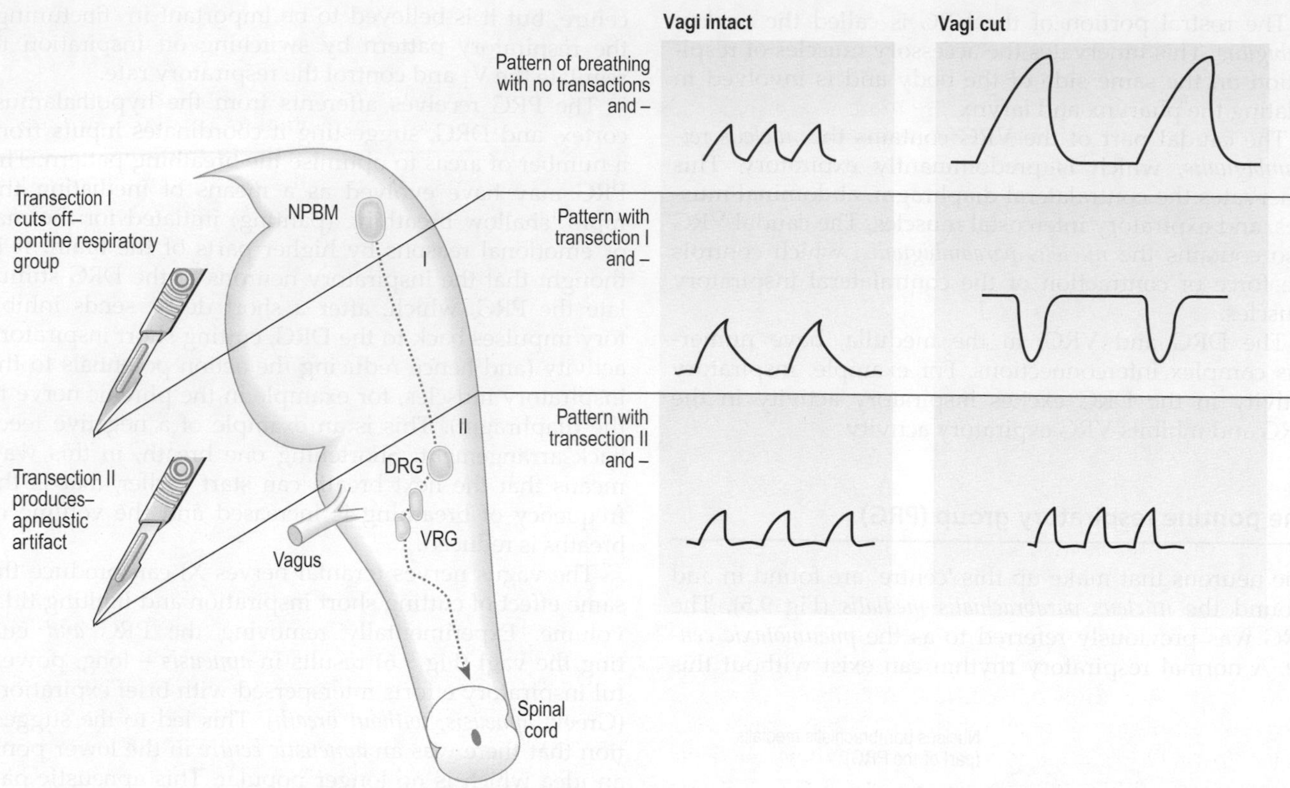

Fig. 9.6 Breathing patterns after brainstem and vagal transections. Experiments such as transecting the nerve pathways in the brain have been used to isolate different effects of parts of the brain on the pattern of breathing. Such experiments are very disruptive, and the results should be interpreted with caution.

called 'Ondine's curse', after the folk tale of the mortal man who betrayed an ondine or water-nymph. She put a curse on the man that if he did not remember to keep his vital functions (e.g. heartbeat and breathing) going, they would stop. Of course, when he fell asleep, he died. In addition to describing central hypoventilation after stroke, the term 'Ondine's curse' can be used to describe a rare congenital central hypoventilation syndrome wherein babies are born with a permanent defect in automatic respiration. This causes apnoea or hypoventilation during sleep and can require diaphragmatic pacing or nocturnal, non-invasive, ventilatory support.

In addition to the voluntary control of breathing arising from the cerebral cortex, there are multiple other complex reflexes which control and coordinate breathing to allow phonation, swallowing, coughing, and sneezing (see later).

Pattern of breathing in chronic obstructive pulmonary disease

A respiratory cycle consists of a breath in and a breath out. The durations of the two phases of breathing (inspiratory time (t_I) and expiratory time (t_E)) can change independently of each other. Both are influenced by the volume of the lungs. When V_T increases, t_E shortens first, with t_I remaining fairly constant until a threshold

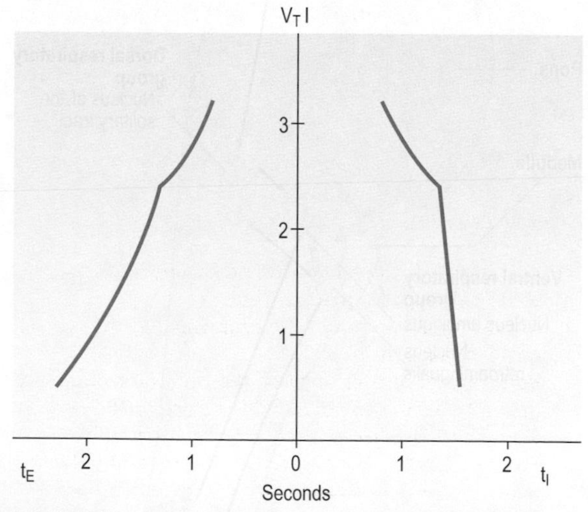

Fig. 9.7 Breathing pattern in man. Tidal volume (V_T) increases while inspiratory duration (t_I) and expiratory duration (t_E) decrease as breathing is stimulated to increase minute ventilation. The actual pattern is highly variable between individuals.

is reached, after which it shortens significantly (Fig 9.7). These changes in t_I and t_E are brought about partly by **peripheral mechanoreceptors** sensing the lungs being stretched with increasing V_T and feeding back, via the vagus nerves, to bring about changes in the durations of inspiration and expiration.

The relationship of t_I:V_T reflects the drive to breathe. The relationship between t_I and the total breath duration reflects the way a single breath is divided up into the time to fill the lungs (t_I) and the time to empty back to the start position (t_E). These two phases are, of course, governed by the mechanical properties of the lungs and airways.

The relationship among V_T, t_I, and t_E shown in Figure 9.7 is disrupted in disease. In chronic obstructive pulmonary disease (COPD), for example, there is reduced respiratory efficiency caused by ventilation–perfusion mismatching and stiffening lungs. As the airflow limitation progresses, there is a compensatory increased drive to breathe. This initially increases the respiratory rate and V_T (and so the overall minute ventilation increases early in COPD). However, as airway resistance and the work of breathing increase, as the disease progresses, V_T decreases below normal. The only way the patient can now increase their minute ventilation is to increase their frequency of breathing. The problem with this strategy is that the expiratory airflow limitation characteristic of COPD demands that a greater proportion of each breath be devoted to expiration and the fraction of each breath devoted to inspiration be reduced. Air trapping and a subjective sensation of relief when breathing at high volume (which holds the airways open in what has been termed autopositive end-expiratory pressure or 'auto-PEEP') causes the patient with severe COPD to breathe with a rapid, shallow pattern at increased lung volumes. This is an inefficient pattern because the lungs are less compliant at high lung volumes. The pattern of breathing in COPD can therefore place the respiratory muscles at such a mechanical disadvantage that the increased work of breathing can exhaust the patient. Respiratory failure ensues.

Summary 1

- Respiration is tightly controlled by neural and chemical mechanisms.
- Breathing originates in the brainstem, in the central pattern generator.
- Respiratory 'centres' include the pontine respiratory group (PRG) in the pons and the dorsal (DRG) and ventral (VRG) respiratory groups in the medulla.
- The basic pattern generated by the central pattern generator is modified by higher centres in the brain.
- The cerebral cortex allows us to voluntarily override the automatic pattern of breathing.
- Other areas of the brain, for example the hypothalamus and limbic system, can affect breathing patterns in hyperthermia and emotional states (e.g. fear or anger).
- The respiratory pattern is fine-tuned by peripheral receptors sending afferents (mainly via the vagus nerve) to the brain. This improves the efficiency of breathing.
- There are anatomically separate voluntary and involuntary pathways from the brainstem to the respiratory muscles.

Respiratory muscle innervation

We have seen that the CPG produces a basic pattern of breathing. The breathing signal is carried via efferent nerves to the respiratory muscles, or effectors. The muscles of respiration include the diaphragm, intercostals (external, internal, and innermost), abdominal muscles, and accessory muscles (e.g. the sternocleidomastoid in the neck and the muscles of the larynx).

In order for the breathing pattern generated by the medulla to be effected, it must reach the respiratory muscles (Fig. 9.8). Signals travel from the brain via **upper motor neurons** to the spinal cord. This activates **alpha motor neurons**, which are **lower motor neurons** with cell bodies in the anterior horn of the spinal cord. The resulting action potentials from the central nervous system propagate along the alpha motor neuron axons to the group of **extrafusal motor fibres** that each neuron innervates, causing a contraction. One alpha motor neuron plus the muscle fibres it activates are called a ***motor unit***. Each motor unit is activated in an all-or-none fashion, producing synchronised contractions.

The diaphragm is innervated by the phrenic nerve (which originates from the cervical cord at C3–5; hence the saying, 'C3, 4, and 5 keep the diaphragm alive') and the lower intercostal nerves. Each of the two phrenic nerves contains hundreds of motor neurons, corresponding to hundreds of motor units within the diaphragm. The diaphragm is the main effector of the neurally controlled pattern of breathing generated by the medulla.

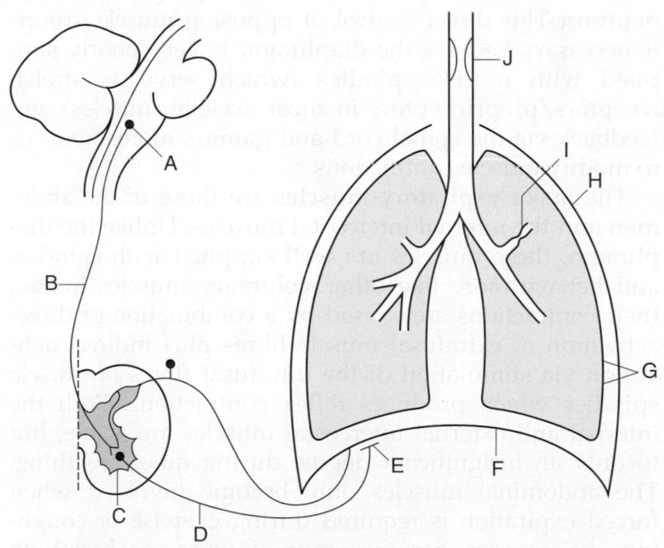

Fig 9.8 Sites at which lesions, drugs, or malfunctions may result in ventilatory failure. (A) Respiratory centre. (B) Upper motor neuron. (C) Anterior horn cell. (D) Lower motor neuron. (E) Neuromuscular junction. (F) Respiratory muscles. (G) Altered elasticity of lungs or chest wall. (H) Loss of structural integrity of chest wall and pleural cavity. (I) Increased resistance of small airways. (J) Upper airway obstruction (From Lumb A. Nunn's Applied Respiratory Physiology. 2011.).

This pattern can vary from quiet breathing in a normal subject, to disordered breathing in disease states, to forceful breathing during exercise, coughing, or sneezing. These different patterns require the production of graded levels of force generation, which is achieved through recruitment of different numbers and types of motor units. Skeletal muscle contains three different types of muscle fibres (type I fibres are slow, fatigue-resistant; IIb are fast, fatiguable; and IIa have intermediate properties). Human respiratory muscle is made up of mostly type I and IIa fibres, with relatively few of the fatiguable IIb fibres; ageing, drugs, and disease can alter the relative proportions. All muscle fibres within a motor unit are homogeneous with respect to their mechanical and fatigue properties. Normal breathing, even under hypoxic or hypercapnic conditions, requires only recruitment of fatigue-resistant motor units; the transdiaphragmatic pressure produced during quiet breathing is less than 10% of the maximum pressure that can be achieved. More forceful expulsive activities, like coughing, sneezing, or breathing against airway obstruction (as in obstructive sleep apnoea – see Chapter 2), all require recruitment of the more fatiguable muscle fibre types. Although these can generate higher transdiaphragmatic pressures through more forceful contractions, this comes at the expense of fatigue; therefore these higher forces cannot be sustained.

The inspiratory motor neurons of the spinal cord are inhibited during expiration and the expiratory motor neurons are inhibited during inspiration. This prevents opposing muscles from contracting simultaneously. In the diaphragm, this inhibition is not brought about by **muscle-spindle** reflexes but is the direct result of the DRG and VRG sequentially activating specific motor neurons. This direct control of opposing muscle groups is necessary because the diaphragm is very poorly supplied with muscle spindles (which serve as stretch receptors/proprioceptors in most skeletal muscles) and feedback via the spinal cord and gamma motor neurons to modify muscle contractions.

The major **expiratory muscles** are those of the abdomen and the internal intercostal muscles. Unlike the diaphragm, these muscles are well supplied with spindles and behave more like other voluntary muscles in that their contractions are caused by a combination of direct activation of extrafusal muscle fibres plus indirect activation via stimulation of the intrafusal fibres of muscle spindles which produces reflex contractions. Both the internal and external intercostal muscles are active, but to only an insignificant degree during quiet breathing. The abdominal muscles only become involved when forced expiration is required during exercise or coughing. As exercise becomes more intense, or breathing becomes more laboured, as in disease, more accessory muscles (e.g. those of the shoulder girdle) are recruited. The muscles of the abdomen and chest are also involved in posture, locomotion, and in the movement of the arms in lifting heavy weights. During almost all of these activities, if not too extreme, it is possible to breathe and vocalise, which involves well controlled modification of airflow.

The **larynx** exhibits movements synchronised with breathing. These movements are brought about by the laryngeal muscles, which are innervated by the superior laryngeal and recurrent laryngeal nerves. These are branches of the vagus nerve. During inspiration, the vocal folds are ***abducted*** (pulled apart) and this reduces the resistance to airflow into the lungs. During expiration the vocal folds ***adduct*** (come together), slowing down the expiratory flow. These movements are automatic – we are not conscious of them – and the nerve impulses that cause them arise from the rostral part of the VRG in the nucleus ambiguous. We can, of course, consciously control our larynx, as in vocalisation. The larynx is therefore almost a model of the control of respiration, with an automatic rhythm that can be consciously overridden.

Neuromuscular disorders

Breathing is initiated by several steps, from the respiratory neurons in the brain, via the spinal cord, through peripheral nerves to the respiratory muscles. At each of these steps and the junctions between them, the process is susceptible to disorder caused by the effects of disease, drugs, or disuse (Fig. 9.8). Conditions affecting the brain, afferent or efferent nerves, or respiratory muscles can cause difficulty breathing or, indeed, respiratory failure. A few examples of these numerous pathologies are listed here:

Central nervous system disorders

Trauma

Trauma, ischaemia, or bleeding in the brain and spinal cord can result in partial or total loss of respiratory function, depending on the degree and site of the lesion. *Hemispheric strokes* can interfere with the voluntary pathways of breathing. *Brainstem strokes* that affect the DRG (see Fig. 9.6) can cause fatal apnoea.

Overdose

A number of recreational and medicinal drugs depress the central drive to breathe and, if taken in overdose, can cause respiratory failure. Opioid-induced respiratory depression is mediated through activation of μ-opioid receptors on neurons in the brainstem respiratory centres.

Poliomyelitis

This is an acute viral infection that can cause destruction of the anterior horn cells of the spinal cord and flaccid paralysis of various muscle groups, including respiratory muscles. About 25% of those infected require mechanical ventilation during the acute stage.

Many recover respiratory muscle strength thanks to the reinnervation of denervated fibres. This disease is now rare due to widespread vaccination.

Spinal cord injury

Spinal cord injury is characterised by motor and sensory loss below the level of the lesion, as well as loss of autonomic control. High cervical spinal cord injuries disrupt the descending upper motor neurons signalling to the phrenic nerve lower motor neurons, thereby disrupting diaphragmatic action. The more caudal intercostal nerve function will also be lost, resulting in significant respiration impairment, manifesting as low lung volumes and weak cough. The mainstays of management include non-invasive respiratory support and assisted cough techniques in patients with lower cervical/thoracic injuries and tracheostomy plus long-term ventilation in higher cervical injuries.

Peripheral nervous system disorders

Diphtheria

The gram-positive bacteria *Corynebacterium diphtheriae* produce an exotoxin that provokes a demyelinating neuropathy, which results in respiratory failure if the respiratory muscles are involved. Antitoxin is the only specific therapy. Like poliomyelitis, this disease is now rare due to widespread vaccination.

Botulism

The anaerobic, gram-positive bacteria *Clostridium botulinum* can be spread in contaminated food or infected wounds. They produce an exotoxin which blocks the release of acetylcholine at the neuromuscular junction. When innervation of the respiratory muscles is involved, artificial ventilation is often required. Treatment includes debridement of infected wounds, penicillin, and antitoxin in the early stages. Recovery may take months, and mortality rates are around 10%.

Guillain-Barré

This is an acute, immune-mediated polyneuropathy that usually follows an infection. It causes ascending, bilateral, symmetrical weakness, which can be accompanied by bulbar weakness; 10%–30% of patients require respiratory support.

Myasthenia gravis

This autoimmune disease causes weakness and increased fatiguability of skeletal muscles. Autoantibodies are produced against the acetylcholine receptors of the neuromuscular junction. The resulting weakness is usually worse during exertion and improved by rest. The resultant respiratory (or bulbar) muscle weakness may necessitate intubation and ventilatory support. Other treatments include acetylcholinesterase inhibitors, immunosuppressive drugs, plasma exchange, and intravenous immunoglobulins.

Respiratory muscle disorders

With respiratory muscle weakness comes a reduction in lung volume, particularly vital capacity and its components. Weakness of the inspiratory muscles leads to a reduction in ventilation and atelectasis (collapse of the alveoli and small airways), which increases ventilation-perfusion mismatch (see Chapter 7). Weakness of the expiratory muscles reduces the efficiency of cough. This is important as it can cause inefficient clearance of mucus and frequent pulmonary infections.

Duchenne muscular dystrophy

This X-linked, recessive, genetic disorder affects the gene for the production of the protein dystrophin, which helps keep muscle cells intact. The disease is characterised by progressive weakness. From the age of 10, vital capacity declines inexorably in these patients. Life expectancy is reduced, with patients commonly dying from respiratory failure secondary to pulmonary infection in their 20s.

Disuse atrophy

Diaphragm strength reduces with disuse, and diaphragm muscle fibre atrophy can be demonstrated as early as 18 hours after onset of artificial ventilation. With ongoing disuse, the proportion of fatigue-resistant type I muscle fibres declines. This makes weaning from a ventilator increasingly difficult as the duration of ventilation increases. To combat this, spontaneous breathing is encouraged as early as possible in most critically ill patients, and newer ventilators have the capacity to sense diaphragmatic activity to synchronise ventilator-delivered breaths with those of the patient.

Respiratory failure is not exclusively caused by disorders in the pathways of neural control of respiration. It may also be caused by abnormalities in the lungs (e.g. airway obstruction, trauma, infection, tumour, acute respiratory disease syndrome), chest wall (e.g. scoliosis, morbid obesity), or the cardiovascular system (e.g. heart failure, hypovolaemia, pulmonary embolism).

Dyspnoea

Dyspnoea is often the only or major symptom patients with lung disease complain of. This condition is difficult to define but is usually described as 'difficulty breathing' or 'air hunger'. The sensation of dyspnoea arises when there is a disproportion between the demand for ventilation and its supply. The sense of respiratory effort, detected as respiratory muscle tension, is not matched by changes in respiratory muscle length and therefore ventilation.

This history of dyspnoea is important in diagnosis. Dyspnoea of sudden onset is often associated with an acute cardiopulmonary event – a pulmonary embolism or left ventricular failure, for example. Chronic dyspnoea of slow onset is usually associated with respiratory disease (e.g. COPD, asthma, pulmonary fibrosis) but can be the result of cardiac diseases, particularly those that cause pulmonary venous congestion.

Summary 2

- The outputs of the respiratory centres are via efferent upper motor neurons which synapse with lower motor neurons (e.g. the phrenic and intercostal nerves), producing motor action potentials in the respiratory muscles (e.g. the diaphragm and intercostals).
- The diaphragm (the main inspiratory muscle) is directly innervated by alpha motor neurons and has few muscle spindles.
- Expiratory muscles are mostly inactive during quiet breathing. They do contain muscle spindles.
- Pathology affecting any part of the neural control pathway, from brainstem to muscles, may cause respiratory disorders.
- Dyspnoea describes a subjective sensation of breathlessness or 'air hunger'.

Afferent inputs to the respiratory centre

The respiratory centres receive a number of afferent inputs (Fig. 9.1) which serve to modify the respiratory pattern arising from the CPG. These afferents originate from various areas within and outside the lungs. Receptors within the lungs provide feedback loops to modify subsequent breaths, while non-pulmonary afferents in the upper airways mediate reflexes that often protect the lungs from damage. The role of chemoreceptors is discussed in Chapter 10. In many animals, the respiratory pattern can form an important part of non-verbal communication, relaying pain or fear, for example. These changes are brought about by afferents from higher regions in the central nervous system. Human reflexive control of breathing is more complex than in most other animals, perhaps to facilitate our unique power of speech.

Pulmonary afferents

The control of the breathing pattern in most mammals is profoundly influenced by inputs travelling in the tenth **cranial nerves** (the vagus nerves). These are two very large nerves which run on either side of the neck, parallel to the trachea. These nerves carry information from other parts of the body, but the information coming from the lungs is of particular importance in the control of breathing. There are three types of receptors in the lung:

1. pulmonary stretch receptors (slowly adapting receptors)
2. irritant receptors (rapidly adapting receptors)
3. J receptors (C-fibre receptors)

The rate of ***adaptation*** describes the way a receptor (in the lungs, or anywhere else in the body) responds to a stimulus. If a constant stimulus is applied to a receptor, it 'gets used to it' and the frequency of the receptor discharge (in action potentials per second) decreases even though the stimulus does not change (Fig. 9.9). The rate at which this happens defines receptors as *slowly adapting* (i.e. the frequency of discharge slowly returns to the rest frequency) or *rapidly adapting* (i.e. the frequency rapidly returns to normal).

1. Slowly adapting pulmonary stretch receptors (PSRs)

These receptors are situated in the airway smooth muscle. The PSRs respond to distension by producing action potentials which travel via large-diameter, myelinated fibres in the vagus nerves to the brain. The PSR discharge is sustained during lung distension as they are slowly adapting receptors. The PSR signals the volume of the lungs at any instant; the greater the volume of the lungs, the higher the frequency of action potentials. It is thought that when the frequency reaches a certain 'threshold', it operates some kind of neural 'off switch' which switches off inspiration (Fig. 9.10).

PSRs play an important role in the control of breathing in animals and are present and active in humans, yet their relevance to the control of quiet breathing in humans is in dispute. The effect of stretch receptors on the pattern of breathing is most dramatically seen in the ***Hering–Breuer inflation reflex*** where lung inflation tends to inhibit further inspiratory muscle activity, particularly in animals (Fig. 9.11). Much larger lung

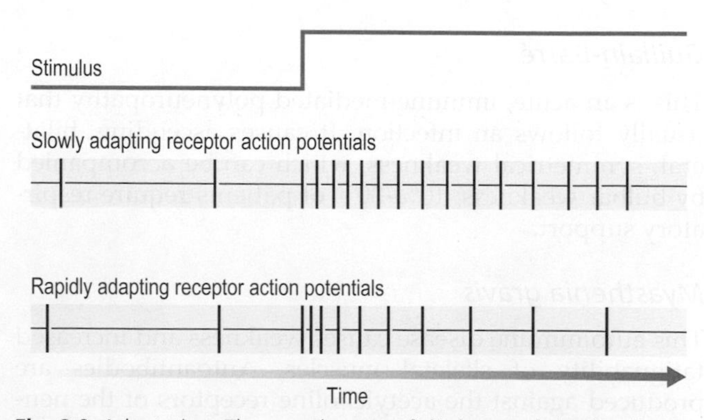

Fig. 9.9 Adaptation: The way the rate of discharge of slowly adapting (pulmonary stretch receptors) or rapidly adapting (pulmonary irritant or deflation) receptors in the lung adapt to a sustained change in stimulation.

inflations (over 1 L) are needed to inhibit inspiration in humans. The Hering–Breuer reflex is more powerful in babies than in adults but is present in adults during sleep. It is important to note that lung inflation does not cause physical obstruction of breathing; inflating the lungs produces a reflex. The subject is not trying to breathe, as demonstrated by the absence of phrenic activity during the lung inflation. Eventually, however, carbon dioxide builds up in the blood and forces breathing to restart (see Chapter 10).

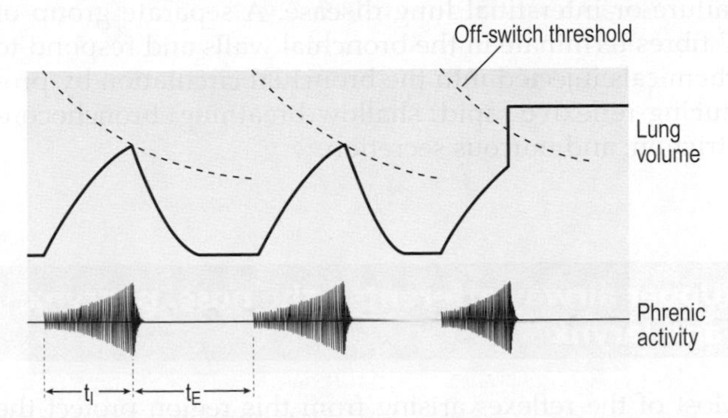

Fig 9.10 The off-switch threshold. Lung inflation is signalled to the brain by pulmonary stretch receptors. When this signal reaches a certain threshold, it switches off inspiration and expiration begins. The brain becomes more sensitive to this signal (the off-switch threshold falls) through a single respiratory cycle. Once the off-switch has operated, its sensitivity is reset to begin a new cycle. If the lungs are artificially inflated to above the threshold, at any time, inspiration is immediately switched off in what is known as the Hering–Breuer inflation reflex.

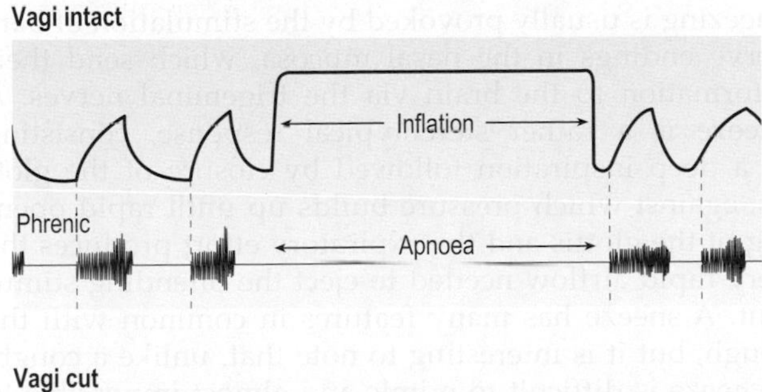

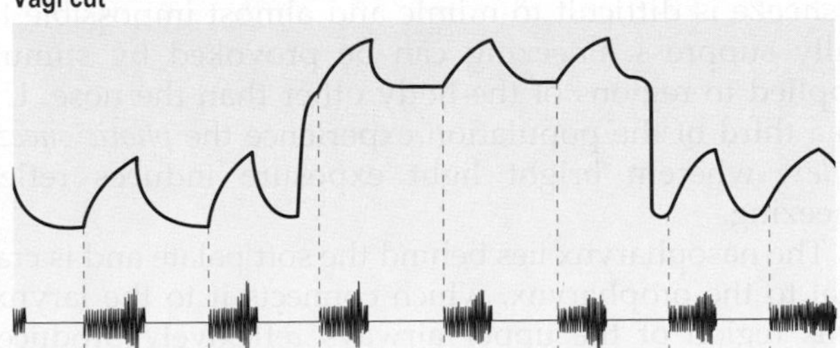

Fig. 9.11 The Hering–Breuer inflation reflex. When the lungs are artificially inflated, increased pulmonary stretch receptor activity (which signals lung volume) operates the inspiratory off-switch and terminates inspiration. This is the Hering–Breuer inflation reflex. The effect is weak in humans and cutting the vagi abolishes this reflex.

PSRs are active throughout the respiratory cycle and are thought to have roles in expiration, too. In addition to terminating inspiration and limiting V_T, PSRs extend expiratory time, as seen in the Hering-Breuer inflation reflex. This aspect of their action is important because the expiratory phase of breathing is usually the longest, at rest, and so it is the most important phase determining the rate of breathing.

The activity of the stretch receptors is not essential for rhythmic breathing: breathing continues even if the vagus nerves are cut. Nevertheless, in animals at least, PSRs modify the pattern of breathing. This modification makes breathing more efficient in terms of the energy required to produce a given ventilation. The stretch receptors 'take note' of the mechanical properties of the lung and inform the central control mechanisms, which alter the pattern of breathing accordingly. For example, if the compliance of the lungs is reduced, stretch receptors will discharge more vigorously (reduced compliance means stiffer lungs which create greater airway wall tension and therefore stimulate the PSR more strongly). The more vigorous discharge will switch off inspiration earlier and breathing will become shallow and rapid. This pattern is the most efficient for stiff lungs.

During exercise, lung inflation is more rapid, which augments stretch receptor activity and may cause them to operate the off switch earlier than normal, which may be one of their roles in humans. PSRs also dilate the airways and accelerate the heart, which may also be an advantage in reducing airway resistance and increasing cardiac output during exercise. Stretch receptors are primarily mechanoreceptors, as their name implies; they are, however, inhibited by an increase in the partial pressure of carbon dioxide. This response to carbon dioxide may play a part in the shortening of expiration seen when inhaled carbon dioxide accelerates breathing.

2. Rapidly adapting (irritant) receptors (RARs)

Pulmonary RARs are free nerve endings lying close to the surface of the airway epithelium, concentrated at points where the airways divide. Also called *irritant receptors*, they are powerfully stimulated by inhaled dust, smoke, noxious gases, and cold air, to produce action potentials which are relayed to the brain via small-diameter, myelinated fibres in the vagus nerves. Even if the stimulus is sustained (e.g. ongoing smoke inhalation), the RAR discharge frequency rapidly returns to the baseline level (see Fig. 9.9).

The stimulation of pulmonary RARs reflexively produces two very different patterns of breathing:

1. Rapid, shallow breathing, resulting mainly from a shortening of expiration.
2. Long, deep, **augmented breaths**, that is sighs, in which inspiration is about twice as long as normal (Fig. 9.12).

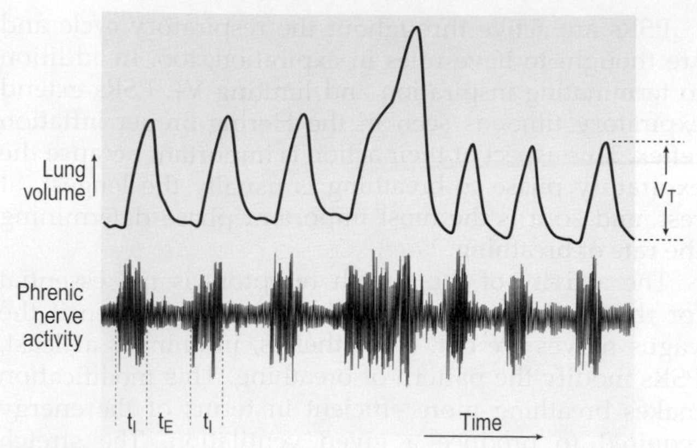

Fig. 9.12 An augmented breath. These 'sighs' occur every few minutes in man and help to reinflate collapsed areas of the lung. They are provoked by increased activity in rapidly adapting pulmonary receptors which pass to the brain via the vagus nerves.

These augmented breaths are periodically taken by mammals (every 5–20 minutes in resting humans) to reverse the slow collapse of the lungs (**atelectasis**) that takes place during quiet breathing.

Until recently, it seemed paradoxical that stimulating these receptors could produce both rapid, shallow breathing and the diametrically opposite pattern of the deep, slow, augmented breaths. The explanation for this seems to be that each augmented breath is followed by a 'refractory period' of at least 2 minutes, during which another augmented breath cannot occur and during which time rapid, shallow breathing, resulting from shortened expirations, intervenes. Your chances of provoking a sigh therefore depend on how recently the last one occurred.

RARs have a role in initiating the first, deep gasps of newborn infants, contributing to the initiation of inspiration in adult breathing, and are also possibly involved in a form of positive feedback during the accelerated breathing of exercise. RARs have another mechanoreceptor function – they are stimulated by changes in lung compliance, as in lung disease or **pneumothorax**, for example. In this scenario, the receptors are probably stimulated by the rate of change in lung volume, which is related to the rate of airflow into or out of the lungs. RARs may therefore be responsible for the changed patterns of breathing seen in lung disease, the sensation of **dyspnoea**, reflexive bronchial constriction, and the increased airway mucus secretion that accompanies many of these pathologies.

3. C-fibre receptors (J receptors)

These are the endings of small-diameter, non-myelinated afferent nerve fibres (*C fibres*), which travel from the lungs to the brain via the vagus nerves. Some C-fibre receptors are found in the alveolar walls, close to the pulmonary capillaries, hence the alternative name ***J (juxta-capillary) receptors***. C-fibre receptors are stimulated by increases in interstitial fluid (oedema) and by histamines, bradykinins, and prostaglandins released during lung damage. The reflex response to vigorous stimulation of these receptors is apnoea, followed by rapid, shallow breathing, hypotension, bradycardia, laryngospasm and a relaxation of the skeletal muscles due to the inhibition of spinal motor neurons. C-fibre receptors may also play a role in the dyspnoea and rapid shallow breathing seen in patients with heart failure or interstitial lung disease. A separate group of C fibres terminate in the bronchial walls and respond to chemicals injected into the bronchial circulation by producing reflexive rapid, shallow breathing; bronchoconstriction; and mucous secretion.

Upper airway afferents – the nose, pharynx, and larynx

Most of the reflexes arising from this region protect the lower airways against the ingress of foreign objects and damaging gases and vapours. These various reflexes arise from the upper airways and many have secondary effects on other systems. The cardiovascular system and the skeletal muscles associated with posture, for example, are affected by a sneeze.

Sneezing

Sneezing is usually provoked by the stimulation of bare nerve endings in the nasal mucosa, which send their information to the brain via the trigeminal nerves. A sneeze is a rather stereotypical response, consisting of a deep inspiration followed by closure of the glottis, against which pressure builds up until rapid opening of the glottis and the expiratory effort produces the very rapid airflow needed to eject the offending stimulant. A sneeze has many features in common with the cough, but it is interesting to note that, unlike a cough, a sneeze is difficult to mimic and almost impossible to fully suppress. Sneezing can be provoked by stimuli applied to regions of the body other than the nose. Up to a third of the population experience the *photic sneeze reflex*, wherein bright light exposure induces reflex sneezing.

The nasopharynx lies behind the soft palate and is cranial to the oropharynx, which connects it to the larynx. This region of the upper airways reflexively produces sniffs and related inspirations and the more powerful aspiration reflex. This consists of powerful inspiratory efforts, with the glottis held open. These efforts tend to pull any material blocking the nasopharynx into the oropharynx, to be swallowed or spat out.

Coughing

The upper airways, particularly the larynx and upper trachea, contain superficially situated **rapidly adapting nerve endings,** which provoke cough. Unlike the RARs deeper in the lungs that produce rapid, shallow breathing, cough receptors produce a reflex similar to a sneeze, involving a slow, deep inspiration followed by an explosive expiration. Cough receptors provide a clear demonstration of the undemocratic nature of the neural control of breathing: the stimulation of a single cough receptor will overpower the activity of all the other receptors in the lungs to produce a cough.

Distinct from the cough reflex is the ***expiration reflex.*** Irritation of the larynx causes rapid, forceful expiration from the lung volume at the time when irritation occurred. There is no preceding inspiration. This prevents solids or liquids at the laryngeal inlet from being aspirated; instead, they are forcefully expelled.

Laryngospasm

Reflexive adduction of the vocal cords can occur with mechanical stimulation of the larynx (e.g. by insertion of an endotracheal tube with insufficient anaesthesia). This is mediated by irritant receptors similar to those found in the lungs.

Swallowing

Although usually associated with food, the swallowing reflex can be initiated by other stimuli applied to the dorsum of the tongue, soft palate, and epiglottis. During swallowing, respiration is inhibited in whatever phase of breathing the swallowing is initiated. This aspect of the reflex prevents the inhalation of food. It is interesting that, in newborns, water, sugar solutions, and milk can provoke swallowing, but saline and amniotic fluid will not. The advantage of this to an individual who has spent the last 9 months surrounded by amniotic fluid are obvious. The anatomy of a baby's upper airways predisposes the child to nose breathing, which is an advantage when suckling. (It was once thought that babies were obligate nose breathers, but this is not the case.) When one considers that babies may swallow four times per second while suckling, at the same time as breathing, the very precise integration of these reflexes becomes clear.

Musculoskeletal afferents

Unlike the diaphragm, the skeletal muscles of the chest wall have **muscle spindles** as part of a spinal feedback mechanism. This muscle–spindle mechanism seems to provide a rapid load-detecting system. Any increase in load caused by decreased compliance or increased resistance applied to the respiratory system is rapidly compensated for by an increased drive to the intercostal muscles, which maintains ventilation.

There is still much debate about what exactly causes the increase in ventilation that occurs during exercise. Reflexes from active or passive movements of the limbs are thought to contribute, particularly during the early stages of exercise.

Somatic and visceral reflexes

Visceral and somatic pain generally produce opposite effects on the pattern of breathing. Stretching the intestine or distending the gallbladder or bile ducts inhibits breathing, whereas somatic pain generally causes brief apnoea, followed by rapid, shallow breathing.

A shower of cold water on the bare skin produces a gasp and an increase in minute ventilation by a mechanism that is independent of the unpleasant nature of the experience. Immersing the face in water, particularly cold water, causes apnoea and cardiovascular changes which are called the ***'diving reflex'***; these are seen in more exaggerated form in diving mammals, such as seals.

Cardiovascular afferents

Arterial hypertension can cause reflex hypoventilation or apnoea through stimulation of aortic and carotid baroreceptors. Conversely, hypotension can provoke hyperventilation.

Summary 3

- Human breathing is more voluntarily and less reflexively controlled than that of other animals.
- Afferent nerves from the lungs and from non-pulmonary receptors relay information to the brain to modify the output of the CPG.
- PSR, RAR, and C-fibre receptor activities travel from the lungs to the respiratory centres via the vagus nerve.
- PSRs terminate inspiration and limit V_T.
- RARs produce rapid, shallow breathing and are responsible for sighs.
- Upper airway afferents protect the lungs and have roles in cough, sneeze, laryngospasm, and swallow reflexes.
- Musculoskeletal, somatic, visceral, and cardiovascular afferents can also modify breathing patterns.

Case 9.1 Coning

In addition to providing the link between the spinal cord and the cerebral hemispheres, the brainstem contains essential centres controlling respiration and consciousness. 'Coning' refers to herniation of the brain stem through the foramen magnum at the base of the skull. This occurs as a result of raised intracranial pressure, and results in pressure damage to the vital brainstem. Coning is quickly followed by *brainstem death*, wherein the ability to breathe and be conscious are permanently lost.

John Thompson is a 21-year-old man who was riding his bicycle to work early one dark and wet morning. Although he had bought a cycle helmet, he very rarely wore it and today was no exception. Unfortunately, John was involved in an accident. He turned out of a side-street without looking properly and a car driving at speed hit him from the side, throwing him from his bicycle. John's right leg was broken in two places in the collision, and he struck his head hard on the nearby kerb. John lay unconscious on the road in a pool of blood.

An ambulance arrived quickly, and John was rushed to a nearby trauma centre hospital. Upon arrival, John was found to be deeply unconscious and had a low blood pressure. Because of his reduced conscious level, an endotracheal tube was passed into his trachea and his lungs were artificially ventilated. His leg fractures were stabilised, and he was given blood and other fluids intravenously to increase his blood pressure to normal values. Following this, he was taken to the computed tomography scanner and a brain scan was performed.

In this case we will consider:

1. How raised intracranial pressure occurs, and why it is dangerous.
2. How raised intracranial pressure can be treated.
3. Brainstem death.

How raised intracranial pressure occurs, and why it is dangerous

The scan showed that John had suffered a severe head injury. His skull was fractured and there was extensive evidence of damage to the brain. There were areas of severe bruising to his brain and there had been bleeding into the intracerebral ventricles. The scan also suggested that because of his brain injuries, the pressure inside his skull was high. John was taken to the intensive care unit, sedated, and artificially ventilated. The neurosurgeons inserted a tiny intracranial pressure monitor into the brain through a small hole drilled in his skull. This showed that the pressure within John's skull (intracranial pressure) was very high.

There are many causes of raised intracranial pressure, including brain injury and brain tumours. Raised intracranial pressure is a very serious condition, which can be fatal. The skull is a rigid box containing brain tissue, blood, and cerebrospinal fluid (CSF). The sum of these three volumes is constant; an increase in one component must be compensated by a decrease in one or both remaining components. This is known as the *Monro-Kellie Doctrine*. The volume of the brain may be increased by, for example, bleeding, swelling, tumours, or CSF obstruction. Once the other components can no longer compensate, the volume within the skull increases, followed by an inevitable increase in pressure within the skull. Raised pressure on the brain can result in a reduction in its blood supply. This, in turn, can lead to ischaemia, which can cause swelling of the brain tissue, leading to a further increase in the intracranial pressure. A 'vicious circle' of increasing intracranial pressure can, therefore, be set up.

Treatment of raised intracranial pressure

John's traumatic brain injury was treated with measures to avoid further brain damage by avoiding further increases in intracranial pressure (carbon dioxide level control, avoidance of venous congestion and hyperthermia, optimising analgesia and sedation, osmotherapy) and drugs to augment his mean arterial blood pressure in order to maintain blood supply to the brain. Despite the best efforts of everyone in the intensive care unit, John's condition continued to deteriorate over the following days, and it became increasingly difficult to control his intracranial pressure.

Brainstem death

The largest 'hole' in the skull is the foramen magnum, through which the spinal cord passes. Just above the foramen magnum lies the medulla, in which are contained the respiratory regions. If there is a sudden, large rise in or a prolonged increase in the intracranial pressure, the brainstem is squashed against the edges of the foramen magnum. The rim of the foramen magnum and the nearby skull bones compress the brainstem, reducing the blood supply to the structures it contains (see Fig. 9.3). Once the blood supply to the brainstem ceases, vital structures within it, which are essential to maintaining life, are permanently damaged, leading to death.

After several days, the intensive care doctors decided that John's brainstem was probably no longer functioning. To confirm this, the doctors performed a series of *brainstem death tests*, looking for signs of activity in the cranial nerves (which are found in the brainstem). The final test involved disconnecting John from the ventilator, having oxygenated his lungs with 100% oxygen. During this 'apnoea test' John's lungs were connected to a continuous low flow of oxygen (to avoid desaturation during the test). John did not make any respiratory effort, even after his blood carbon dioxide had been allowed to rise to a level that would be sufficient to stimulate ventilation. After the brainstem death tests had been repeated by the doctors, John was pronounced dead.

Brainstem death tests confirm that the vital areas in the brainstem that are responsible for breathing and consciousness have been irreparably damaged. The heart can function independently of nervous control from the brainstem, such that with ongoing artificial ventilation John's heart would continue to beat. However, he could never be liberated from life support and under these circumstances continuing with intensive care is futile. The diagnosis of brainstem death was explained to John's family and the life-sustaining treatments were subsequently withdrawn, allowing his heart to stop beating.

References and further reading

Berlowitz, D.J., Wadsworth, B., Ross, J., 2016. Respiratory problems and management in people with spinal cord injury. Breathe (Sheff) 12, 328–340.

Dallak, M.A., Pirie, L.J., Davies, A., 2007. The influence of pulmonary receptors on respiratory drive in a rabbit model of pulmonary emphysema. Respir. Physiol. Neurobiol. 156, 33–39.

Davies, A., Roumy, M., 1982. The effect of transient stimulation of lung irritant receptors on the pattern of breathing in rabbits. J. Physiol. 324, 389–401.

Eyzaguirre, C., Zapata, P., 1984. Perspectives in carotid body research. J. Appl. Physiol. Respir. Environ. Exerc. Physiol. 57, 931–957.

Fogarty, M.J., Mantilla, C.B., Sieck, G.C., 2018. Breathing: Motor control of diaphragm muscle. Physiology (Bethesda) 33, 113–126.

Khurana I., Khurana A., Kowlgi N., 2020. Regulation of respiration. In: Textbook of Medical Physiology, 3ed. Elsevier.

Lumb, A., 2011. Ventilatory failure. In: Nunn's Applied Respiratory Physiology. Churchill Livingstone.

Lumb, A.B., Thomas, C.R., 2020. Control of breathing. In: Nunn and Lumb's Applied Respiratory Physiology, ninth ed. Elsevier.

Murphy, P.B., Kumar, A., Reilly, C., et al., 2011. Neural respiratory drive as a physiological biomarker to monitor change during acute exacerbations of COPD. Thorax 66, 602–608.

Severinghaus, J.W., Mitchell, R.A., 1962. Ondines curse: failure of respiratory centre automaticity while asleep. Clin. Res. 10, 122.

Yuki, N., Hartung, H.P., 2012. Guillain–Barré syndrome. N. Engl. J. Med. 366, 2294–2304.

10

CHEMICAL CONTROL OF BREATHING

Chapter objectives

After studying this chapter, you should be able to:

1. Explain the different roles of chemical and neural control of breathing.
2. Define hypoxaemia and hypercapnia.
3. Describe the location and stimulus of the central and peripheral chemoreceptors.
4. State the effects of changes in $PaCO_2$; PaO_2, and $[H^+]$ on breathing.
5. State the relative potency of the above stimuli.
6. Explain how the adaptation of chemoreceptors affects breathing in chronic obstructive pulmonary disease.
7. Describe how anaesthesia affects ventilatory responses to hypoxaemia and hypercapnia.

Introduction

The respiratory system functions to maintain oxygen (O_2) and carbon dioxide (CO_2) at optimal levels in the blood. O_2 consumption and CO_2 production vary according to metabolic rate, and so the breathing pattern and rate must also vary to keep the arterial partial pressures of O_2 (**PaO_2**) and CO_2 (**$PaCO_2$**) within normal ranges. This matching requires monitoring of the chemical composition of arterial blood through sensors called ***chemoreceptors***. The chemoreceptors signal the brain to bring about changes in ventilation (see Fig. 9.1). This process is referred to as the 'chemical control of breathing'.

All control of breathing is fundamentally neural. The chemoreceptors that detect changes in the external environment and the composition of the blood and cerebrospinal fluid comprise the central processors in the brain and the outputs that activate the muscles of breathing are all nerves. However, for ease of understanding, the 'neural' mechanisms involved in the fine control of breathing (see Chapter 9) are discussed separately from the 'chemical' control mechanisms discussed in this chapter.

'Neural control' of breathing refers to the ventilatory pattern produced in the brainstem (modified by pulmonary and non-pulmonary afferent nerves) and transmitted via efferent nerves to produce activity in the respiratory muscles. This neural control differs from the chemical control of breathing with regard to response speed. Neural mechanisms respond in fractions of a second and change the size and duration of individual breaths based on afferent information from the lungs and other sites in the body. Chemical control is normally much slower in its response, changing breathing minute by minute. In essence, chemical control determines **minute ventilation**, whereas neural control determines the most efficient *pattern* to achieve that ventilation with the minimum expenditure of work.

Chemoreceptors can be classified by their anatomical location. Those within the central nervous system are called **central chemoreceptors** and those outside are **peripheral chemoreceptors**. Central chemoreceptors are most sensitive to excess CO_2; peripheral chemoreceptors are most sensitive to a lack of O_2. The whole chemoreceptor system is shown schematically in Figure 10.1.

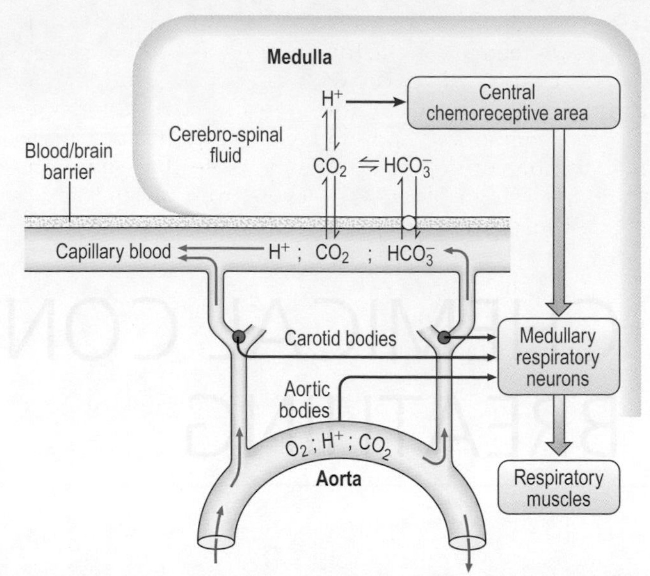

Fig. 10.1 A schematic of the chemoreceptors and structures associated with the chemical control of breathing.

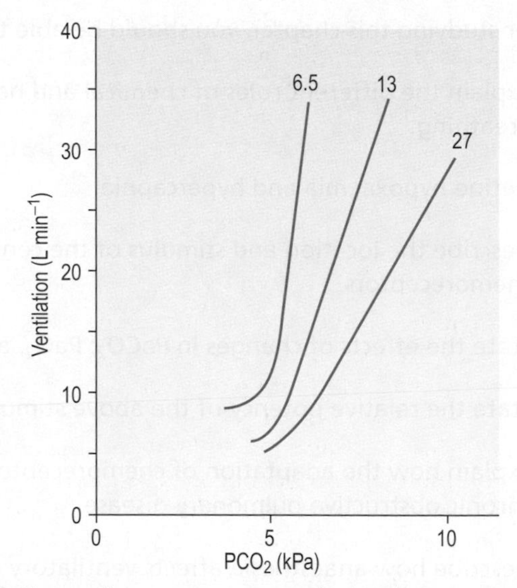

Fig. 10.2 The ventilatory response to asphyxia. The response to varying levels of carbon dioxide at fixed levels of oxygen is shown. This relationship might be equally well demonstrated with fixed levels of carbon dioxide and varying levels of oxygen (Fig. 10.5). PCO_2, partial pressure of carbon dioxide.

Hypercapnia

CO_2 is an acidic gas. **Hypercapnia** (or hypercarbia) refers to high blood CO_2 levels (>6 kPa; >45 mm Hg), while low levels (<4.7 kPa; <35 mm Hg) are called **hypocapnia** (also known as hypocarbia).

The $PaCO_2$ of the blood reaching the brain is the major chemical factor regulating ventilation. Both central and peripheral chemoreceptors have a role in the response to $PaCO_2$ changes. The central chemoreceptors are slower to respond, but account for 80% of the respiratory response, while the peripheral chemoreceptors respond more quickly but only account for 20% of the response.

Ambient air normally contains very little CO_2 (0.03%) and, unlike reductions in PaO_2, any increase in inhaled CO_2 stimulates breathing in a linear manner (Fig. 10.2). On average, increasing a person's PCO_2 by 0.3 kPa will double their minute ventilation. At high $PaCO_2$ levels, that is around 13.3 kPa (100 mm Hg), respiratory fatigue starts to occur, and at higher levels (around 26 kPa or 200 mm Hg) CO_2 *narcosis* can occur, wherein breathing is no longer stimulated, conscious levels drop, and coma and death may ensue. The actual degree of ventilation produced at any PCO_2 level will depend on a number of factors, including respiratory muscle strength, degree of hypoxaemia, and individual or drug-induced variations in chemoreceptor sensitivity. Note that small and acute *decreases* in blood CO_2 levels from normal values (e.g. those caused by singing) do not depress breathing, as demonstrated by the horizontal lower part of the $PCO_2/\dot{V}_E$ curve (Fig. 10.2).

Central chemoreceptors

Anatomy

The central chemoreceptors reside near the ventral surface of the medulla, near the exit of the 9th and 10th cranial nerves (Fig. 10.3A). They are anatomically distinct from the medullary respiratory centres, but they do have connections to the central pattern generator (see Chapter 9). Application of hydrogen ions (H^+) or dissolved CO_2 to the central chemoreceptor area produces an increased frequency of discharge in those neurons and stimulates breathing within seconds. Research has elucidated that the specific stimulus to the central chemoreceptor neurons is intracellular H^+ concentration ($[H^+]$), which is determined primarily by the PCO_2 of the cerebrospinal fluid (CSF).

Function

Central chemoreceptors take a few minutes to respond to changes in $PaCO_2$ because they are separated from the blood by the **blood–brain barrier**. This is a unique physiological barrier which tightly regulates the movement of substances between the blood and the brain (Fig. 10.3B). The blood–brain barrier is composed of specialised capillary endothelial cells (joined by tight junctions), a basement membrane, and astrocytes. The activity of the blood–brain barrier makes the CSF bathing the brain and spinal cord the most closely controlled environment in the body. Lipid-soluble molecules, such as O_2 and CO_2, diffuse freely between the blood plasma and the brain. In contrast, ions such as H^+ and bicarbonate (HCO_3^-) move under strict control and are often pumped against their concentration gradients by active transport when it is necessary to control the environment of the brain.

The central chemoreceptors are surrounded by the brain extracellular fluid (ECF). When blood PCO_2 rises, CO_2 diffuses from the cerebral blood vessels into the CSF. This displaces the reaction:

$$CO_2 + H_2O \leftrightarrow H_2CO_3 \leftrightarrow HCO_3^- + H^+$$

to the right, producing H^+, which stimulate the central chemoreceptors. This causes an increase in ventilation,

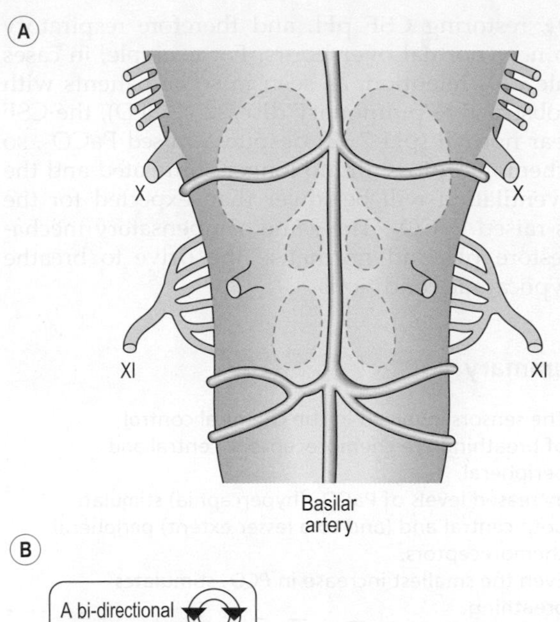

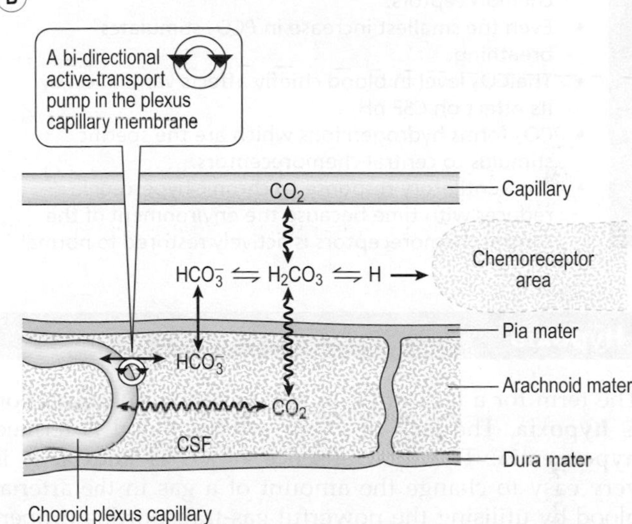

Fig. 10.3 Central chemoreceptive areas of the brain. (A) These are not the traditional 'respiratory centres' dealt with in Chapter 9. (B) Their environment is closely controlled by the blood–brain barrier which is permeable to the passive diffusion of carbon dioxide and actively transports bicarbonate ions. CSF, cerebrospinal fluid.

which lowers the blood PCO_2 back towards normal. It is difficult to see, at first glance, why the above reaction, which produces both acid (H^+) and base (HCO_3^-), acidifies a solution (but remember, it is the *ratio* of $[H^+]/[HCO_3^-]$ that determines acidity, and there is a lower concentration of H^+ than HCO_3^- in plasma; therefore, the addition of one of each of the ions has a proportionately bigger effect on $[H^+]$ (see Chapter 8). Note that increases in arterial $[H^+]$ do not affect the central chemoreceptors, if the $PaCO_2$ is kept constant, because the blood–brain barrier is relatively impermeable to H^+.

The ion-pumping activity of the blood–brain barrier is particularly important in compensating for chronic disturbances in the composition of the CSF, such as occur in chronic lung disease. If the CSF PCO_2 remains at a raised level, there will be a compensatory increase in HCO_3^-, restoring CSF pH, and therefore respiratory drive, to near normal over hours. For example, in cases of chronic CO_2 retention, as seen in some patients with chronic obstructive pulmonary disease (COPD), the CSF pH is near normal (pH 7.32) despite a raised $PaCO_2$, so central chemoreceptors are no longer stimulated and the minute ventilation will be lower than expected for the patient's raised $PaCO_2$. The same compensatory mechanisms restore pH and normalise the drive to breathe under hypocapnic conditions.

Summary 1

- The sensors involved in the chemical control of breathing are chemoreceptors: central and peripheral.
- Increased levels of $PaCO_2$ (hypercapnia) stimulate both central and (and to a lesser extent) peripheral chemoreceptors.
- Even the smallest increase in PCO_2 stimulates breathing.
- The CO_2 level in blood chiefly affects ventilation by its effect on CSF pH.
- CO_2 forms hydrogen ions which are the specific stimulus to central chemoreceptors.
- The ventilatory response to chronic hypercapnia reduces with time because the environment of the central chemoreceptors is actively restored to normal.

Hypoxia

The term for a lack of O_2 in any gas mixture or solution is **hypoxia**. The lack of O_2 in arterial blood is termed **hypoxaemia**. The total absence of O_2 is **anoxia**. It is very easy to change the amount of a gas in the arterial blood by utilising the powerful gas-transporting properties of the lungs. Simply giving a subject a gas mixture to breathe will result in his or her arterial blood taking on the composition of that gas mixture within remarkably few breaths. The rate at which equilibrium is reached depends on the solubility of the gas in body fluids, and this has important consequences in anaesthesia. However, for the gases we are concerned with here, equilibrium is approached within a few dozen breaths.

Hypoxaemia produces a compensatory increase in ventilation mediated through the peripheral chemoreceptors.

Peripheral chemoreceptors

Anatomy and histology

The peripheral chemoreceptors comprise the **carotid bodies** and the **aortic bodies**, both of which lie close to the output of the left ventricle and thereby sense hypoxaemia in the blood leaving the heart.

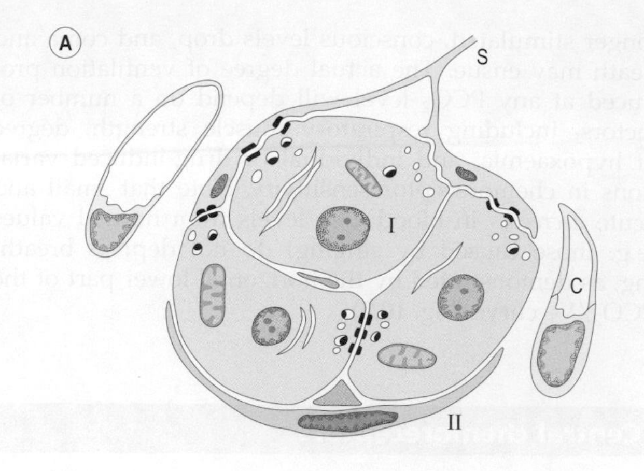

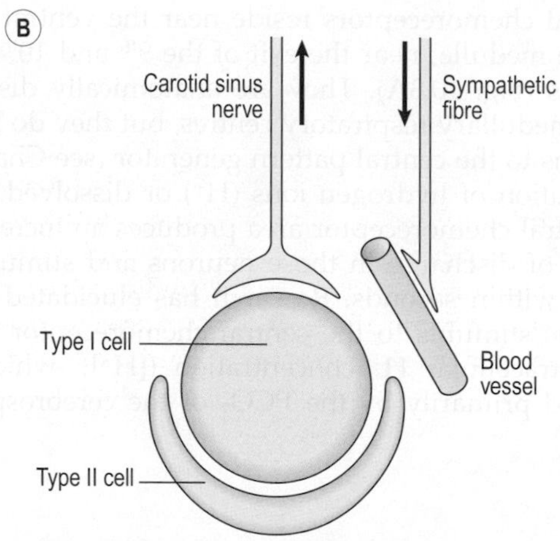

Fig. 10.4 (A) Sketch of cells of the carotid body. I, *type I* cell; II, *type II* sustentacular cell; C, capillary; S, sensory nerve. (B) Schematic of the cell types and nerve fibres of the carotid body.

In humans, it is the carotid bodies that are mainly responsible for the respiratory response. They are small (3–5-mm diameter) nodules of ***glomus*** tissue (from Latin: a skein or ball of thread, i.e. a knot of capillaries) situated near the bifurcation of each common carotid artery in the neck. The carotid bodies must not be confused with the **baroreceptor** region of the carotid arteries which regulates blood pressure.

The function of the carotid bodies is related to their unusual structure. They have an extremely high metabolic rate (about three times that of the brain) and the highest perfusion per gram of tissue of any organ in the body. The chemoreceptor tissue is made up of type I (or glomus) cells which respond to hypoxaemia by releasing excitatory neurotransmitters (e.g. acetylcholine and dopamine), which in turn stimulate nearby carotid sinus nerve endings, leading to an increase in discharges to the brain (Fig. 10.4A and B). The type I cells are supported by type II (sustentacular) cells, which behave as stem cell precursors for glomus cells under chronic hypoxic conditions.

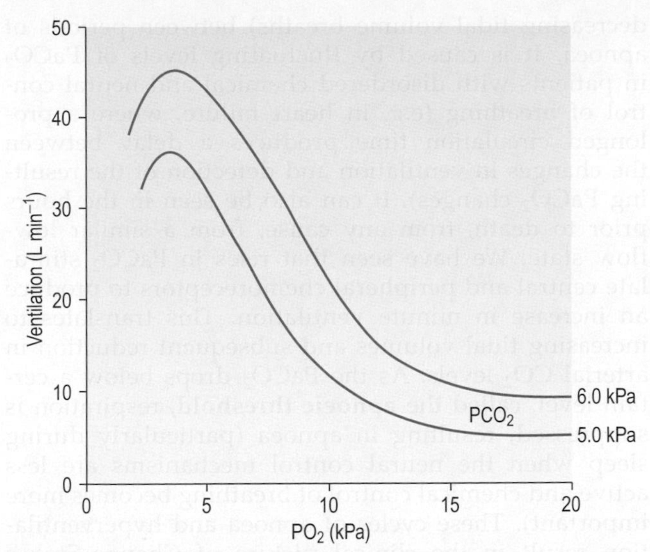

Fig. 10.5 The relationship between minute ventilation and inhaled oxygen tension. The relationship at two levels of carbon dioxide is shown. PCO_2, partial pressure of carbon dioxide; PO_2, partial pressure of oxygen.

The carotid sinus nerve, a branch of the glossopharyngeal nerve, also provides sympathetic and parasympathetic innervation *to* the carotid bodies. A separate supply of sympathetic fibres from the nearby superior cervical ganglion innervates the carotid bodies' blood vessels. Drugs that stimulate the sympathetic ganglia, such as nicotine, can increase ventilation through their effects on the peripheral chemoreceptors.

Function

During **eupnoea,** under normoxic conditions, most of the **drive to breathe** comes from central chemoreceptors, and also from the neural mechanisms associated with wakefulness. However, the peripheral chemoreceptors also contribute to the drive to breathe, as evidenced by the observation that $PaCO_2$ is elevated by up to 0.8 kPa in patients subjected to carotid body denervation.

Peripheral chemoreceptors are stimulated by hypoxaemia, hypercapnia, acidaemia, or hypoperfusion. Stimulation produces an increase in the rate and depth of breathing, but also produces hypertension through peripheral vasoconstriction and increases in heart rate and adrenal secretion.

Hypoxic stimulation

The effect of decreasing a subject's PaO_2 by giving them increasingly hypoxic gas to breathe is shown in Figure 10.5. Activity in the carotid bodies (measured experimentally as the frequency of action potential discharges in the carotid sinus nerve) is low during normoxia, but the discharge frequency starts to increase as PaO_2 drops. This is signalled to the dorsal respiratory group (see Chapter 9) via the carotid sinus nerves/glossopharyngeal nerves and is translated into an increase in minute ventilation to increase O_2 uptake in the lungs. There are a few points to note here:

- PaO_2 must be reduced considerably before there is stimulation of breathing, but then the increase in ventilation is large.
- Very low PO_2 levels depress breathing. This is through a direct effect on the respiratory centres in the brainstem.
- Increasing PaO_2 above normal (13 kPa) by inhaling O_2-rich mixtures only produces a small reduction in breathing by depressing chemoreceptor activity.
- The carotid bodies respond to $\mathbf{PaO_2}$ rather than the ***total blood oxygen content.*** This means conditions like carbon monoxide poisoning and anaemia have little effect on ventilation through the peripheral chemoreceptors.
- On a cellular level, hypoxia inhibits the activity of O_2-sensitive potassium channels on the glomus cell membrane. This alters the membrane potential of the cell, opening calcium channels. The resulting calcium influx stimulates excitatory neurotransmitter (e.g. acetylcholine and adenosine triphosphate) release. These neurotransmitters stimulate the carotid sinus neurons. Drugs like doxapram, which inhibit the potassium channels, produce an increase in the rate and depth of breathing through the same mechanism.

We have seen that hypoxaemia has to be quite pronounced before it produces an effect on breathing (Fig 10.5). Why is there such a modest response to the lack of such a vital substance?

The answer is that it would be a waste of time having a more sensitive detector of O_2 levels because the shape of the oxyhaemoglobin dissociation curve would defeat its sensitivity. You can see from the oxyhaemoglobin dissociation curve (see Chapter 8) that even if PO_2 is reduced to 8 kPa, the haemoglobin is still 90% saturated. Also, PO_2 can rise to infinity and haemoglobin can only be 100% saturated. This useful situation means that ventilation of the lungs can halve or double without the amount of O_2 being carried changing very much. But, by the same token, a mechanism that relied on O_2 saturation to control breathing under normal circumstances would lack sensitivity, because saturation does not change much over a large range of partial pressures.

The importance of the peripheral chemoreceptors lies in the fact that they are the only mechanism in the body by which low O_2 tension can stimulate breathing, and when tension falls sufficiently, this stimulation is very vigorous.

Hypoxic stimulation of breathing is opposed by changes in CO_2 and H^+ levels because, as breathing begins to be stimulated, CO_2 is washed out of the blood, the arterial $[H^+]$ falls, and the drive to breathe (from

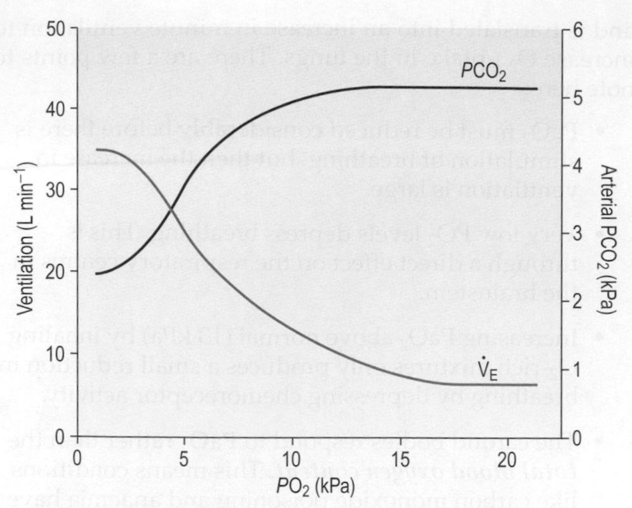

Fig. 10.6 The hypocapnic brake. Increased *ventilation* caused by hypoxia washes carbon dioxide out, the reduced partial pressure of carbon dioxide (PCO_2) reduces drive to breathe; thus, the overall response is less than if the PCO_2 was maintained. PO_2, partial pressure of oxygen.

these two sources) is reduced, producing what is sometimes called the ***hypocapnic brake*** (Fig. 10.6). Just how powerful a drive to breathe hypoxia can be is demonstrated by abolishing this braking effect by adding CO_2 to the inspired air to keep its levels constant in the blood. With a constant PCO_2 level, hypoxia produces 10 times the effect produced if CO_2 is allowed to be washed out.

Hypercapnic stimulation

Hypercapnia stimulates peripheral chemoreceptor activity, probably by increasing [H^+] within the glomus cells in the same way that an increased intracellular acidity increases central chemoreceptor activity, but the peripheral chemoreceptors are not as sensitive to increases in $PaCO_2$. The position of the central chemoreceptors behind the blood–brain barrier results in the following two key differences in their stimulation:

- Peripheral chemoreceptors respond more quickly. The carotid and aortic bodies respond to changes in CO_2 and H^+ levels within seconds, whereas the central chemoreceptors rely on CO_2 diffusion across a barrier and hence take minutes to respond.
- Increasing arterial [H^+] does not have a great effect on central chemoreceptors (because the blood–brain barrier is relatively impermeable to ions) but does stimulate peripheral chemoreceptors.

Cheyne–Stokes breathing

Cheyne–Stokes breathing is a specific form of waxing and waning respiration, characterised by a crescendo-decrescendo pattern of breathing (increasing and decreasing tidal volume breaths) between periods of apnoea. It is caused by fluctuating levels of $PaCO_2$ in patients with disordered chemical and neural control of breathing (e.g. in heart failure, where a prolonged circulation time produces a delay between the changes in ventilation and detection of the resulting $PaCO_2$ changes). It can also be seen in the hours prior to death, from any cause, from a similar low-flow state. We have seen that rises in $PaCO_2$ stimulate central and peripheral chemoreceptors to produce an increase in minute ventilation. This translates to increasing tidal volumes and subsequent reduction in arterial CO_2 levels. As the $PaCO_2$ drops below a certain level, called the **apnoeic threshold**, respiration is suppressed, resulting in apnoea (particularly during sleep when the neural control mechanisms are less active and chemical control of breathing becomes more important). These cycles of apnoea and hyperventilation result in the clinical picture of Cheyne–Stokes breathing.

Long-term hypoxic stimulation

The response of the body to sustained hypoxia of the kind one encounters at high altitudes or when the lungs are so damaged by disease that they cannot efficiently transfer O_2 to the blood differs from the acute response described above.

The ventilatory response to hypoxaemia depends on the duration of hypoxia. For example, in adult human subjects, hypoxia lasting for about an hour produces an immediate increase in ventilation (within 3–5 minutes) followed by a decrease to a steady state level that is higher than the control, normoxic level. This occurs even when $PaCO_2$ is kept constant; this phenomenon is called ***hypoxic ventilatory decline***. This may be due to hypoxic central nervous system depression. As the duration of hypoxia increases, so does ventilation (Fig. 10.7). The rate of ventilation then stabilises at a value greater than the response to acute hypoxia. This is thought to be due to an increased sensitivity of the carotid body.

In even longer-lasting hypoxaemia, such as that seen in people living at high altitudes, the peripheral chemoreceptor response is modified by CSF and renal compensatory mechanisms. This is known as ***ventilatory acclimatisation***. Reduced PaO_2 causes stimulation of the peripheral chemoreceptors, which in turn increase ventilation. This hyperventilation washes CO_2 from the blood and CSF, and they become more alkaline, reducing the drive to breathe (mainly at the central chemoreceptors) below the increased level that is appropriate for the reduced atmospheric PO_2. After a day or two, the active transport system of the blood–brain barrier returns the [H^+] of the CSF to normal. This restored drive from increased CO_2/[H^+] levels again increases ventilation. Within a few weeks at a high altitude, the

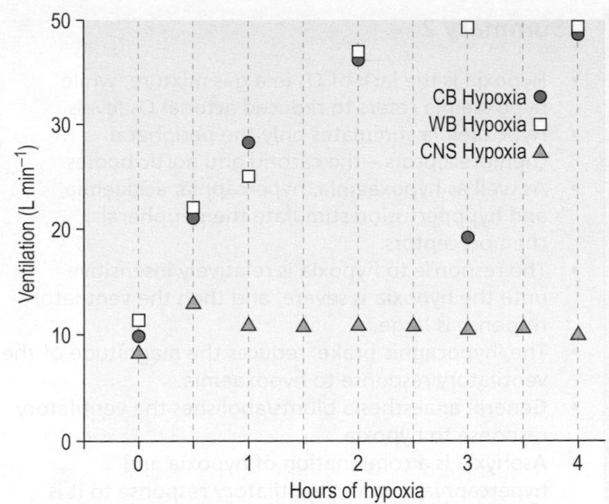

Fig. 10.7 Ventilatory acclimatisation to hypoxia. This type of acclimatisation is called acclimatisation to short-term hypoxia, although it takes place over hours, to distinguish it from long-term acclimatisation that occurs over years or a lifetime. The graph shows that *hypoxia* of the carotid body (CB) has the same effect as whole body hypoxia (WB) while hypoxia of the central nervous system (CNS) has little effect.

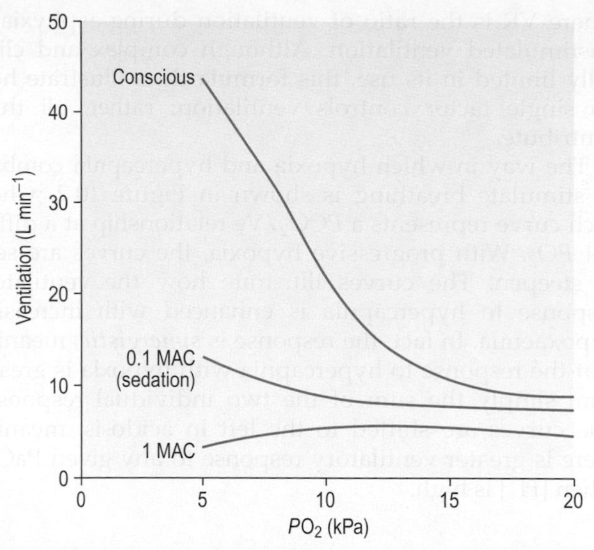

Fig. 10.8 Effect of anaesthesia on hypoxic response. General anaesthesia can almost abolish sensitivity to hypoxia. Response to carbon dioxide is maintained. MAC, minimal alveolar concentration; PO_2, partial pressure of oxygen.

kidneys excrete extra HCO_3^- and restore blood $[H^+]$, which, together with the hypoxic drive to the peripheral chemoreceptors, stimulates breathing to an appropriate level.

Some unfortunate patients with prolonged hypoxaemia due to respiratory disease do not make this compensation, particularly if they are of the type picturesquely described as a 'blue bloater'. This description relates to patients with COPD who have marked arterial hypoxaemia and CO_2 retention but do not seem to be breathless. They are blue because they are cyanosed and bloated by congestive heart failure. These patients have adapted to high $PaCO_2$, and so the majority of their drive to breathe comes from the hypoxaemia detected by the peripheral chemoreceptors. These individuals are particularly at risk if they receive O_2 therapy, as dangerous hypoventilation and type II respiratory failure can ensue if their vital hypoxic drive to breathe is abolished.

Effects of anaesthesia on chemical control of breathing

Anaesthesia involving muscle relaxant drugs abolishes all chemical and neural responses to ventilation as the final effectors, the respiratory muscles, are paralysed. Patients can continue to breathe spontaneously under general anaesthesia which does not involve muscle relaxant drugs. However, anaesthetic drugs affect the normal ventilatory responses to hypoxaemia. The peripheral chemoreceptors are extremely sensitive to inhalation anaesthetics (Fig. 10.8), such that with an increasing depth of anaesthesia, the response to hypoxia is abolished ('MAC' refers to minimal alveolar concentration and is a measure of the depth of anaesthesia). However, the ventilatory response to hypercapnia is maintained. The consequences of this for patients with lung disease who are receiving anaesthesia are important. They cannot respond when challenged by hypoxia and, if of the 'blue bloater' type, they have already lost their CO_2-based drive to breathe, will stop breathing when the anaesthesia abolishes their drive from hypoxia. You can see from Figure 10.8 that quite low levels of anaesthesia, of the order of those found in the postoperative period, when the patient appears able to look after himself, can seriously blunt the response to hypoxia. Hence the need for close intra- and postoperative monitoring of patients receiving general anaesthesia. Note that deep anaesthesia abolishes all ventilatory efforts, probably by a direct effect on the brainstem respiratory centres.

Asphyxia

It is rare for the arterial PO_2, PCO_2, or $[H^+]$ of a healthy individual to change without changes in the other two. The stimulus to breathe that builds up during asphyxia, or when you hold your breath, involves changes in all three of these variables.

The overall effects of changes in arterial PO_2, PCO_2, and [H+] are described by a formula devised by Gray, in 1945:

$$VR = 0.22\ [H^+] + 0.26\ PCO_2 - 18 + 105 / 10^{0.038}\ PO_2$$

where VR is the ratio of ventilation during asphyxia to unstimulated ventilation. Although complex and clinically limited in its use, this formula does illustrate how no single factor controls ventilation; rather, all three contribute.

The way in which hypoxia and hypercapnia combine to stimulate breathing is shown in Figure 10.2, where each curve represents a PCO_2/V_E relationship at a different PO_2. With progressive hypoxia, the curves are seen to steepen. The curves illustrate how the ventilatory response to hypercapnia is enhanced with increasing hypoxaemia. In fact, the response is ***synergistic***, meaning that the response to hypercapnia with hypoxia is greater than simply the sum of the two individual responses. The curves are shifted to the left in acidosis, meaning there is greater ventilatory response to any given $PaCO_2$ when $[H^+]$ is high.

Summary 2

- Hypoxia is the lack of O_2 in a gas mixture, while hypoxaemia refers to reduced arterial O_2 levels.
- Hypoxaemia stimulates only the peripheral chemoreceptors – the carotid and aortic bodies.
- As well as hypoxaemia, hypercapnia, acidaemia, and hypoperfusion stimulate the peripheral chemoreceptors.
- The response to hypoxia is relatively insensitive until the hypoxia is severe, and then the ventilatory response is large.
- The 'hypocapnic brake' reduces the magnitude of the ventilatory response to hypoxaemia.
- General anaesthesia blunts/abolishes the ventilatory response to hypoxia.
- Asphyxia is a combination of hypoxia and hypercapnia, and the ventilatory response to it is greater than the response to the sum of its parts.

Case 10.1

Chemical control of breathing: 1

Chronic obstructive pulmonary disease

Mrs Andrews is a 69-year-old lady who suffers from COPD. This has been brought about by many years of heavy smoking – Mrs Andrews smokes 30 cigarettes per day and has done so since she was a teenager. Mrs Andrews has a cough that is usually productive of white sputum. She often feels breathless and 'wheezy' and takes two bronchodilator drugs via an inhaler. She frequently suffers from chest infections that are usually treated with antibiotics by her doctor.

One winter, Mrs Andrews contracted a particularly severe chest infection. She had a cough productive of large volumes of green sputum and became very breathless. Her general practitioner decided to admit her to the hospital for treatment.

In the hospital, Mrs Andrews was found to be cyanosed and her arterial blood gases indicated that she was hypoxic with a PaO_2 of 6.2 kPa. Her blood gases also indicated that her $PaCO_2$ was raised, at 7.3 kPa. Initially, she was given oxygen to breathe. Although this resulted in the PaO_2 increasing to 10.8 kPa, it also resulted in an increase in $PaCO_2$ to 8.4 kPa. At this stage, she was becoming very breathless, and the effort of breathing was starting to exhaust her. The decision was taken to artificially ventilate her lungs while she received treatment for her infection, and she was taken to the intensive care unit.

In this case we will consider:

1. What causes COPD.
2. The clinical features of COPD.
3. O_2 therapy and COPD.

What causes chronic obstructive pulmonary disease?

COPD is nearly always the result of long-term smoking. It results in changes throughout the respiratory system, from the large airways to the alveoli, as a result of prolonged irritation by smoke.

In the larger airways, there is inflammation of the airway mucosa, accompanied by an increase in the thickness of the airway wall and an increase in the mucus-secreting glands. Smaller airways are also inflamed and may be significantly narrowed or obstructed by secretions. This narrowing and obstruction of the smaller airways results in the characteristic increase in airway resistance that is a defining feature of COPD.

There is a generalised loss of lung tissue with the destruction of alveoli and pulmonary capillaries and the loss of supporting connective tissue. The loss of alveoli and capillaries results in a very significant impairment of gas exchange as a result of a severe mismatch between ventilation and perfusion. The loss of connective tissue means that there is a generalised increase in the lung volume as a whole, but very little of this additional volume is ventilated. The loss of connective tissue also tends to worsen the narrowing of the smaller airways. This is because these airways rely on tension in the surrounding connective tissue to keep their lumens patent; unlike the larger airways, they do not have cartilage or other supportive tissue in their walls.

COPD used to be termed 'chronic bronchitis and emphysema', a name which related to the airway inflammation (chronic bronchitis) and the loss of alveolar tissue (emphysema). However, the newer term emphasises the usually single aetiology behind the condition as well as emphasising the airways obstruction, which is a cardinal feature of the condition.

Case 10.1 Chemical control of breathing: 1 – cont'd

Clinical features of chronic obstructive pulmonary disease

COPD is characterised by a chronic, productive cough. The sputum is generally white, but during periods of airway infection it may become thick and green coloured. As the disease progresses, patients become increasingly breathless upon exertion and, in severe cases, may become breathless at rest. Upon examination, patients with COPD often have a hyperinflated chest and may have an audible wheeze. They may be centrally cyanosed and may exhale through pursed lips in an attempt to increase their airway pressure and therefore keep their smaller airways open. Upon auscultation, there may be widespread wheeze throughout the chest and coarse crackles may also be heard. In the early stages of the disease, spirometry usually reveals an obstructive pattern with a reduction in the forced expiratory volume in one second, but in more severe cases, a restrictive pattern with a reduction in forced vital capacity is seen. Chest X-rays reveal a hyperinflated chest and may show changes due to lung infection, if this is present.

The impaired gas exchange that occurs as a result of COPD means that there is a reduction in PaO_2. Initially, the $PaCO_2$ is normal, as an increase in minute ventilation can compensate, to some extent, for the failing lung function. However, in severe cases and during acute exacerbations of the disease, the $PaCO_2$ starts to rise.

Treatment of COPD is largely symptomatic. Patients are encouraged to give up smoking, often with only limited success. Acute infections are treated with antibiotics, when required. Patients often derive some benefit from inhaled bronchodilators, such as the beta-adrenergic agonist salbutamol, and anticholinergic drugs, such as ipratropium. Whereas in asthmatic patients, beta-adrenergic agents are generally thought to be more effective bronchodilators than anticholinergics, in patients with COPD, these two types of agents are often equally effective. Patients may administer bronchodilators via an inhaler device, but they may require a nebuliser to obtain an adequate dose of bronchodilator drug during the later stages of the disease. In some patients, inhaled steroids may also bring about an improvement. In very severe cases of COPD, gas exchange is so impaired that the patient needs additional O_2 on a long-term basis, including O_2 therapy at home.

Oxygen therapy and COPD

Why did Mrs Andrews' $PaCO_2$ start to rise when she received O_2 therapy? We have seen that in normal individuals, the $PaCO_2$ is what determines ventilation on a minute-to-minute basis. A rise in $PaCO_2$ is detected by the central chemoreceptors (and, to a lesser extent, by the peripheral chemoreceptors) and this provokes an increase in minute ventilation that, in turn, tends to bring the $PaCO_2$ back towards normal. In a small subgroup of patients with severe COPD, this mechanism for controlling ventilation fails. In these patients, the $PaCO_2$ is higher than normal, and their ventilatory response to CO_2 is very much reduced or even absent. For these individuals, the ventilatory response to hypoxia is vital. The chronic hypoxia resulting from COPD is their 'stimulus' to breathe. If these patients are given supplementary oxygen to breathe, their PaO_2 rises and the magnitude of this stimulus is reduced, and their minute ventilation may start to decline. This will, in turn, result in an increase in PCO_2. In very severe cases, the increase is $PaCO_2$ may be so large that it actually results in a further decrease in ventilation (remember that although CO_2 usually *stimulates* ventilation, at very high concentrations it can act on the respiratory centres to *inhibit* ventilation).

In a small number of patients with COPD, O_2 therapy may therefore result in an increase in $PaCO_2$, and occasionally this increase can be dangerous. It is important to stress, however, that this occurs only in a small minority of COPD patients. It does mean, though, that O_2 therapy in these patients has to be administered with care (using Venturi masks that administer a known concentration of O_2) including regular monitoring of blood gases. However, hypoxia is usually more dangerous than a rise in CO_2, which, in any case, usually takes a while to happen. For this reason, it is very important that O_2 therapy not be withheld from patients with COPD. Where an increase in $PaCO_2$ is provoked by O_2 therapy, the patient will often require artificial ventilation, as occurred in Mrs Andrews' case.

References and further reading

Brown, J.P.R., Grocott, M.P.W. 2013. Humans at altitude: physiology and pathophysiology. BJA Educ. 13 (1), 17–22.

Fitzgerald, R.S., Eyzaguirre, C., Zapata, P. 2009. Fifty years of progress in carotid body physiology. In: Gonzalez, C., Nurse, C.A., Peers, C. (Eds.), Arterial Chemoreceptors, vol. 648. Springer, Dordrecht, p. 19.

Global Initiative for Chronic Obstructive Lung Disease (GOLD). Global Strategy for the Diagnosis, Management and Prevention of Chronic Obstructive Pulmonary Disease. 2020 Report. http://www.goldcopd.org.

Lumb, A., Thomas, C. 2020. Control of breathing. In: Nunn and Lumb's Applied Respiratory Physiology, ninth ed. Elsevier.

Martin, D., Windsor, J. 2008. From mountain to bedside: understanding the clinical relevance of human acclimatisation to high-altitude hypoxia. Postgrad. Med. 84 (998), 622–627.

Naughton, M.T. 1998. Pathophysiology and treatment of Cheyne-Stokes respiration. Thorax 53 (6), 514–518.

West, J.B. 1990. Ventilation/Blood Flow and Gas Exchange, fifth ed. Blackwell Science, Oxford.

11

LUNG FUNCTION TESTS

Chapter objectives

After studying this chapter, you should be able to:

1. Appreciate that lung function tests quantify disability of function. Diagnoses are usually based on the patient's clinical history.
2. Explain spirometry and outline the changes in static and dynamic measurements caused by restrictive and obstructive disease.
3. Describe how flow/volume loops are obtained, and the changes caused by chronic obstructive pulmonary disease.
4. Outline the principles of plethysmography.
5. Explain blood gas analysis.
6. Describe washout techniques for measuring ventilation/perfusion ($\dot{V}/\dot{Q}$) inequalities
7. Explain the need for functional testing.

Introduction

Lung function tests enable quantitative measurements to be made of the effect of disease on the functioning of the respiratory system. These tests range from the relatively simple to those undertaken in a specialised lung function laboratory. Most tests involve comparing the results obtained from a patient to standard results from comparable healthy subjects and are often presented as the absolute value alongside the percentage of the predicted value for that subject.

Measuring lung volumes and capacities

Spirometry

The simple spirometer described in Chapter 5 (Fig. 5.2) provides much useful information about a patient's lungs. Its use allows the measurement of the following static lung volumes: **vital capacity (VC), tidal volume, inspiratory reserve, and expiratory reserve volumes**. Large people have larger lungs than small people, and age exerts a deleterious effect on lung function. Extensive study of these relationships has provided us with tables which, for example, relate height to VC (see Appendix), allowing the comparison of expected and actual values obtained by testing a subject.

Measurements made using a spirometer may be classified as:

- ***Static***, where the only consideration is the volume exhaled, or
- ***Dynamic***, where the time taken to exhale a certain volume is being measured.

Forced vital capacity and forced expired volume in one second

Although measurements such as inspiratory reserve volume and expiratory reserve volume can be informative, the most usual and useful static spirometric test is the ***forced vital capacity*** (FVC). This is 'forced' because the subject must breathe in and out to the full extent that they are able (Fig. 11.1). This test can be classed as static because it does not involve an element of time, but it is often combined with a dynamic test, the ***forced expired volume in one second*** (FEV_1). Here, the subject inhales as much as they can and then exhales as forcefully as they can. The volume breathed out in 1 second is the FEV_1.

An FEV_1 is commonly expressed as a percentage or ratio of the FVC. This takes into account the problem that a small person (with small but perfectly healthy lungs) would be unable to breathe out the same volume in a second as a larger person whose lungs may not be so healthy. The FEV_1/FVC ratio is the ratio of the forced expiratory volume in the first one second to the forced vital capacity of the lungs. The normal value for this ratio is greater than 0.75–0.85 (i.e. one expects a healthy person to force out at least 75% of their vital capacity in 1 second). Using this percentage alone can create problems in restrictive lung diseases (diseases that restrict the expansion of the lungs). In these diseases both the VC and the FEV_1 are reduced; therefore in those cases, that percentage may remain normal. For this reason, both absolute values and percentages are measured.

Characteristic traces in normal subjects and patients with obstructive (e.g. chronic obstructive emphysematous or bronchitic lung disease) or restrictive (e.g. fibrotic) lung diseases are shown in Figure 11.1.

Obstructive patterns of lung disease can be described as reversible (typical in asthma) or irreversible (typical in chronic obstructive pulmonary disease (COPD)).

Helium dilution, nitrogen washout, and plethysmography

Because a subject cannot breathe out their **residual volume** (RV), dilution and plethysmographic methods must be used to measure the residual volume and the capacities that include the RV. These are the **total lung capacity** (TLC), ***functional residual capacity*** (FRC) and *the* RV itself. The most usual approach is to measure the FRC and use this to derive the others. The TLC and FRC are frequently increased in diseases such as asthma, bronchitis, and emphysema, in which both increased airway resistance and gas trapping occur. Increased FRC and TLC, in these patients, is the result of reduced lung recoil and breathing at increased lung volumes in an attempt to keep the airways open. Restrictive lung diseases decrease the TLC, FRC, RV, and VC, with the RV frequently being the first to be affected. Care should be taken in interpreting results from obese patients, where the outward recoil of the chest wall is reduced, resulting in lower FRC values.

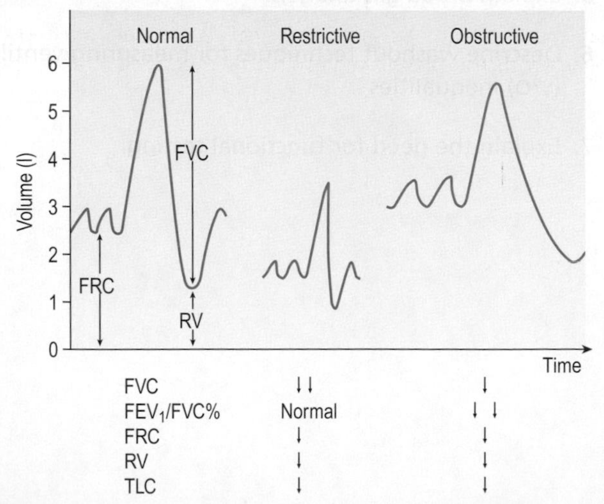

Fig. 11.1 Spirometry. Changes in lung volumes measured by spirometry that occur due to *restrictive* or *obstructive* disease. FEV_1, forced expiratory volume in 1 second; FRC, functional residual capacity; FVC, forced vital capacity; RV, residual volume; TLC, total lung capacity.

To measure the FRC, the helium dilution method can be used. The patient breathes out to FRC and is then connected to a spirometer of known volume containing helium at a known concentration. The patient breathes normally for an appropriate length of time and the dilution of the helium by the FRC in the lungs is measured. Oxygen is added at the same rate as it is used up to keep the overall volume in the lungs plus spirometer constant (Fig. 11.2).

Alternatively, a **nitrogen wash-out technique** may be used. Here, the subject breathes, from FRC, from a bag containing a known volume of 100% oxygen. They then breathe out into the bag. Because the air in the FRC contained approximately 80% nitrogen, the dilution of this by the known volume of pure oxygen in the bag enables the volume to be calculated.

The total body **plethysmograph** is described in Chapter 4 and consists of an airtight box in which the subject sits. To understand the principles on which this instrument works, consider the subject's chest as a syringe with the diaphragm represented by the plunger. Understanding Boyle's law (see Appendix) is helpful in understanding this instrument: $P \propto 1/V$, where P = pressure and V = volume.

The subject first pants against a closed shutter, that is, the neck of the syringe is blocked.

The technique is as shown in Figure 11.3, where a large, enclosed volume of gas (the contents of the box) surrounds a small, enclosed volume of gas (the air in the lungs) which increases and decreases in volume as it is compressed or decompressed. This change in volume of the syringe compresses and decompresses the air in the box, and the pressure in the box varies inversely with the pressure in the lungs. Measuring the pressure changes in the box while the subject pants against a closed shutter enables us to calculate the pressure within the lungs and, therefore (using Boyle's law), calculate lung volume.

Plethysmography is used to measure lung volumes in patients with severe airflow obstructions in preference to the helium dilution or nitrogen washout techniques. This is because, in these patients, the air trapping is so severe that the helium cannot get to the collapsed, closed-off volumes in the lungs, which are therefore not taken into account. In plethysmography, however, these closed-off volumes are still subject to the gas laws (see Appendix) on which this technique is based.

The principle of the relationship between box pressure and airway pressure does not depend on the 'syringe', which represents the lungs being closed. In Figure 11.3B, the narrow tube represents the resistance of the airways and, despite air being forced into or out of the syringe, the relationship between this driving pressure and box pressure still holds. In this case, by measuring the driving alveolar pressure (by measuring box pressure) and flow (using a pneumotachograph), we can also measure airway resistance.

Although plethysmography offers an accurate way to measure a number of pulmonary variables, one of its major limitations is that many subjects object to being locked inside an airtight box!

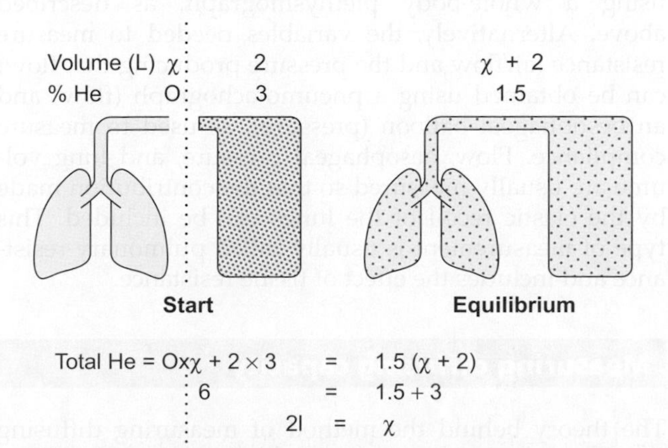

Fig. 11.2 Helium (He) dilution. Helium dilution is used to measure lung *volumes* that cannot be measured by direct spirometry (functional residual capacity and residual volume).

Measuring Flow

Peak expiratory flow is the maximum expiratory flow (expressed as $L\ s^{-1}$ or $L\ min^{-1}$) that a subject can produce. Of course, this is dependent on the subject's motivation, even with healthy lungs. The advantage of the peak flow measurement is that it can be made using a simple apparatus into which the subject blows against a paddle or propeller, which then records flow. Although not precise, this has been found to be a useful domiciliary measurement for patients with asthma, with the patient keeping a diary of their progress.

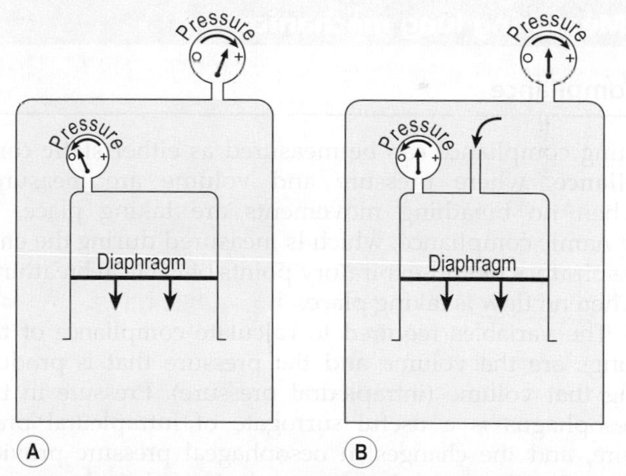

Fig. 11.3 The principle of the plethysmograph. The plethysmograph is an airtight box in which the subject sits. It can be used to measure air *pressure* within the subject's lungs. To understand the principle on which it works, consider the subject's chest as a 'syringe' in which the diaphragm represents the plunger, and the 'neck' of the syringe represents the conducting airways of the lungs. In (A) the neck of the syringe is closed off (mouth closed). Lowering the plunger reduces the *pressure* in the lungs and compresses the air in the box, raising its *pressure*. Raising the plunger has the opposite effect. By measuring airway *pressure* and box *pressure* simultaneously, while the subject pants against a closed shutter, the relationship between box and lung pressures can be established. This relationship holds even when air is flowing in to or out of the lungs (B) and enables us to measure air *pressure* within the lungs simply by measuring box *pressure*.

Clinical skill - performing a PEFR measurement

The subject is provided with a simple flow meter device which records airflow in $L \cdot s^{-1}$ or $L \cdot min^{-1}$. Advise the subject to take a deep breath and then blow into the mouthpiece as quickly and as hard as possible. Tell the subject that they must not put their tongue in front of the mouthpiece. The test is repeated three times, with the 'best of three' recorded. A result of 400–600 $L \cdot min^{-1}$ is regarded as a normal result.

To further assess flow, flow-volume loops can be produced. With the subject breathing through a pneumotachograph (Fig. 4.13), which measures flow and by integrating that flow to provide volume, the loops of inspiratory and expiratory flow–volume relationships can be recorded (Fig. 11.4). These loops are constructed by having the patient breathe from TLC down to RV several times. They are particularly useful in assessing COPD, where the inspiratory part of the loop has a normal shape, although being of reduced volume, while the expiratory part of the loop has a characteristic 'scooped out' shape as flow is restricted by airway collapse.

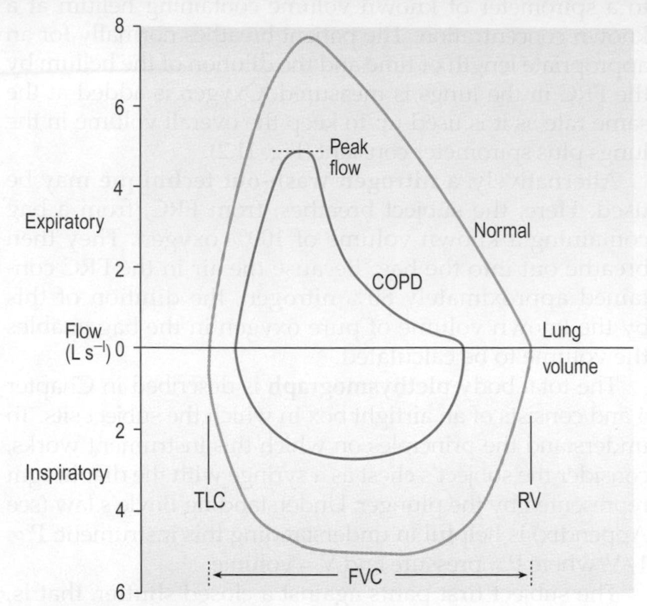

Fig. 11.4 Flow/volume loops. Plotting *flow* against *volume* while a patient takes a maximum inspiration and maximum expiration through a pneumotachograph produces a loop, the shape of which is useful in diagnosis. COPD, chronic obstructive pulmonary disease; FVC, forced vital capacity; TLC, total lung capacity; RV, residual volume.

Measuring lung mechanics

Compliance

Lung compliance can be measured as either **static compliance**, where pressure and volume are measured when no breathing movements are taking place, or dynamic compliance, which is measured during the end-inspiratory or end-expiratory points of cyclical breathing, when no flow is taking place.

The variables required to calculate compliance of the lungs are the volume and the pressure that is producing that volume (intrapleural pressure). Pressure in the oesophagus is a useful surrogate of intrapleural pressure, and the changes in oesophageal pressure provide a good estimate of the changes in intrapleural pressure. Intraoesophageal pressure is measured by introducing a catheter and small air-filled balloon, attached to a pressure transducer, into the oesophagus via the nose. Because intraoesophageal pressure rises as the balloon descends, the pressure reading is conventionally taken when the balloon has been passed 32–35 cm into the oesophagus from the tip of the nose. The subject inhales to TLC in a series of steps, holding their breath for a moment between steps. The volume breathed in at each step is measured, using a spirometer, and the oesophageal pressure at each step is also measured. The subject then breathes out in a series of steps, with the same measurements being made.

Because compliance depends on lung size, the curves are not linear (Fig. 11.5), and there is hysteresis between the inflation and deflation curves, it is conventional to measure volume as a percentage of the predicted TLC and to report compliance on the deflation limb of the curve 1 L above the predicted FRC.

Resistance

The usual way of measuring airway resistance involves using a whole-body plethysmograph, as described above. Alternatively, the variables needed to measure resistance (airflow and the pressure producing that flow) can be obtained using a pneumotachograph (flow) and an oesophageal balloon (pressure), as used to measure compliance. Flow, oesophageal pressure, and lung volume are usually measured so that the contribution made by the elastic recoil of the lungs can be included. This type of measurement is usually called pulmonary resistance and includes the effect of tissue resistance.

Measuring diffusing capacity

The theory behind the method of measuring diffusing capacity (which also may be referred to as transfer factor) is outlined in Chapter 6 ('Measuring diffusing capacity'). Diffusing capacity is measured using carbon monoxide

(CO) under steady-state or single-breath methods, both of which require us to know the partial pressure driving CO from the inhaled air into the blood and the rate of uptake of CO. The diffusing capacity, in clinical practice, is usually presented as the absolute value alongside the percentage of the predicted value for that subject.

Steady-state method

The time to which the lung is exposed to CO is easily calculated; the difficulty is determining the driving partial pressure from alveolar air into the blood. In this method, the subject breathes a gas mixture, containing approximately 0.2% CO, until a steady state of removal is reached. The partial pressure of CO in the alveoli fluctuates throughout the respiratory cycle and so cannot be measured directly. It is calculated by partitioning the concentration in the expired gas into alveolar and dead space (which does not take part in gas transfer) compartments. The size of the dead space component is calculated from the amount of CO_2 in the expired air using the relationship:

$$V_D/V_T = (P_ACO_2 - P_ECO_2) = (P_ACO_2 - P_ICO_2)$$

where V_D and V_T are the physiological dead space and tidal volume, and P_I, P_A, and P_E are the partial pressures of CO_2 in the inspired, alveolar, and expired gas, respectively. This method depends on estimating CO_2 in the alveolar gas and, partly because of the inaccuracies this introduces, has been superseded by the single-breath method.

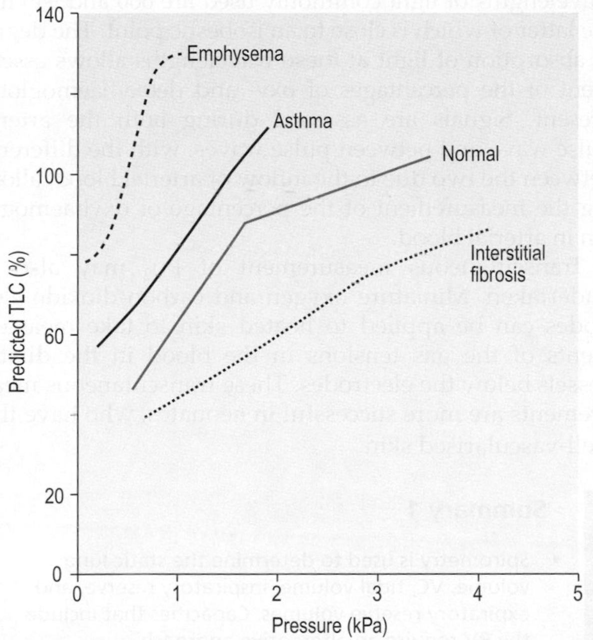

Fig. 11.5 Lung compliance. Compliance is the relationship between *pressure* and volume of the lungs. By measuring intrapleural pressure (as intraoesophageal pressure) and lung volume (as % predicted total lung capacity (TLC)), these characteristic curves are obtained.

Single-breath method

The results obtained using this method are influenced by the volume of the lung taking part and the amount of haemoglobin in the blood (which binds the CO). Diffusing capacity is directly related to lung volume and is greatest at TLC, so it is standard practice to measure the lung volume at which the diffusing capacity was measured by inert gas dilution, often using helium. Diffusing capacity can then be measured as diffusing capacity per litre of alveolar volume, referred to as the diffusion constant, with units of mmol min^{-1} kPa^{-1} L^{-1} (or mL min ^{1} mun Ilg^{-1} L^{-1}) and corrected to a standard blood haemoglobin concentration.

The subject exhales to RV and then inhales a VC breath containing 0.2% of CO and a known percentage (about 10%) of helium. The subject holds their breath for 10 seconds and then breathes out through a gas analyser (Fig. 11.6). The first 750 mL of the expirate is

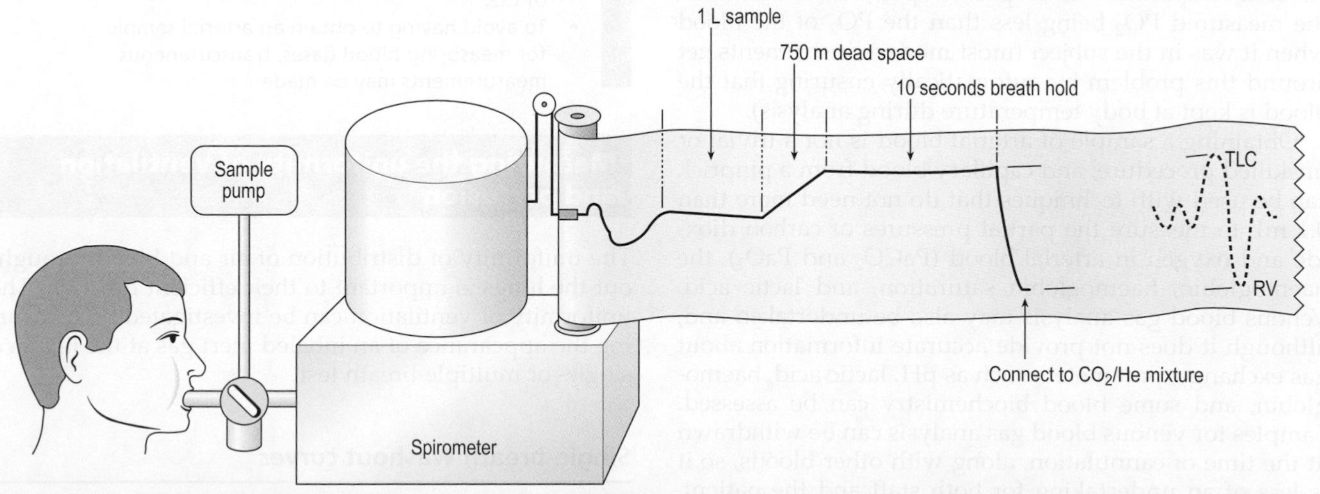

Fig. 11.6 Diffusing capacity. Volume manoeuvres to measure diffusing capacity by the single breath method. The subject breathes out to residual volume and then takes a maximum breath of the carbon dioxide (CO_2)/helium (He) mixture. They hold their breath for 10 seconds and then breathe out past a sample pump. The first 750 mL is rejected to avoid dead space and the next 1 L sampled.

abandoned to clear the dead space and the sample analysed for CO and helium. The dilution of the CO by gas already in the lung is obtained from the fall in helium concentration.

The interpretation of a low diffusing capacity may be difficult because a number of factors, such as uneven ventilation, uneven perfusion, uneven emptying, and diffusion properties, may be involved. This emphasises the fact that lung function tests are more important for quantifying disability than for making a diagnosis. In general, however, diffusing capacity is reduced in emphysema, where the respiratory surface has been lost, but less affected in bronchitis, where there has been little destruction of tissue.

Blood gas analysis

The respiratory system alters arterial blood for the benefit of the tissues it perfuses. Measuring the properties of arterial blood with the subject at rest and, if necessary, during the increased demands of exercise, tells us how effectively the respiratory system performs this function.

During blood gas analysis, PO_2, PCO_2, and pH are measured by bringing the blood into contact with electrodes where the resistance to current or where the accumulation of H^+ is determined by the PO_2, PCO_2, and pH of the blood being tested. By bringing the blood into contact with standard gas mixtures and carrying out a variety of calculations, modern blood gas analysers calculate other variables, such as standard bicarbonate and base excess/deficit.

These instruments have now displaced earlier methods of measuring blood gases and pH, but they still depend on the operator presenting a sample which has been correctly collected. The causes of error in collection are mainly due to contamination of the sample by air, delayed analysis (which results in oxygen being consumed within the stored blood) and, secondarily, the effect of temperature. A drop in temperature can result in the measured PO_2 being less than the PO_2 of the blood when it was in the subject (most modern instruments get around this problem by automatically ensuring that the blood is kept at body temperature during analysis).

Obtaining a sample of arterial blood is not a trivial or unskilled procedure, and capillary blood from a pinprick can be used with techniques that do not need more than 0.1 mL to measure the partial pressures of carbon dioxide and oxygen in arterial blood ($PaCO_2$ and PaO_2), the haemoglobin, haemoglobin saturation, and lactic acid. Venous blood gas analysis may also be undertaken and, although it does not provide accurate information about gas exchange, parameters such as pH, lactic acid, haemoglobin, and some blood biochemistry can be assessed. Samples for venous blood gas analysis can be withdrawn at the time of cannulation, along with other bloods, so it is less of an undertaking for both staff and the patient. A number of non-invasive alternatives have also been developed.

Measuring oxygen levels

Pulse oximetry is a technique used to measure blood oxygen saturation. The underlying principle is that monochromatic light of certain wavelengths is absorbed equally by both oxygenated and deoxygenated blood, whereas at other wavelengths, there is a significant difference in the absorption of light by the two forms of haemoglobin. The wavelengths at which similar absorption takes place are known as isobestic points. Putting this to practical use, light at two different wavelengths is transmitted through an extremity, usually a finger or an earlobe. The two wavelengths of light commonly used are 660 and 940 nm, the latter of which is close to an isobestic point. The degree of absorption of light at these wavelengths allows assessment of the percentages of oxy- and deoxyhaemoglobin present. Signals are assessed during both the arterial pulse wave and between pulse waves, with the difference between the two due to the inflow of arterial blood, allowing the measurement of the percentage of oxyhaemoglobin in arterial blood.

Transcutaneous measurement of Po_2 may also be undertaken. Miniature oxygen and carbon dioxide electrodes can be applied to heated skin to take measurements of the gas tensions in the blood in the dilated vessels below the electrodes. These transcutaneous measurements are more successful in neonates, who have thin well-vascularised skin.

Summary 1

- Spirometry is used to determine the static lung volume, VC, tidal volume, inspiratory reserve, and expiratory reserve volumes. Capacities that include the RV require an alternative approach.
- Estimates of lung mechanics require measurements of pressure, flow, and volume, often made in a plethysmograph.
- Diffusing capacity is measured as the rate of uptake of CO.
- To avoid having to obtain an arterial sample for measuring blood gases, transcutaneous measurements may be made.

Measuring the uniformity of ventilation and perfusion

The uniformity of distribution of air and blood throughout the lungs is important to their efficient function. The uniformity of ventilation can be investigated by measuring the appearance of an inhaled inert gas at the lips in a single- or multiple-breath test.

Single-breath washout curves

In this test, a single breath of 100% oxygen is inspired and the nitrogen concentration is continuously measured at the lips during the following expiration. Better-ventilated regions of the lung will have their RV (which contains air from the breath before the single breath of oxygen) more diluted by oxygen than poorly ventilated regions. In healthy subjects, the residual nitrogen in the expiration starts at zero (dead-space gas, Phase 1; Fig. 11.7).

The nitrogen concentration then increases rapidly after the dead space is cleared (Phase 2) and continues to rise very slightly (Phase 3) to a plateau with a slight slope, due mainly to differences in the ventilation of different regions of the lung. Disease can cause gross abnormalities of regional ventilation which flatten Phase 2 and cause a conspicuous slope of the plateau in Phase 3. In subjects with healthy lungs, there is a slight upturn at the end of the plateau as lung volume approaches RV. This is due to airway closure in the lower lobes causing a disproportionate amount of gas, containing a high percentage of nitrogen, to come from the upper regions. The lung volume at which this starts is the critical **closing volume** (see Chapter 4, 'Emphysema'), which increases in obstructive airway diseases.

Multiple-breath washout curves

In this test, the subject, after breathing room air, is connected to a system of one-way valves which cause inhalation to take place from a reservoir of 100% oxygen and exhalation to be through an nitrogen meter. With each breath, the concentration of nitrogen is seen to fall as the residual nitrogen is washed out of the lungs. This is the same process as repeatedly rinsing a piece of cloth which has been dyed: the colour of the water in each successive rinse becomes lighter and lighter. The concentration of nitrogen falls along an exponential curve. If the log of concentration is plotted against the number of breaths of oxygen taken, the graph is nearly a straight line for healthy subjects, with complete washout of nitrogen in 5–7 minutes (Fig. 11.8).

In subjects with less uniform distribution, as found in disease, the line becomes less steep and more non-linear, and the time for complete washout increases.

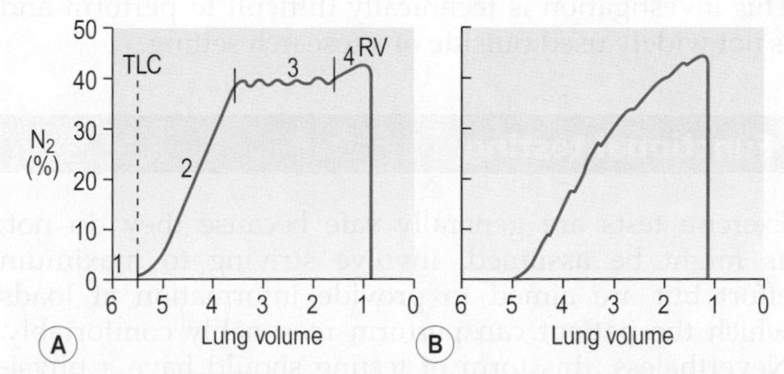

Fig. 11.7 Single-breath washout curves. After taking a breath of 100% oxygen, the subject breathes out past a rapidly responding *nitrogen* (N_2) metre. In healthy subjects, the concentration of *nitrogen* left in the expired air rises rapidly to a plateau (A). In patients with uneven distribution of ventilation the trace is as shown, with no distinct plateau (B).

Inert gas washout

Uneven distribution of blood flow in the lungs is the commonest cause of defective oxygenation of the blood. Unfortunately, uneven perfusion is more difficult to measure than uneven ventilation. Various methods involving the injection of radioactive gases into the blood and measuring their accumulation in the lungs have been developed to measure regional perfusion, but these are research techniques rather than for more widespread use. An important concept in uneven distribution of blood flow is that of the 'virtual shunt'.

This concept deals with the different degrees of uneven distribution as if they were a single 'shunt' of blood from one side of the lungs to the other, without coming into contact with alveolar air (Fig. 11.9). The important point is that a subject with such a shunt will not improve the oxygenation of their arterial blood even if they are given 100% oxygen to breathe. Blood in the shunt cannot be reached by the additional inspired oxygen and continues to create a 'venous admixture' in the arterial blood. Blood in the alveolar capillaries, however, is fully loaded and cannot carry more oxygen. Therefore, because of the flat upper part of the oxygen dissociation curve, the P_AO_2 is considerably depressed, irrespective of whether the subject is breathing air or 100% oxygen. Nomograms were developed in the early 1970s to estimate the 'virtual shunt' that a patient may be suffering from (Fig. 11.10). This 'virtual shunt' is a calculated shunt that is based on the assumption that the arterial/mixed venous oxygen content difference is 50 mL L^{-1}.

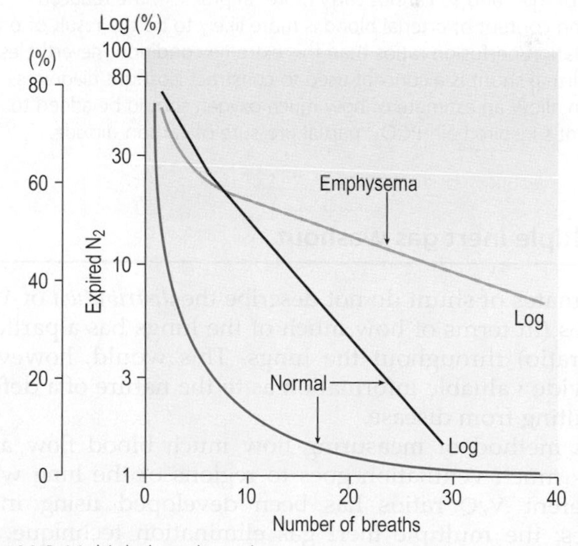

Fig. 11.8 Multiple-breath washout curves. The subject repeatedly inhales from a bag of pure oxygen and exhales past a rapidly responding *nitrogen* (N_2) meter. As the residual *nitrogen* is washed out of the lungs the percentage in each sequential expiration falls, as shown (if the lungs are healthy). If you convert this type of curve to log percent, you get a straight line (which is easier to quantify). The log percent nitrogen plotted against breath number for an emphysematous patient is shown.

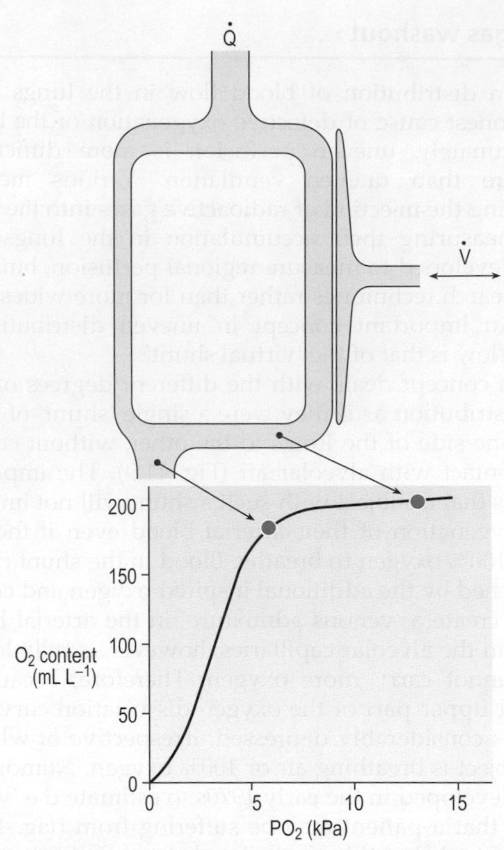

Fig. 11.9 Virtual shunt. If blood 'shunts' past or through the lungs without coming into contact with an effective respiratory zone it constitutes a venous admixture to the arterial blood. Adding *oxygen* (O_2) to the inspired air does not help this situation because this only brings oxygen into contact with blood which is already fully loaded with oxygen and so cannot carry more. In practice, the reduced oxygen content of arterial blood is more likely to be the result of poor ventilation/perfusion ratios than this extreme condition; nevertheless, the virtual shunt is a concept used to construct isoshunt diagrams which allow an estimate of how much oxygen should be added to a patient's inspired air. PCO_2, partial pressure of carbon dioxide.

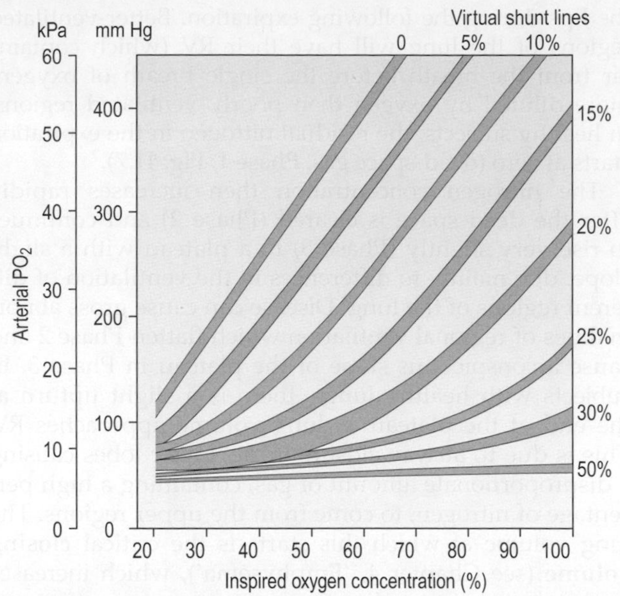

Fig. 11.10 Isoshunt diagram. Using the concept of a *virtual shunt*, based on an assumed arterial/mixed venous blood *oxygen* content difference of 50 mL L^{-1}, it is possible to construct isoshunt diagrams which, assuming the shunt remains the same, relate arterial oxygen partial pressures (PaO_2) to inspired oxygen concentration.

Multiple inert gas washout

Estimates of shunt do not describe the *distribution* of V̇/Q̇ ratios (in terms of how much of the lungs has a particular ratio) throughout the lungs. This would, however, provide valuable information as to the nature of a defect resulting from disease.

A method of measuring how much blood flow and how much ventilation goes to regions of the lung with different V̇/Q̇ ratios has been developed using inert gases: the multiple inert gas elimination technique. In this method, the lung is considered to consist of a number of compartments (usually 50), based upon varying V̇/Q̇ ratios. Each compartment is considered independent of all others. A mixture of several (usually six) inert gases of different solubilities is continuously infused into the blood, and their concentrations are measured or calculated in the expired air and arterial and venous blood. The gases will partition themselves between the alveolar air and the blood of each compartment. The retention (ratio of arterial to venous concentration) and excretion (ratio of expired to venous concentration) of each gas is plotted against the solubility of the gas in question. The retention/solubility plot yields the distribution of blood flow with respect to V̇/Q̇ and, independently, the excretion/solubility plot yields the distribution of ventilation with respect to V̇/Q̇. A plot for a normal subject is shown in Figure 11.11A. Note that the V̇/Q̇ ratios for the lung compartments are on a log scale, which spreads out the low V̇/Q̇ ratios. The distribution of ratios for the patient in Figure 11.11B shows many compartments with low V̇/Q̇ ratios, and 5% of the total blood flow (calculated separately) going to unventilated compartments (shunt). This investigation is technically difficult to perform and is not widely used outside of a research setting.

Functional testing

Exercise tests are generally safe because they do not, as might be assumed, involve striving to maximum effort but are aimed to provide information at loads which the patient can perform reasonably comfortably. Nevertheless, this form of testing should have a physician in attendance as cardiac dysrhythmias are not infrequent. Walking with the patient or asking them to climb stairs are traditional guides to incapacity and the assessment of fitness for surgery but they lack sensitivity and

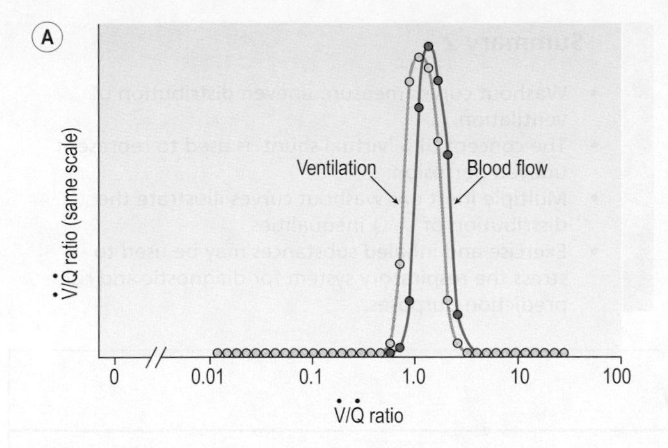

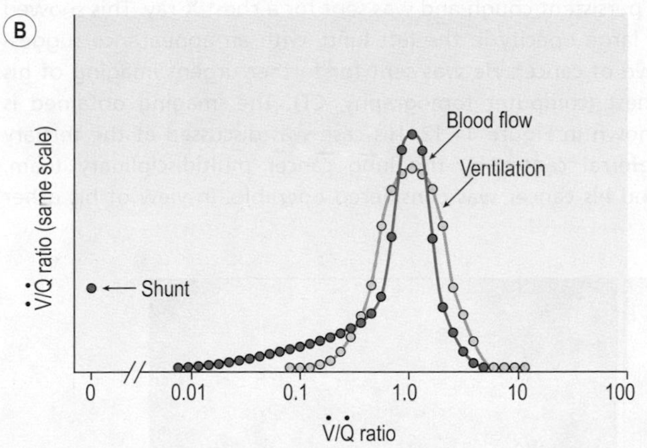

Fig. 11.11 Multiple inert gas washout. The lung is considered for analysis as consisting of 50 compartments which are based upon *ventilation/perfusion* ($\dot{V}/\dot{Q}$) ratios rather than anatomical divisions. A mixture of (usually 6) inert gases, dissolved in saline, is continuously infused into a vein. At equilibrium, the retention or excretion of each gas, when plotted against its solubility, yields the quantitative distribution of perfusion or *ventilation* against the $\dot{V}/\dot{Q}$ ratio for that particular compartment. A plot for a normal subject is shown in A and one for a patient in B. In B, 5% of the total *blood flow* is shunted (i.e. the $\dot{V}/\dot{Q}$ ratio is 0) and many compartments have low $\dot{V}/\dot{Q}$ ratios (A) Normal subject. (B) Patient with $\dot{V}/\dot{Q}$ mismatch.

specificity. More objective tests include the 6-minute walk test (a simple test carried out to determine the distance an individual can walk on a flat surface in six minutes) or the incremental shuttle walk test (a subject walks between cones placed 10 m apart and increases their pace every minute according to an audio prompt). Cardiopulmonary exercise testing is, however, considered the gold standard for assessing cardiopulmonary fitness and function.

Cardiopulmonary exercise testing

Cardiopulmonary exercise testing (CPET) is a dynamic, non-invasive assessment of the cardiopulmonary system at rest and during exercise. Validated indications for performing CPET are to investigate whether a patient who is short of breath has an underlying cardiac or respiratory cause, to monitor the functional status of a patient with known cardiac disease, or to inform the management of perioperative risk in patients being considered for major elective surgery.

CPET is usually conducted on a cycle ergometer, with each test taking approximately 15 minutes. Data are collected from the patient's expired gases using a rapid gas analyser and a pressure differential pneumotachograph, with additional continuous 12-lead electrocardiograms, oxygen saturations, and non-invasive blood pressure monitoring. Measurements are taken at rest, during unloaded cycling, pedalling against a continuously increasing resistance, and during the recovery phase immediately after exercise. By adding the individual's height, weight, age, and gender, computer software is used to predict normal values against which an individual is assessed. Thousands of data points are generated and are represented graphically in a standard format called the nine-panel plot. Examples of data reviewed include the work rate, oxygen uptake, carbon dioxide production, ventilatory measurements (such as ventilatory efficiency for carbon dioxide defined as the minute ventilation per unit CO_2 production, termed $\dot{V}E/\dot{V}CO_2$), and cardiovascular variables (such as heart rate, changes in blood pressure, and ST-segment changes).

Deficiencies in anaerobic threshold (the point at which metabolism switches from aerobic to anaerobic), peak recorded oxygen uptake per minute, and $\dot{V}E/\dot{V}CO_2$ are all associated with increased perioperative morbidity and mortality. Patients with impaired heart valves reach maximum heart rates at lower-than-normal workloads. Patients with airflow obstruction have higher-than-expected minute ventilation for the level of exercise, which reflects wasted ventilation and leads to poor $\dot{V}E/\dot{V}CO_2$. Patients with restrictive lung diseases respond in the same way, except that their increased minute ventilation is made up of a pattern of high frequency and low tidal volume.

Bronchial challenge tests

A bronchial challenge test (also referred to as an airway provocation test) may be used to assist in the diagnosis of asthma. Tests of bronchial responsiveness exploit the fact that asthmatics show abnormally large bronchoconstrictor responses to the inhalation of specific allergens and non-specific chemical and physical stimuli; even the exercise test, described previously, or the inhalation of cold air may trigger an attack. The chemical provocation agents most commonly used are histamine, methacholine, and mannitol, which are administered using a nebuliser or inhaler. Baseline spirometry is performed prior to the administration of the challenge test. The provocation agent is then administered and, after a minute, the spirometry is repeated. The procedure is repeated at intervals using an increased concentration of the provocation agent until the FEV_1 falls by more than 20%. The concentration which produces a 20% fall is then interpolated and this provocation concentration is reported (the PC 20). Clearly, any significant bronchoconstriction must be managed pharmacologically before the subject can be discharged home.

Summary 2

- Washout curves measure uneven distribution of ventilation.
- The concept of a 'virtual shunt' is used to represent uneven perfusion.
- Multiple inert gas washout curves illustrate the distribution of $\dot{V}/\dot{Q}$ inequalities.
- Exercise and inhaled substances may be used to stress the respiratory system for diagnostic and risk prediction purposes.

Case 11.1 Referral and assessment for major surgery

Mr Bennett is 75 and lives with his brother. He enjoys playing bowls and is an active participant in the social aspects of the club. He smokes around 10 cigarettes per day, as he has for the past 60 years. He has a number of other medical problems, including type 2 diabetes and he had a myocardial infarction 12 years ago, after which he underwent coronary artery stenting. He presented to his general practitioner with a persistent cough and was sent for a chest X-ray. This showed a large opacity in the left lung, with an appearance suggestive of cancer. He was sent for further urgent imaging of his chest (computer tomography, CT). The imaging obtained is shown in Figure 11.12. His case was discussed at the tertiary referral centre by the lung cancer multidisciplinary team, and his cancer was considered operable. In view of his other

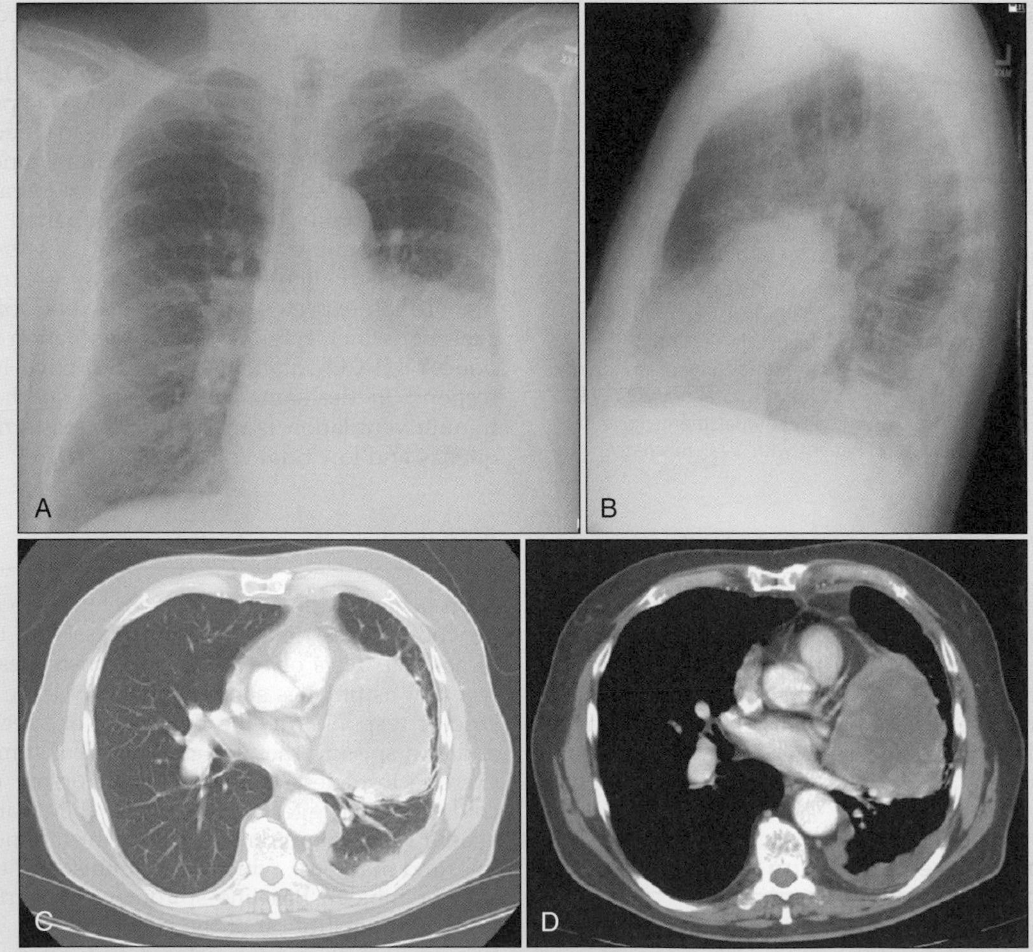

Fig. 11.12 Imaging findings in lung cancer. (A) Posteroanterior and (B) lateral chest radiographs indicating locally advanced disease. (C) and (D) are computed tomography (CT) images. Note that the CT images are interpreted as if looking up from a supine patient's feet (From Niederhuber J. et al. Abeloff's Clinical Oncology. 2020.).

Case 11.1 Referral and assessment for major surgery – cont'd

medical problems, he was referred to preoperative assessment services. This included nurses (specialising in preoperative assessment and enhanced recovery), surgeons, anaesthetists, and because of his age, geriatricians. He was given smoking cessation advice and was referred to smoking cessation services. Much work has been done in recent years in attempting to evaluate a patient's baseline health, predict their risk of perioperative complications when considering major surgery, and investigate approaches to modifying this risk to improve surgical outcomes. This is currently a very active area of research.

A full medical history was taken from Mr Bennett and he was seen by a geriatrician who carried out a holistic assessment. His cardiovascular function and current regime of medications was found to be optimal. Following this, he underwent spirometry and transfer factor testing. His FEV_1 was found to be 75% of that predicted for people of similar age and height and his diffusing capacity for carbon monoxide was 60% of predicted. These results suggest that he would be at moderate to high risk of perioperative complications; therefore, he was referred for CPET.

He was rather apprehensive about getting on an exercise bike as he had not cycled in years, but he managed to complete the test. His results were analysed, and he was found to have a peak recorded oxygen uptake per minute of 14 mL O_2 kg^{-1} min^{-1}, a $\dot{V}E/\dot{V}CO_2$ of 41 and his anaerobic threshold occurred at 10 mL O_2 kg^{-1} min^{-1}. Imaging and calculations were carried out to estimate his predicted postoperative FEV_1 (i.e. his predicted FEV_1 following surgical resection). This was found to be around 50% of that predicted for people of similar age and height. These results suggested that he would be at high risk of developing perioperative complications, including postoperative pulmonary complications (e.g. pneumonia) or cardiovascular complications (e.g. myocardial infarction or stroke). However, his results were sufficiently good to allow him to undergo lung resection surgery, if that decision aligned with his wishes.

After a long and detailed discussion among Mr Bennett, the surgeon, and the anaesthetist about the pros and cons of undergoing this surgery, a decision was reached that lung resection would be undertaken. However, because of Mr Bennett's physical condition, if the required surgery was found to be more extensive, on the day, a full resection of that lung (pneumonectomy) would not be attempted because of the very high risk of postoperative complications.

Mr Bennett underwent his lung resection surgery uneventfully and was managed postoperatively in a high dependency unit. With support and intervention (nicotine replacement patches), he had been able to reduce the number of cigarettes smoked each day and had stopped altogether by the day of surgery. He was advised to take deep breaths regularly and to carry out breathing exercises. He managed to do these, although he found pain a limiting factor to fully engaging in these exercises. On Day 2, he was noted to have lower than expected oxygen saturations (92% on 2 L of oxygen via nasal cannulae), a respiratory rate of 28 per minute, and a temperature of 38°C. A chest X-ray indicated a right lower lobe pneumonia, for which he was commenced on antibiotics, given increased supplemental oxygen (40% via a facemask), and regular chest physiotherapy. After 48 hours, he began to improve and was discharged from the hospital after 10 days. He subsequently underwent a course of chemotherapy to help prevent recurrence. He felt fatigued and not really able to engage in his usual activities for around 9 months following this. However, he slowly improved and made sufficient recovery, with the support of family and cancer services, to return to the activities he enjoys. He remains an ex-smoker.

The decision to proceed with major surgery of any nature must be made after carefully weighing the risks and benefits. In-depth discussion of the procedure and potential risks should be undertaken with the patient, and all decisions should be made by the patient in conjunction with specialist clinicians. Tests and investigations, as discussed in this chapter, play important roles in informing the decisions made.

References and further reading

Chambers, D.J., Wisely, N.A. 2019. Cardiopulmonary exercise testing – a beginners guide to the nine-panel plot. BJA. Educ. 19, 158–164.

Lumb, A., Thomas, C. 2020. Diffusion of respiratory gases. In: Lumb, A.B., Thomas, C.R. (Eds.), Nunn's Applied Respiratory Physiology. Elsevier, London, pp. 111–121.

Niederhuber, J., Armitage, J., Doroshow, J., et al., 2020. Cancer of the Lung. In: Abeloff's Clinical Oncology, sixth edition. Elsevier.

Ntima, N., Lumb., A.B., 2019a. Physiology and conduct of pulmonary function tests. BJA Educ. 19, 198–204.

Ntima, N.O., Lumb, A.B. 2019b. Pulmonary function tests in anaesthetic practice. BJA Educ. 19, 206–211.

Parasuraman, S.K., Schwarz, K., Gollop, N.D. 2015. Healthcare professional's guide to cardiopulmonary exercise testing. Brit. J. Cardiol. 22, 156.

Wanger, J., et al. 2005. Standardisation of the measurement of lung volumes. Eur. Resp. J. 26, 511–522.

BASIC SCIENCE APPENDIX

States of matter

The matter in the world around us can be considered to be made up of particles (*molecules*) which exist in three *states:* solids, liquids, and gases. The respiratory system involves all three.

Solids

The molecules are strongly attached to each other and are very tightly packed. Their movement within the solid is highly constrained. Very few molecules escape from the surface of a solid.

Liquids

The molecules are freer to move within the bulk of the liquid, and the most rapidly moving may escape into the space above the liquid to form a gas which exerts a *vapour pressure.* Molecules in a liquid are, however, quite powerfully attracted to each other and those on the surface of a liquid are attracted into the bulk of the liquid by those underneath. This effect forms a skin, which has *surface tension* (Fig. A1). This is why drops of rain form spheres and drops of liquid on a surface that is not wetted by the liquid do not spread out to form a thin film. Of particular interest to us is the situation when a liquid forms a bubble or lines the tiny bubbles (alveoli) of the lungs (see 'Surface tension and bubbles' below).

Gases

Molecules are free to move throughout the vessel containing them, which they do at considerable speed; molecules of room air move at around 500 m s^{-1}. Because they are so far apart, the attraction between gas molecules is relatively weak. The impact of these molecules on the walls of the vessel containing the gas exerts a pressure, which depends on the temperature (which determines the velocity of the molecules) and the number of molecules present.

An interesting fact is that in a mixture of gases, each of the constituents of the mixture behaves entirely independently of the other gases and exerts its pressure as if the others were not there. This *partial pressure* that a particular gas in a mixture exerts is part of the total pressure exerted by the mixture and is numerically proportional to the amount of the gas present. For example, it is intuitively obvious that in a cylinder containing only oxygen (100% O_2), 100% of the pressure is due to O_2. It is

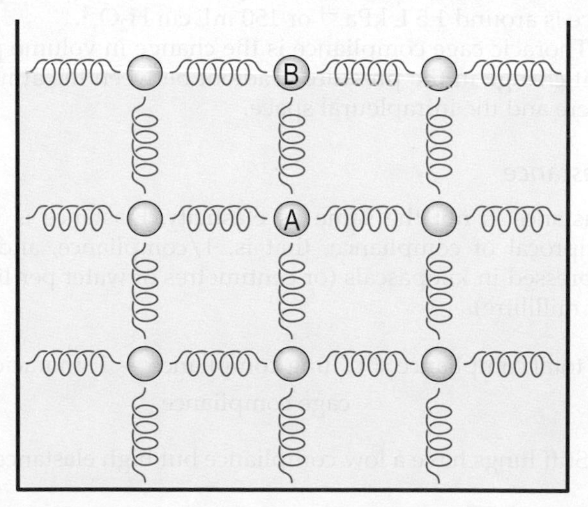

Fig. A1 The origin of surface tension. Molecules attract each other. In a liquid they have freedom to move in any direction within the bulk of the liquid. Molecule A is equally attracted in all directions, so any slight imbalance will cause it to move. Molecule B, on the surface, is attracted only below and to the sides, which keeps it on the surface of the liquid. The forces in the horizontal plane give the surface tension, like a sheet being pulled at all corners.

not so obvious that in a cylinder containing, say 25% O_2, 25% of the total pressure, whatever that may be, is due to O_2 (see 'Dalton's law' later in this appendix).

The molecules of a liquid that escape into the space above the liquid exert a partial pressure. This pressure is proportional to temperature because the higher the temperature, the more molecules have enough energy to escape. However, unlike the partial pressure of gases, this *vapour pressure* is independent of the total pressure over the liquid. This effect is particularly important in terms of the effects of water and volatile anaesthetics. Water at body temperature exerts a partial pressure of 6 kPa. That means that within the lungs, where the air is saturated with water, if the atmospheric pressure is 100 kPa (the value at sea level), there is only

$$100 - 6 = 94 \text{ kPa}$$

remaining to be made up by the other gases of the atmosphere. This is not a problem at sea level, but when ascending to a higher altitude, the temperature inside the lungs stays around the same and so water in the lungs still exerts 6 kPa but the total pressure falls so that the component due to water has a bigger effect (being unaffected by the total pressure). This is particularly important in terms of O_2 supplies to the body.

Compliance, elastance, and elasticity

Compliance

Compliance is defined as a change in volume per unit change in pressure.

For lung compliance, this is the change in lung volume per unit change in the transmural pressure gradient and is usually expressed as litres (or millilitres) per kilopascal (or centimetres of water). Normal lung compliance is around 1.5 L kPa^{-1} or 150 mL cm H_2O^{-1}.

Thoracic cage compliance is the change in volume per unit change in the pressure gradient between the atmosphere and the intrapleural space.

Elastance

Elastance is not the same as elasticity. Elastance is the reciprocal of compliance, that is, 1/compliance, and is expressed in kilopascals (or centimetres of water per litre (or millilitre).

$$1/\text{total compliance} = 1/\text{lung compliance} + 1/\text{thoracic cage compliance}.$$

Stiff lungs have a low compliance but high elastance.

Elasticity

One of the properties of solids, which is important in understanding how the respiratory system works, is *elasticity*. The definition of an elastic material or object is one which returns to its original shape when a distorting force is removed. Perfectly elastic bodies obey Hook's law, that the force (F) applied to a body is directly proportional to its extension (x) (or compression):

$$F = K x \text{ (where K is the stiffness constant)}$$

An important concept is that energy is stored in a distorted elastic body and is released to return it to its original shape.

When we distort a body:

Stress is the force (F) per unit area (a) applied to the body (and has the units N m^{-2}).

Strain is the increase in length per unit length produced by a stress (as increases in both length (e) and unit length (l) have the same dimensions, strain is dimensionless).

Hook's law can be expressed in a different way for a body made of a particular material, where K = a constant (**Young's modulus**):

$$\frac{\text{Stress}}{\text{Strain}} = \frac{F/a}{e/l} = K$$

Be careful not to confuse the terms elastic and elasticity. A material is said to be perfectly elastic if it gives up all the energy put into it by distorting forces to return to its original shape, without sequestering any as heat. A high modulus of *elasticity* on the other hand is frequently a property of materials that, in everyday speech, we do not usually refer to as elastic. Young's Modulus (in N m^{-2}) for steel is 2×10^{11}; for rubber is 2×10^6; and for elastin, a component of connective tissue, is 6×10^5.

The highly elastic nature of steel is clearly seen if a steel ball is dropped on a steel plate. The ball returns to nearly the height from which it was dropped, showing it has given up almost all the kinetic energy which was used to distort it on impact with the plate in returning to its original shape. That is one of the reasons why the balls in the 'Newton's Cradle' executive desk-top toy are made of steel, not putty.

It is the elasticity of the respiratory system that brings about normal quiet expiration by restoring the lungs and chest wall to the end-expiratory position. This elasticity is reduced in fibrosing lung diseases where the lungs are scarred and stiff, making breathing more difficult. In emphysema, the elasticity changes to make the lungs more 'floppy', which causes them to collapse, trapping air in the lungs.

The Gas Laws

Just as the elastic properties of solids can be mathematically defined, the pressure, volume, and temperature of a fixed mass of gas are related, with mathematical precision, by what are known as the Gas Laws. It is these laws by which we measure loss of lung function in disease:

Charles' law. The volume (V) of a mass of gas at constant pressure varies directly with (is proportional to) its absolute temperature, $V \propto T$.

Boyle's law. The pressure (P) of a mass of gas at constant temperature is inversely proportional to its volume (V):

$$P \propto 1/V$$

These two laws can be combined to describe the relationship between pressure, temperature, and volume of a mass of gas under different conditions. This is called *the general gas equation*:

$$P_1 V_1/T_1 = P_2 V_2/T_2$$

where 1 and 2 are the two different conditions being considered.

The general gas equation is invaluable when we wish to take into account what happens to a volume of inhaled cold air when it is warmed in the lungs. This correction is essential when measuring the amount of gas breathed in during lung function tests (see Chapter 11) because the temperature and pressure at which the exhaled gas was measured will vary depending on the temperature of the room and barometric pressure on the day. The temperature of the gas within the lungs, however, will be at a fairly constant body temperature of 32°C. The general gas equation is also used when we wish to calculate what is happening in a plethysmograph (see Chapters 4 and 11).

Dalton's law of partial pressure. Each gas in a mixture of gases exerts the same pressure as it would if it alone occupied the same volume as the mixture. This is another way of saying that gases in a mixture have no effect on one another. An alternative way of expressing the partial pressure (P) of a gas which makes up a percentage of a mixture, which exerts a total pressure (T), is:

$$P = \% \times T$$

If the atmosphere exerts 100 kPa and contains 21% O_2, the partial pressure of O_2 is:

$$100 \text{ kPa} \times 21/100 = 21 \text{ kPa}$$

This law is fundamental to understanding the monitoring of patients in intensive care and those being anaesthetised, as well as in diagnosing many lung diseases. The composition of gases administered to patients and the composition of the gases sampled from patients' lungs are frequently reported in terms of partial pressures.

Graham's law of diffusion. Describing the fact that lighter molecules travel faster than heavier ones, Graham's law states that the rates of diffusion (D) of two gases at the same temperature and pressure are inversely proportional to the square roots of their molecular weights (MW).

$$D_1/D_2 = \sqrt{MW_2}/\sqrt{MW_1}$$

where 1 and 2 refer to the two gases and √ indicates the square root.

Because the molecular weights of the three main gases in the air (O_2, nitrogen, and carbon dioxide (CO_2)) are around 32, 28, and 44 daltons, respectively, their rates of diffusion in the gases in the alveoli of the lungs are similar. This does not mean that the ease with which the respiratory gases are taken up and released by the blood is the same because other factors are involved (see later in the appendix).

Fick's law of diffusion. The rate of diffusion of a substance through a membrane is proportional to the area of the membrane (A), the solubility (S) of the substance in the membrane, and the partial pressure gradient ΔC; it is inversely proportional to the thickness of the membrane (t) and the square root of the substance's MW:

$$\text{Rate of diffusion} = \frac{A \times S\ (\Delta C)}{t\sqrt{MW}}$$

Evolution has resulted in the lung exploiting Fick's law by evolving a thin wall with a large area between air and blood and a system of ventilation and perfusion that ensures a steep concentration gradient. CO_2 is 24 times more soluble in tissue fluid than O_2 and even though it has a greater MW, it will diffuse 20 times more rapidly down the same concentration gradient. This is why, when the respiratory membrane, across which diffusion takes place in the lungs, is reduced or damaged by disease, the uptake of O_2 is usually impeded before the loss of CO_2.

Henry's law. This describes diffusion across a gas–liquid interface. It states that, at equilibrium, the amount of gas dissolved in a given volume of the liquid at a given temperature is proportional to the partial pressure of that gas in the gas phase above the liquid.

The situation under physiological situations is slightly more complicated because, although the amount of a single gas dissolved is always proportional to its partial pressure, obeying Henry's law, different gases have different solubility coefficients and therefore different absolute amounts dissolve at the same partial pressure (more CO_2 than O_2, for example).

Also complicating the situation is the fact that a gas taken up in chemical combination with other substances in the solution is 'locked away' and not involved in the equilibrium. Only that in free solution is considered. For example, O_2 must dissolve in blood plasma before it can reach its carrier in the blood, haemoglobin. The solubility coefficient for O_2 in blood without haemoglobin is very much lower than with haemoglobin. This storage phenomenon alters the amount carried. It does not alter the partial pressures involved and, at equilibrium, the partial pressure of a gas dissolved in a solution is the same as the partial pressure of the gas above the solution.

The flow of gases

The flow of fluids (liquids and gases) takes place from a region of high pressure to a region of low pressure. During this flow, pressure falls because energy is being used up to produce the flow. This use of energy is the result of *viscosity*, which Sir Isaac Newton described as a 'lack of slipperiness' between concentric layers of the fluid. Flow can be generally considered as one of two types, ***laminar*** or ***turbulent***. In laminar flow, the fluid moves parallel with the walls of the conducting tube in organised layers called laminae. The action is something like the closing of an old-fashioned telescope where the tubes slide one within the other. It is also the flow observed in a gently flowing river. The 'lack of slipperiness' means there is a resistance to flow which depends on the rate of flow ($\dot{V}$), the viscosity of the fluid (η), the length of the tube containing the fluid (l), and the radius of the tube (r).

Poiseuille's law states that in a situation where the tube is relatively long and smooth, a pressure difference (ΔP) between its ends will produce a flow:

$$\dot{V} = (\Delta P)\,\pi r^4/8\,\eta l$$

This law strictly applies to straight, circular, rigid tubes of considerable length with smooth walls in which the flow is constant. This does not apply to many tubes in the body, although it makes an approximation of what is happening under many circumstances, such as the flow in the airways of the lungs and in blood vessels. This law is of importance in understanding what happens to asthmatic patients during an attack: the smooth muscle constricts the airways, reduces their radius, and so has a profound effect on the airflow through them.

Laminar flow becomes turbulent in the long, straight, smooth tube mentioned above when the flow exceeds a certain rate. In a perfect tube, it is possible to calculate when this will happen by calculating *Reynolds' number (Re)*:

$$Re = \rho\, vD/\eta$$

where ρ is the density of the fluid, v is the velocity of flow, and D is the diameter of the tube. When Re exceeds 2000, flow is more likely to be turbulent.

Long, straight, round, smooth tubes do not exist in the body and therefore turbulent flow often occurs. In turbulent flow, a significant percentage of the movement of the fluid is not aligned with the axis of the conducting tube; eddies occur with flow moving at all angles, even backward, against the general direction of flow. Turbulent flow is seen in a rushing mountain stream. It is more difficult to propel a turbulent stream of fluid than a laminar one. If all other things are kept the same, to double the laminar flow, the driving pressure must be doubled; to double a turbulent flow, the pressure must be squared. Turbulence is very important in causing particles to be deposited in the nose, which helps to protect the lungs from pollution.

Surface tension and bubbles

The respiratory surfaces of our lungs are moist; they are lined with a film of liquid which exhibits the properties of surface tension. The tubes and surfaces are curved (the major respiratory surfaces, the alveoli, are roughly spherical). This causes them to behave like bubbles. A bubble remains as a sphere because the air pressure inside it is

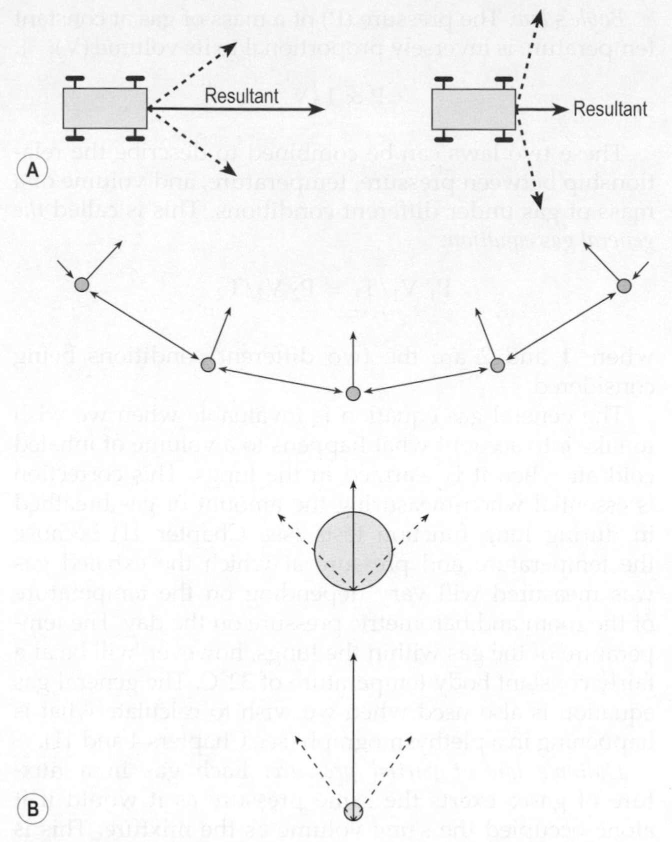

Fig. A2 Pressure in a bubble. If two people are pulling a cart with ropes (A), part of the tension in the ropes is exerted in the direction in which they want the cart to move. This is called the *resultant* of the two tensions or forces. The nearer they are to the required direction, the greater the effect (no-one would attempt to move something by pulling at right angles to the direction you want it to go). The same effect exists in a bubble (B) where the pull between the molecules at its surface would cause the molecules to move in, collapsing the bubble, if not for the excess pressure inside the bubble resisting the movement. You can see there is a bigger *resultant* (pressure) in a smaller bubble.

greater than the pressure outside. This excess pressure resists the tendency of the bubble to collapse due to surface tension. In the case of a bubble, unlike the flat liquid surface considered in Figure A2, the attraction between the molecules is resolved towards the centre of the curvature.

Laplace's law states that the pressure (P) inside a sphere of liquid, with a surface tension (T), is inversely proportional to the radius (R) of the sphere:

$$P = 2T/R$$

The excess pressure (P) inside a bubble is:

$$P = 4T/R$$

because there are two air/liquid surfaces to a bubble.

For a cylinder, like the airways of the lungs, where the surface only curves in one dimension and has only one air liquid surface:

$$P = T/R$$

The relationship between pressure and surface tension has important consequences for the compliance of the lung (see Chapter 3) and is of particular importance in the treatment of premature babies whose lungs tend to collapse because they are not yet making sufficient surfactant to reduce surface tension.

Measuring gas volumes

The air around us is relatively cool and dry compared with the air in our lungs. From the laws listed above, we expect the temperature and/or pressure of a volume of gas we inhale to change when it passes into the conditions inside our lungs. This creates difficulties when we are accurately measuring the size of a breath (it has a different volume before and after you have breathed it in).

It is less important which measuring system is used, as long as it is made clear which is being used. The two most usual systems of expressing volume in respiratory physiology are: **B**ody **T**emperature and **P**ressure, **S**aturated with water vapour (BTPS), which is the condition of air within the lungs or immediately after leaving them, and **St**andard **T**emperature and **P**ressure **D**ry (STPD), which refers to the condition when the gas has all water vapour removed and is measured at 0°C (273 K) and 100 kPa (1 atmosphere, 1 bar, 760 mm Hg). Although expressing the properties of a fixed amount of gas using these two systems would result in very different figures, this difference does not affect the systems described in this book. Therefore it is not mentioned further except to repeat the warning that, when carrying out quantitative measurements, it is essential to specify the conditions under which the measurements are being made.

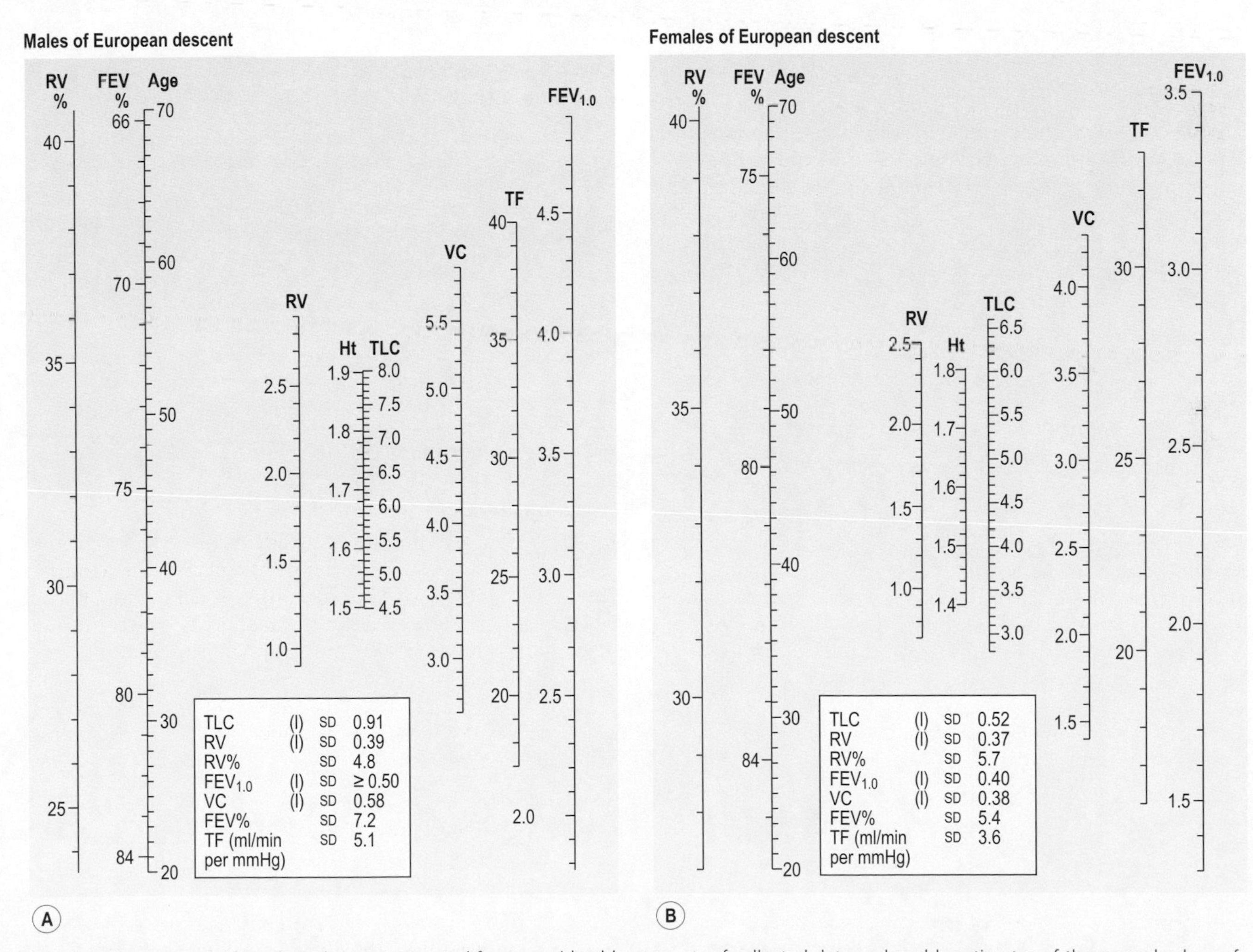

Fig. A3 Normograms. These have been constructed from considerable amounts of collected data and enable estimates of the normal values of lung variables by drawing a line from the age and height of the subject to the scale of the variable required. (A) Normal adult males of Western European descent. The percent residual volume and the percent forced expiratory volume are related only to age; the total lung capacity is related only to height. (B) Normal adult females. The residual volume percent and the forced expiratory volume percent are related only to age. FEV, forced expiratory volume; Ht, height; RV, residual volume; TF, transfer factor; TLC, total lung capacity; VC, vital capacity.

α_1-antitrypsin – any of a group of glycoproteins migrating in the α_1 region on serum protein electrophoresis and capable of inhibiting trypsin and other such proteolytic enzymes.
acetylcholine – an important neurotransmitter. It is produced by the vagus and other parasympathetic nerves.
acidaemia – an abnormally low blood pH (less than pH 7.35).
acidosis – an abnormal process which lowers the arterial pH if there are no compensatory changes in response to it.
adenosine triphosphate – a phosphate donor in biochemical systems. It functions as an energy store and is used up in muscular work, ion pumping, and many other energy-requiring reactions.
adrenaline – a proprietary name for epinephrine.
aerosol – a suspension in the air or other gaseous medium of minute solid and/or liquid particles having a negligible falling velocity.
afferent – leading *towards* a region or structure of interest, for example, afferent nerves transmit sensory information from the peripheries to the spinal cord or brainstem.
airway resistance – the resistance to flow of gas presented by the airways of the lungs. Analogous to the electrical resistance of a wire to the flow of current.
alkalaemia – an abnormally high blood pH (greater than 7.45).
alkalosis – an abnormal process which raises the arterial pH if there are no compensatory changes in response to it.
alpha motor neurons – large, multipolar, lower motor neurons (nerves) from the central nervous system which innervate extrafusal skeletal muscle fibres and initiate their contraction.
alveolar-arterial PO_2 gradient (A-a difference) – measures the difference in oxygen partial pressures in the alveoli and arteries to provide an estimate of the degree of shunt and ventilation–perfusion mismatch. A normal A-a gradient for a young, nonsmoking adult is 5–10 mm Hg.
alveolar dead space – that alveolar region of the lung that is ventilated but not perfused. This is not an absolute state. Alveoli may be relatively underperfused for their ventilation. This type of dead space should be minimal in healthy subjects.
alveolar gas equation – defines the relationship between the alveolar concentration of a gas, its inspired concentration, its output or uptake, and alveolar ventilation.
alveolar gas pressure – refers to the combined partial pressures of all the gases in the alveoli.
alveolar sac – the last generation of air passages in the lungs. They are similar in structure to alveolar ducts, except they are blind ended. Both ducts and sacs bear about half of the total alveoli, each.
alveolar ventilation – the rate of air flow (mL min^{-1}) that the gas exchange areas of the lung encounter during breathing.
alveoli – the blind-ended terminal sacs of the airways where the majority of gas exchange takes place, and where the majority of the lung volume resides.
anatomical dead space – the volume of an inspired breath which does not mix with gas in the alveoli. It is equivalent to the volume of the conducting airways which do not take part in gas exchange and is around 150 mL.
anoxia – lack of oxygen in the circulating blood or in the tissues.
aortic body – peripheral chemoreceptors situated near the aortic arch.
apneustic – prolonged breath-holding at full inspiration.
apnoeic threshold – the arterial carbon dioxide tension below which spontaneous breathing ceases.
aspiration – the act of drawing foreign material into the lungs.
atelectasis – alveolar collapse. Can occur in large areas of lung.
augmented breath – a sigh, a deep breath having an inspiratory duration about one and a half times normal.
baroreceptor – a sense organ responsive to the stretch of large blood vessel walls, signalling blood pressure.
base – a substance that can combine with protons and neutralise acids.
blood–brain barrier – the functional isolation of the cerebrospinal fluid from the blood plasma.
Bohr shift – shift of the oxyhaemoglobin dissociation curve caused by a change in pH (due mainly to carbon dioxide) which facilitates oxygen loading in the lung and unloading at the tissues.
bronchi – airways between the trachea and the alveoli.
bronchial tree – a phrase that draws attention to the similarity of the branching of the conducting airways of the lung to that of a deciduous tree in winter.
bronchiolus – one of the numerous subdivisions of the intrapulmonary secondary bronchi in which the diameter diminishes to 1 mm or less.
bronchoconstriction – narrowing of a bronchus caused by contraction of the bronchial smooth muscle.
bronchopneumonia – inflammation of the lung producing patchy and often widespread consolidation.
buffer – a system that keeps the concentration of some constituent relatively constant, (usually hydrogen ions).
canaliculus – a small groove or channel (plural, canaliculi). A very narrow, fine canal or channel.
carbaminohaemoglobin – the normal complex of haemoglobin with carbon dioxide that transports carbon dioxide in the blood.
carbonic anhydrase – an enzyme found in red blood corpuscles which accelerates the equilibrium of the reaction CO_2+ H_2O= H_2CO_3.
carina – the ridge between the proximal ends of the two principal bronchi.
carotid body – peripheral chemoreceptors situated near bifurcation of the common carotid artery.
cartilage – a relatively non-vascular, specialised connective tissue comprising cartilage cells and young chondrocytes, occupying lacunae in a matrix of amorphous ground substance surrounding a network of collagen fibres.

GLOSSARY

central chemoreceptors – chemosensitive regions of the medulla whose activity promotes breathing. (See peripheral chemoreceptors.)
central pattern generator – neural networks in the pons and medulla, as yet poorly defined anatomically, which generate the basic pattern of breathing.
chloride shift – the movement of chloride ions into or out of red blood corpuscles to compensate for the movement of bicarbonate ions and to maintain electrical neutrality.
closing capacity and volume – as lung volume is reduced towards residual volume, there is a point at which the airways begin to close, this is called the closing capacity. The closing volume is the closing capacity minus the residual volume.
compliance – the ease of stretching of the lungs or chest wall. Reciprocal of elastance. Units 5 L kPa^{-1} or L cm^{-1} H_2O.
conductance – the ease with which a gas or liquid can be made to flow down a tube. Reciprocal of resistance.
conducting airway – those airways involved in the conduction of air to the respiratory regions of the lung. They largely make up the anatomical dead space.
cor pulmonale – right heart failure secondary to a primary respiratory disorder.
countercurrent – two streams flowing in opposite directions in such a way as to maximise the exchange of chemicals or heat.
cranial nerves – 12 paired nerves arising directly from the brain to form part of the peripheral nervous system.
cyanosis – blue/grey/purple colour of the skin caused by the presence of abnormal amounts of deoxygenated haemoglobin.
dead space – the volume of a breath that does not participate in gas exchange. Physiologic or total dead space is the sum of the anatomical and alveolar dead space.
degranulation – the process of shedding granules from the cell cytoplasm to the exterior.
detoxification – the inactivation of the toxic properties of substances in the body by enzymic action.
diaphragm – the dome-shaped, musculofibrous partition between the thoracic and abdominal cavities.
diffusing capacity – the ability (capacity) of the lungs to allow gas to diffuse from the air to the blood and vice versa.
diffusion – the process whereby a substance is transported along a concentration gradient by the random movement of molecules.
double Bohr shift – a Bohr shift (see above) occurring in both foetal and maternal blood caused by the same carbon dioxide produced by the foetus and enhancing its supply of oxygen.
drive to breathe – physiological changes (e.g. increased carbon dioxide or decreased oxygen) which increase ventilation.
dynamic airway collapse – collapse of the airways provoked by the phenomena which bring about flow, thus increasing flow (e.g. a cough provokes more collapse).
dynamic compliance – compliance measured while breathing is taking place.
dyspnoea – the sensation of breathlessness or 'air hunger'.
ectoderm – outer embryonic layer giving rise to the skin and neural tissue.
efferent – leading *away from* a structure or region of interest, for example, efferent nerves carry information from the central nervous system to the peripheral effector organs.
elastance – the reciprocal of compliance.
elastic recoil – the ease with which the lungs rebound after being stretched.
elasticity – the tendency to return to the normal shape when a distorting force is removed.
elastin – an elastic protein.
emphysema – a condition where there is dilatation of the pulmonary alveoli distal to the terminal bronchioles with destruction of their walls.
empyema – an accumulation of pus in the pleural space.
endoderm – the inner layer of the embryo, giving rise to the primitive intestine and the yolk sac.
epiglottis – an unpaired, leaf-like plate of elastic fibrocartilage situated behind the root of the tongue and the hyoid bone, and in front of and overhanging the inlet of the larynx.
equal pressure point – during forced expiration, that point in the airways at which the intraluminal pressure equals the external lung pressure and where collapse is likely to occur.
erythrocyte – an anucleate cell, normally the most common formed element in circulating blood, filled with haemoglobin and shaped as a biconcave disk. Also red cell, red blood cell, red corpuscle, red blood corpuscle.
eupnoea – normal or quiet breathing at rest.
expiratory flow limitation – expiration is brought about by forces that tend to collapse the airways. With age and some diseases, the airways collapse more easily than normal, tending to limit expiratory flow.
expiratory muscle – expiration is passive in quiet breathing. Forceful expiration, as in exercise, enlists muscles which directly or indirectly compress the chest. These include the **rectus abdominus, external intercostals, external obliques, internal obliques,** and **transversalis.**
expiratory reserve volume – that part of the functional residual capacity that can be voluntarily exhaled.
extrafusal muscle fibres – skeletal muscle fibres, innervated by alpha motor neurons, which contract allowing skeletal movement.
forced expiratory volume in 1 second (FEV_1) – the volume of air that a subject can blow out in 1 second making a maximum effort from a maximum inspiration. This lung function test is used to assess airway resistance.
forced vital capacity (FVC) – the largest breath a subject can take making maximal effort.
free radical – a highly reactive radical frequently of oxygen.
functional residual capacity – that volume of air remaining in the respiratory system at the end of quiet expiration, around 2.5 L.
generation – order of airways within the bronchial tree. The most usual convention is to call the trachea generation 0, the main bronchi generation 1, the lobar bronchi generations 2 and 3, the segmental bronchi generation 4, and so on to the alveolar sacs, which are generation 23.

haemoglobin – a complex molecule by which most of the oxygen in the blood is carried.
haemothorax – the presence of blood in the pleural space.
Haldane effect – displacement of the carbon dioxide dissociation curve upwards in deoxygenated blood, enabling blood to carry more carbon dioxide from the tissues.
heat of vaporization – the amount of heat required to change 1 g of the substance in question from the liquid to the gaseous state. The latent heat of vaporization is high in the case of water, which makes the evaporation of water a good way to keep cool.
helium dilution method – a method of measuring residual volume (RV), functional residual capacity (FRC, which is RV+ ERV, expiratory reserve volume) or total lung capacity. The subject breathes out to the volume being evaluated, (e.g. RV or FRC) and then breathes from a bag containing a known volume and concentration of helium. The dilution of the helium enables the volume (e.g. RV or FRC) to be calculated.
Henderson–Hasselbalch equation – equation relating blood pH to blood carbon dioxide and bicarbonate levels.
hilum/hila – small gap/s or hollow/s in an organ where vessels, nerves, and ducts enter or leave.
homeostasis – the relative stability of the internal environment of a normal organism, which is preserved through feedback mechanisms despite the presence of influences capable of causing profound changes.
hypercapnia – an elevated level of carbon dioxide in the blood.
hypocapnia – an abnormally low concentration of carbon dioxide in the blood.
hypotension – abnormally low tension or pressure, especially blood pressure.
hypoventilation – insufficient ventilation of the alveoli of the lungs to maintain normal levels of oxygen and/or carbon dioxide in arterial blood.
hypoxaemia – reduced oxygen concentration in arterial blood.
hypoxia – inadequate oxygen supply in the body or tissues.
hypoxic pulmonary vasoconstriction – reflexive contraction of the pulmonary vascular smooth muscle in response to a low, local, partial pressure of oxygen.
hysteresis – characteristic 'loop'-shaped graph describing the relationship between two variables, where the value of one variable at a given value of the second depends on whether the latter is increasing or decreasing.
immunoglobulin – a family of proteins having antibody activity. There are five classes of immunoglobulins (IgA, IgD, IgE, IgG, IgM).
impaction – the collision of a moving particle with another or a stationary object.
impedance – the mechanical load of the respiratory system in response to ventilation. It can be thought of as the 'hindrance' to ventilation and results from a number of sources, for example, elastic resistance of lung tissue or chest wall, resistance from surface forces at the gas–liquid interface, and frictional resistance to airflow.
in parallel – elements (tubes or components) of a circuit are in parallel when they are connected to each other and the rest of the circuit at both ends.
in series – elements (tubes or components) are in series when they are connected 'one after the other'. Flow is therefore the same in all series elements.
inspiratory reserve volume – the volume which can be additionally inspired after a normal inspiratory breath.
intercostal – between the ribs.
interstitial fluid – the fluid in the interstices or interspaces of a tissue or organ.
intrapleural pressure – the pressure within the pleural cavity.
intrapleuralspace – between the pleura; a potential space which, in health, contains only 10–20 mL of fluid, in total.
irritant receptor – free endings of small myelinated afferent nerves found in the airway walls. They provoke cough, rapid shallow breathing, and augmented breaths, depending on their site and the stimulus they receive (also called rapidly-adapting receptor; deflation receptor).
laminar flow – the condition when fluid moves parallel to the walls of the conducting tube in an organised pattern, as if in layers.
LaPlace relationship – relates excess pressure (P) within a bubble to it radius (R) and the surface tension (T) of the liquid of which it is made. P52T/R.
laryngospasm – reflexive spasm of the laryngeal sphincter, particularly the glottic sphincter, typically initiated by the threat of inhalation of foreign material.
larynx – a tubular organ which extends vertically from the root of the tongue, opposite the hyoid bone, to the trachea and is composed of a framework of cartilage held together by ligaments and membranes.
leukotrienes – a group of icosanoid compounds derived from 5-hydroperoxy-6,8,11,14-icosatetraenoic acid (and ultimately from arachidonic acid) that are mediators of the inflammatory reaction.
loading region – the flat upper portion of the oxyhaemoglobin dissociation curve. This region of the curve represents conditions in the lung where oxygen is loaded into blood.
lower motor neuron – the efferent neuron that connects the central nervous system with a muscle. The lower motor neuron is part of the peripheral nervous system.
lung volumes – internationally agreed names for the volumes that make up breathing and other respiratory manoeuvres. Lung capacities are the sum of two or more lung volumes.
macrophage – a cell found in many tissues in the body which is derived from the blood monocyte and which has an important role in host defence mechanisms. It phagocytises and kills many bacteria.
mechanoreceptor – receptors which are sensitive to mechanical stimulation. In the respiratory system, these include receptors in the chest wall and diaphragm, as well as the slowly and rapidly adapting receptors in the airways which are sensitive to stretch as well as to the mechanical stimulation of the respiratory mucosa.

mediastinum – a median septum or partition between two parts of a cavity or an organ.
medulla oblongata – the caudal portion of the brainstem that extends between the pons and the most rostral part of the cervical spinal cord.
mesoderm – one of the three primary germ layers of the embryo. From this layer are derived the majority of the skeletal system, the lungs, the circulatory system, musculature, the excretory system, and most of the reproductive system.
methaemoglobin reductase – an erythrocyte enzyme that converts methaemoglobin to haemoglobin while oxidising nicotinamide adenine dinucleotide phosphate (NADPH).
minimal air – the small amount of air left in the lungs if they are taken out of the body and allowed to collapse.
minute ventilation (V_E) – the volume breathed out per minute.
mixed venous blood – blood in the/sampled from the pulmonary artery.
motor cortex – posterior part of the frontal lobe of the brain, anterior to the central sulcus, from which impulses for voluntary movement arise.
mucopolysaccharide – a polysaccharide that contains amino sugars or monosaccharides. They occur alone or in combination with proteins.
multiunit smooth muscle – smooth muscle made up of individual fibres not connected by gap junctions.
muscle spindle – a proprioceptor which detects striated muscle length and rate of shortening.
nitrogen wash-out technique – a technique used to measure either the residual volume, functional residual capacity, or total lung capacity. These all contain a fraction that cannot be measured by spirometry (the residual volume).
oxyhaemoglobin dissociation curve – graph with oxygen partial pressures on the x-axis and oxygen saturation on the y-axis; has a classic S, or sigmoidal, shape.
PaO_2 – partial pressure of oxygen in arterial blood.
$PaCO_2$ – partial pressure of carbon dioxide in arterial blood.
parietal pleura – the outer membrane attached to the inner surface of the thoracic cavity.
partial pressure – this is applicable to a gas in a gas mixture. The partial pressure is the pressure the gas would exert if it occupied the volume alone.
peak expiratory flow – the maximum expiratory flow ($L\ s^{-1}$) that a subject can produce.
perfusion – passage of blood through the circulation to an organ or tissue.
peripheral mechanoreceptors – receptors which are sensitive to mechanical stimulation. In the respiratory system, these include receptors in the chest wall and diaphragm and the slowly and rapidly adapting receptors in the airways which are sensitive to stretch and the mechanical stimulation of the respiratory mucosa.
pharynx – the space behind the nose and the mouth leading to the larynx and the oesophagus.
phosphoric acid – an important intracellular buffer. Also, an acid which is excreted by the kidneys as part of maintaining acid/base balance.
phrenic nerve – the nerve which originates from the cervical spinal cord and innervates the diaphragm.
physiological dead space – the volume of gas in the respiratory system which does not equilibrate with blood. It includes the volume of the conducting airways (the anatomical dead space) plus an additional volume relating to alveoli which have better ventilation than perfusion, the alveolar dead space.
pK – this is the pH at which a buffer system has both the buffer salt and the acid half dissociated. This is the ideal state for resisting changes of pH in either direction.
pleural effusion – the presence of fluid in the pleural space.
plethysmograph – an instrument used to measure and record variations in the volume of the lungs.
pneumotachograph – instrument for measuring gas flow.
pneumotaxic centre – respiratory area of the pons whose discharge is thought to cut short inspiration.
pneumothorax – gas entering into the intrapleural space causing the underlying lung to collapse.
pons – area of the brainstem above the medulla.
prostaglandins – regulatory substances derived from arachidonic acid which have a range of actions on nearby organs, for example, prostaglandins released from cells in the immune system can cause bronchoconstriction or bronchodilatation in the respiratory system.
proton – positively charged subatomic particle found in the nucleus of an atom. A term often used synonymously with hydrogen ion, H^+ (when the electron is removed from a hydrogen atom, all that remains is a proton).
pulmonary circulation – the blood vessels carrying deoxygenated blood from the right ventricle to the lungs and oxygenated blood back from the lungs to the left atrium.
pulmonary hypertension – raised blood pressure in the pulmonary arteries: the mean pulmonary artery pressure is greater than 25 mm Hg, at rest, or greater than 30 mm Hg, during exercise.
pulse oximetry – a method of monitoring the oxygenation of the peripheral blood. Light is shone through a peripheral extremity, such as a finger or earlobe, and the pattern of light absorption indicates the degree of haemoglobin saturation.
radial traction – in the respiratory system, radial traction is the outward pull of the lung parenchyma which tends to 'hold open' smaller airways and alveoli.
rapidly adapting nerve ending – a nerve ending whose response to a stimulus decreases quickly with time, even though the stimulus is still present.
rapidly adapting receptor – receptors in the airways which respond to dynamic changes in lung volume or to irritants in the respiratory tract.
recoil pressure – the alveolar pressure minus the intrapleural pressure. Recoil pressure is also sometimes termed distending pressure or transpulmonary pressure.
recruitment – the process in the pulmonary circulation whereby additional blood vessels open up and carry blood when there is an increase in cardiac output.
refractory period – the quiescent period following activation during which tissue, such as nerves and muscles, cannot be fully stimulated again.

Reid Index – the proportion of the total airway thickness that is made up of mucous glands. It is normally less than 40%.
residual volume – the volume of gas that is left in the lungs at the end of maximum expiration, around 1 L.
respiratory airway – airways from which alveoli branch directly.
respiratory exchange ratio – ratio of carbon dioxide output to oxygen input (also called respiratory quotient).
shunt – deoxygenated blood which passes from the right hand (venous) side of the circulation to the left, without becoming oxygenated in the alveoli. By doing so, it reduces the oxygen content of arterial blood.
shunt equation – equation used to calculate the shunt fraction or venous admixture.
shunt fraction – the amount of blood passing through the lungs that does not meet ventilated areas of the lung, expressed as a fraction of total blood flow through the lungs.
sickle cell disease – inherited abnormality of haemoglobin characterised by a change in the shape of red blood corpuscles (sickling) in response to hypoxia. So called because the shape of the deformed blood corpuscles is thought to resemble a sickle.
smooth muscle – involuntary muscle such as that found in the bronchial walls, digestive system, etc.
spirometer – instrument for measuring and recording lung volumes.
standard bicarbonate – the theoretical concentration of bicarbonate in the plasma at a normal carbon dioxide partial pressure, calculated from the pH and the measured (actual) carbon dioxide partial pressure.
sternum – the 'breastbone' situated in the front of the ribcage, in the midline, and to which the costal cartilages attach.
strong acid – in physiological terms, an acid which dissociates almost completely at body pH, making it a poor buffer.
surface tension – surface tension results from greater than normal attraction between molecules on the surface of a liquid. This force tends to cause droplets of liquid to assume a spherical shape and also tends to cause alveoli, which are lined by a thin film of liquid, to collapse.
surfactant – phospholipid secreted by type II alveolar cells which reduces the surface tension of the alveoli and increases lung compliance and stability; dipalmitoyl phosphotidylcholine.
sympathetic nervous system – part of the involuntary nervous system. Fibres from the sympathetic nervous system innervate organs which are not under voluntary control, such as the heart, airways, digestive organs, etc.
systemic circulation – blood vessel system carrying oxygenated blood from the left ventricle to the body and deoxygenated blood from the body back to the right atrium.
tension – blood gas tension refers to the partial pressure of gases in blood.
thalassaemia – inherited group of diseases characterised by reduced production of one or more of the molecules making up haemoglobin. This can lead to severe anaemia in badly affected individuals.
thebesian veins – veins of the myocardium which drain blood into the underlying atrium or ventricle.
tidal volume – that volume of air passing into the respiratory system during each breath.
tidal breathing – inhalation and exhalation of the tidal volume, only (around 500 mL). This is quiet breathing and is also sometimes referred to as 'normal' breathing.
time constant – this term describes the rate at which the functional units of the lungs inflate and deflate. One time constant is the time taken for a lung unit to complete 63% of its maximal inflation.
total cross-sectional area – the sum of the cross-sectional areas of all the airways at a given distance into the lung.
total lung capacity – the sum of the residual volume, the expiratory reserve volume, the tidal volume, and the inspiratory reserve volume, that is, the volume of gas that is in the lungs at maximum inspiration.
trachea – the 'windpipe'; the tube which connects the larynx to the two main bronchi.
transfer factor – in respiratory physiology, the transfer factor for a gas is the rate of movement of the gas across the alveolar membrane divided by the difference in the partial pressures of the gas across that membrane.
transmural pressure – in respiratory physiology, this usually refers to the difference between the alveolar gas pressure and the intrapleural pressure.
turbinates – bony, mucosa-covered projections into the nasal cavity. There are three on each side. Sometimes also called conchae.
turbulent – flow of a fluid through a vessel whereby the particles making up the fluid move in lines that are not parallel.
upper motor neurons – nerves that convey information from the cerebral cortex to the spine.
vagus nerve – parasympathetic nerve which arises from the brainstem and which innervates many of the internal organs, including those of the respiratory system.
vapour pressure – the gas pressure exerted by a vapour.
vasoconstriction – the reduction in diameter of a blood vessel as a result of the action of smooth muscle in its walls.
vasodilation – the increase in diameter of a blood vessel as a result of the relaxation of the smooth muscle in its walls.
venous admixture – the theoretical volume of mixed venous blood that would need to be added to blood leaving the alveoli per unit time in order to produce an oxygen content equal to that actually seen in aortic arterial blood.
ventilation – the volume of air leaving the respiratory system.
ventilation/perfusion ratio – for any given part of the respiratory system, the ratio of gas leaving the region per unit time divided by the blood flow through that region.
vasoactive intestinal polypeptide – A neurotransmitter found in the respiratory system.
visceral pleura – the innermost of the two layers of pleura, that is, the one lying directly over the lung.
vital capacity – the maximum volume of air that can be passed into or out of the respiratory system in one breath.

vocal folds – also called vocal cords. Paired folds of tissue in the larynx which vibrate when air passes between them, producing a sound from which the voice is generated.
volatile acid – acid that is formed by the solution of a gas in water. The most important volatile acid in respiratory physiology is carbonic acid, formed when carbon dioxide dissolves in water.
voluntary control – the ability to control an organ at will. Skeletal muscles are under voluntary control, smooth muscles of the respiratory tract are not.
weak acid – an acid that only partially dissociates in solution.
West zones – physiological concept dividing the lungs into areas dependent on the interplay between alveolar pressure, arterial pressure, and venous pressure.
work of breathing – the energy exerted by the respiratory system on its surroundings per unit time. It is not equal to the total energy used by the respiratory system because not all of that energy is transferred to its surroundings.
Young's modulus – a measure of the ability of a material to withstand changes in length when under lengthwise tension or compression. Also referred to as the **modulus of elasticity.**

Index

Note: Page numbers followed by 'f' indicate figures, 't' indicate tables and 'b' indicate boxes.

A

Abducted, 128
Acidaemia, 112
Acid-base balance, 111–114
  acidaemia, 112
  acidosis, 115
  alkalaemia, 112
  alkalosis, 115
  arterial blood gases, interpretation of, 117b–119b
  bicarbonate as a buffer, 113–114
  blood, 116b–117b
  blood buffering, 112–113
  buffers, 112
  calculation, 115
  clinical measurements, 115–119
  Davenport diagram, 115
  fixed/nonvolatile acids, 112
  Henderson–Hasselbalch equation, 114
  illustration of, 115
  little chemistry, 111–112
  normal plasma hydrogen ion concentration, 112
  phosphates as buffers, 113
  pK of a buffer, 113
  proteins as buffers, 113
  strong acid, 112–113
  volatile acids, 112
  weak acid, 112–113
Acidosis, 115
Acute respiratory distress syndrome, 31
Adducted, 128
Afferent, 122
Age, 31
Airflow
  asthma, 44
  bringing about, 44–45

Airflow *(Continued)*
  factors affecting flow, 45–46, 46f
  impedance, 44
  laminar flow, 45, 45f
  respiratory system, 59b–60b
  turbulent flow, 45, 45f
Air pollution, 23
Airway resistance, 31, 46–48
  sites, 46–48
Airways, 10
  histological structure of, 14–16, 15f
Alkalaemia, 112
Alkalosis, 115
Allergic rhinitis, 12
Alpha motor neurons, 127
Alveolar-arterial PO_2 gradient, 95
Alveolar gas equation, 67
Alveolar membrane, 81
Alveolar ventilation, 66
Alveoli liquid lining, surfactant in, 36–37, 36f–37f
Aminophylline/theophylline, 57
Anatomical/alveolar dead space, 64–65, 64f
Anatomical shunt, 94
Anticholinergic drugs, 57
Aorta, 8b
Aortic bodies, 140
Arterial blood gases, interpretation of, 117b–119b
Asphyxia, 143–145
Asthma, 31, 44, 54–57
  bronchitis, 57
  bronchoconstriction relief, 56–57
    aminophylline/theophylline, 57
    anticholinergic drugs, 57
    corticosteroids, 57
    leukotriene receptor antagonists, 57
  chronic obstructive pulmonary disease (COPD), 57

Asthma *(Continued)*
  diagnosis, 54–55
  emphysema, 57–60
  factors affecting bronchomotor tone, 55–56
    carbon dioxide, 56
    circulating catecholamines, 55
    eosinophils, 56
    mast cell degranulation, 56
    neutrophils, 56
    nonadrenergic noncholinergic systems (NANC), 56
    parasympathetic nerves, 55
    rapidly adapting pulmonary receptors, 56
    slowly adapting pulmonary receptors, 56
    sympathetic nerves, 55
  pathophysiology, 54–55
  principles of treatment of, 56–57
  radial traction, 57–58
  sodium cromoglicate, 57
Atmosphere to alveoli, 67–68
Auscultation, 6b

B

Baroreceptor, 140
Basic science
  bubbles, 162–163
  compliance, 160
  elastance, 160
  elasticity, 160
  flow of gases, 161–162
  gas laws, 160–161
  gas volumes, 163
  states of matter
    gases, 159–160
    liquids, 159, 159f

Basic science (Continued)
solids, 159
surface tension, 162–163
Young's Modulus, 160
Bicarbonate, carbon dioxide in, 109
Biologically active substances, 24
Blood, 83b
buffering, 112–113
capacity, 25
filtration, 24
Blood flow distribution, lungs, 89–92
cor pulmonale, 91
dead space, 90
gravity, 89–90
hypoxic pulmonary vasoconstriction (HPV), 90–91
pulmonary hypertension, 91
pulmonary vessels innervation, 91–92, 91f
regional differences in ventilation, 92, 92f
vasoconstrict, 90
vasodilate, 90
Blood fluidity, 24–25
Blood gas analysis, 152
Blood plasma, 81
Blood transport gases, 102
Bohr equation, 65–66
Breathing
abducted, 128
adduct, 128
afferent, 122
alpha motor neurons, 127
asphyxia, 143–145
central chemoreceptors, 138–140
anatomy, 139, 139f
function, 139–140, 139f
central control of, 123
central pattern generator (CPG), 123
chemical control anaesthesia, 143, 143f
Cheyne–Stokes breathing, 142
apnoeic threshold, 142
chronic obstructive pulmonary disease (COPD), 126f, 126–127, 144b–145b
causes, 144b–145b
clinical features of, 144b–145b
oxygen therapy, 144b–145b
conscious control, 125–126
economy of energy, 122–123
expiratory muscles, 128
extrafusal motor fibres, 127
hypercapnia, 138–139
hypocapnia, 138
hypoxia, 140
larynx, 128
long-term hypoxic stimulation, 142–143
lower motor neurons, 127
mechanics of, 20–21
medullary respiratory centres, 124–125
dorsal respiratory group (DRG), 124
pontine respiratory group (PRG), 125f, 125
ventral respiratory group (VRG), 124–125
minute ventilation, 122, 138
motor unit, 127
muscle-spindle reflexes, 128
musculoskeletal afferents, 133
Breathing (Continued)
cardiovascular afferents, 133
coning, 134b
somatic and visceral reflexes, 133
neuromuscular disorders, 128–130
central nervous system disorders, 128–129
disuse atrophy, 129
Duchenne muscular dystrophy, 129
dyspnoea, 129–130
peripheral nervous system disorders, 129
respiratory centre, afferent inputs to, 130
respiratory muscle disorders, 129
peripheral chemoreceptors, 138, 140–142
anatomy, 140–141
aortic bodies, 140
baroreceptor, 140
carotid bodies, 140
eupnoea, 141
function, 141–142
glomus tissue, 140
histology, 140–141
hypercapnic stimulation, 142
hypoxic stimulation, 141–142
total blood oxygen content, 141
peripheral mechanoreceptors, 126
pulmonary afferents, 130–132
C-fibre receptors (J receptors), 132
rapidly adapting (irritant) receptors (RARs), 131–132
slowly adapting pulmonary stretch receptors (PSRs), 130–131
respiratory muscle innervation, 127–128
upper airway afferents, 132–133
coughing, 133
laryngospasm, 133
larynx, 132–133
nose, 132–133
pharynx, 132–133
sneezing, 132
swallowing, 133
upper motor neurons, 127
Bronchial challenge tests, 155–157
Bronchial circulation, 86, 86f, 94
Bronchitis, 57
Bronchoconstriction relief, 56–57
aminophylline/theophylline, 57
anticholinergic drugs, 57
corticosteroids, 57
leukotriene receptor antagonists, 57
Bronchomotor, 19–20
Bubbles, 162–163
Buffers, 112
Phosphates, 113
pK of, 113
proteins as, 113

C

Carbamino Hb, 106
Carbon dioxide, 56, 83–84
combined with proteins, 109–110
dissociation curve for, 111
transport, 109–111
Carboxyhaemoglobin (HbCO), 108
Cardiopulmonary exercise testing (CPET), 155
Cardiovascular afferents, 133
Carotid bodies, 140
Carriage of gases
acid–base balance, 111–114
acidaemia, 112
acidosis, 115
alkalaemia, 112
alkalosis, 115
arterial blood gases, interpretation of, 117b–119b
bicarbonate as a buffer, 113–114
blood, 116b–117b
blood buffering, 112–113
buffers, 112
calculation, 115
clinical measurements, 115–119
Davenport diagram, 115
fixed/nonvolatile acids, 112
Henderson–Hasselbalch equation, 114
illustration of, 115
little chemistry, 111–112
normal plasma hydrogen ion concentration, 112
phosphates as buffers, 113
pK of a buffer, 113
proteins as buffers, 113
strong acid, 112–113
volatile acids, 112
weak acid, 112–113
bicarbonate, carbon dioxide in, 109
blood transport gases, 102
carbamino Hb, 106
carbon dioxide
combined with proteins, 109–110
dissociation curve for, 111
transport, 109–111
carboxyhaemoglobin (HbCO), 108
cyanosis, 105
dissolved carbon dioxide, 109
double Bohr shift, 107–108
DPG, 106–107
foetal haemoglobin (HbF), 107–108, 108f
gas exchange in the lungs, 110
haemoglobin, 103–107
oxygen combination with, 103–104
haemoglobin variants, 107–109
Hb content, 104–105
Hb saturation, 105
hydrogen ion concentration, 106
methaemoglobin (Met-Hb), 108
myoglobin, 107, 108f
oxygen transport, 102–103
oxyhaemoglobin dissociation curve, 104–106
displacement, 106–107
partial pressure, 104–105
sickle cell disease (HbS), 108–109
temperature, 106
thalassaemia, 109
transported carbon dioxide quantities, 110–111
Central chemoreceptors, 138–140
anatomy, 139, 139f
function, 139–140, 139f

Central nervous system disorders, 128–129
overdose, 128
poliomyelitis, 128–129
spinal cord injury, 129
trauma, 128
Central pattern generator (CPG), 123
C-fibre receptors (J receptors), 132
Chemical control anaesthesia, 143, 143f
Chest inspection, 6b
Cheyne–Stokes breathing, 142
apnoeic threshold, 142
Chronic obstructive pulmonary disease (COPD), 126f, 57, 126–127, 144b–145b
causes, 144b–145b
clinical features of, 144b–145b
oxygen therapy, 144b–145b
Ciliated epithelium, 15
Compliance, 150, 160
Conditioning air, 21
Conductance, 49–50
Coning, 134b
Conscious control, 125–126
Corticosteroids, 57
Coughing, 5, 133
Cyanosis, 6b, 105

D

Davenport diagram, 115
Dead space, 14, 64, 93–94
alveolar gas equation, 67
alveolar ventilation, 66
anatomical/alveolar dead space, 64–65, 64f
atmosphere to alveoli, 67–68
Bohr equation, 65–66
factors affecting, 66–69
Fowler's method, 65
regional differences, 68–69, 69f
respiratory exchange, 66
ventilation regional variation, 69–75
airway smooth muscle tone, 70
pathological changes, 70–75
pneumonia, 73b–74b
pneumothorax, 71b–73b
posture, 70
Diaphragm, 8b, 17–18, 17f–18f
Dichotomous branching, 13–14
Diffusion, 3, 21–22
alveolar membrane, 81
blood plasma, 81
capacity, 150–152
carbon dioxide, 83–84
factors affecting, 78–79
gas exchange, 83b
surface area available for, 79–81
haemoglobin, 81
idiopathic pulmonary fibrosis
clinical features of, 84b
diagnosis, 84b
treatment of, 84b
inadequate diffusion, 82–83
measuring capacity, 81–82
partial pressure, 78
Dissolved carbon dioxide, 109
Disuse atrophy, 129
Double Bohr shift, 107–108
DPG, 106–107
Driving pressure, 88–89
Drugs, 5
Duchenne muscular dystrophy, 129
Dynamic lung compliance, 39, 39f
Dyspnoea, 129–130

E

Economy of energy, 122–123
Elastance, 30, 160
Elasticity, 160
Embryology, 10
Emphysema, 31, 57–60
Empyema, 17
Environment, defences against, 21
Eosinophils, 56
Eupnoea, 141
Expiratory flow limitation, 48–49
Expiratory muscles, 128
Expiratory reserve volume (ERV), 63
Extrafusal motor fibres, 127
Exudates, 17

F

Finger clubbing, 6b
Fixed/nonvolatile acids, 112
Flow of gases, 161–162
Flow-related airway collapse, 48–49
Folds/cords, 12
Forced vital capacity (FVC), 148
Fowler's method, 65
Functional residual capacity (FRC), 50, 148
Functional testing, 154–157
bronchial challenge tests, 155–157
cardiopulmonary exercise testing (CPET), 155

G

Gas exchange, 83b
surface area available for, 79–81
Gas laws, 160–161
Gas transport, 3
Gas volumes, 163
Glomus tissue, 140

H

Haemoglobin, 81
Haemoptysis, 5
Haemothorax, 17
Heart, 8b
Helium dilution, 148–149
Henderson–Hasselbalch equation, 114
Homeostasis, 2
Hypercapnia, 138–139
Hypercapnic stimulation, 142
Hypocapnia, 138
Hypoxia, 140
Hypoxic stimulation, 141–142

I

Idiopathic pulmonary fibrosis
clinical features of, 84b
diagnosis, 84b
treatment of, 84b
Impaction, 21–22
Impedance, 44
Inadequate diffusion, 82–83
Inert gas washout, 153
Inertia, 46
Infective rhinitis, 12
Inhaled particles, 21–23
Inspiratory reserve volume (IRV), 63
Interrupter technique, 52–53
Intrathoracic airways, 13–14

L

Laminar flow, 45, 45f
Laryngospasm, 12, 133
Laryngotracheal bud, 10
Larynx, 12, 46–48, 128, 132–133
Leukotriene receptor antagonists, 57
Liquid lining, 34–35, 35f
Little chemistry, 111–112
Long-term hypoxic stimulation, 142–143
Lower motor neurons, 127
Lung compliance, 30
acute respiratory distress syndrome, 31
age, 31
airway resistance, 31
asthma, 31
disease effects, 31
elastance, 30
emphysema, 31
factors affecting, 30
lung volume, 31
measuring compliance, 38–39
dynamic lung compliance, 39, 39f
static compliance, 39–42
static lung compliance, 38–39, 38f
new-born, respiratory distress syndrome of, 31
physical basis of, 33–38
alveoli liquid lining, surfactant in, 36–37, 36f–37f
liquid lining of, 34–35, 35f
lung tissue elasticity, 34
nature of bubbles, 35–36
opening and closing, 37–38
surface of liquids, 35, 35f
pneumonia, 31
posture, 31
pulmonary blood volume, 31
pulmonary fibrosis, 31
static compliance, 30
thoracic cage, 31–32

Lung compliance *(Continued)*
total compliance, 32–33
intrapleural pressure, 32–33, 32f
vital capacity, 31
Lung function tests
blood gas analysis, 152
diffusing capacity, 150–152
functional testing, 154–157
bronchial challenge tests, 155–157
cardiopulmonary exercise testing (CPET), 155
inert gas washout, 153
lung mechanics
compliance, 150
resistance, 150
static compliance, 150
major surgery, referral and assessment for, 156b–157b
measuring flow, 149
peak expiratory flow, 149
multiple-breath washout curves, 153–154
multiple inert gas washout, 154, 154f
oxygen levels, measuring, 152
PEFR measurement, clinical skill–performing, 150
perfusion, 152–153
single-breath method, 151–152
single-breath washout curves, 152–153
steady-state method, 151
ventilation, 152–153
volumes and capacities
forced vital capacity (FVC), 148
functional residual capacity (FRC), 148
helium dilution, 148–149
nitrogen washout, 148–149
nitrogen wash-out technique, 149
plethysmograph, 149
plethysmography, 148–149
spirometry, 148
Lungs, 8b
mechanics
compliance, 150
resistance, 150
static compliance, 150
non-respiratory functions of, 24–25
blood capacity, 25
blood filtration, 24
blood fluidity, 24–25
cooling, 25
structure of, 25b
voluntary control of breathing, 25
tissue elasticity, 34
volume, 31
volumes, 62–63
Lymphatics, 19

M

Massive pulmonary embolism, 96b–98b
Mast cell degranulation, 56
Medullary respiratory centres, 124–125
dorsal respiratory group (DRG), 124
pontine respiratory group (PRG), 125f, 125
ventral respiratory group (VRG), 124–125
Metabolic activity, 23–24
Microcirculation, 18–19
Minute ventilation, 62, 122, 138
Mixed venous blood, 88
Motor unit, 127
Mouth and nose, 11–12, 11f
Multiple-breath washout curves, 153–154
Multiple inert gas washout, 154, 154f
Muscle-spindle reflexes, 128
Musculoskeletal afferents, 133
cardiovascular afferents, 133
coning, 134b
somatic and visceral reflexes, 133

N

Nature of bubbles, 35–36
Nerves, 19–20
bronchomotor, 19–20
parasympathetic nerves, 19–20
sympathetic nerves, 19
visceral afferents, 19–20
Neuromuscular disorders, 128–130
central nervous system disorders, 128–129
disuse atrophy, 129
Duchenne muscular dystrophy, 129
dyspnoea, 129–130
peripheral nervous system disorders, 129
respiratory centre, afferent inputs to, 130
respiratory muscle disorders, 129
Neutrophils, 56
New-born, respiratory distress syndrome of, 31
Nitrogen washout, 148–149
Nonadrenergic noncholinergic systems (NANC), 56
Normal plasma hydrogen ion concentration, 112
Nose, 46–48, 132–133

O

Ohm's law, 46
Oxygen
carbon dioxide diagram, 93–94
levels, measuring, 152
therapy, 144b–145b

P

Parasympathetic nerves, 19–20, 55
Parenchyma, 16–17
Partial pressure, 78
Pathophysiology, 54–55
Peak expiratory flow, 149
PEFR measurement, clinical skill–performing, 150
Percussion, 6b
Perfusion, 86, 89–92, 152–153
Peripheral chemoreceptors, 138, 140–142
anatomy, 140–141
aortic bodies, 140
baroreceptor, 140
carotid bodies, 140
eupnoea, 141
function, 141–142
glomus tissue, 140
histology, 140–141
hypercapnic stimulation, 142
hypoxic stimulation, 141–142
total blood oxygen content, 141
Peripheral mechanoreceptors, 126
Peripheral nervous system disorders, 129
botulism, 129
diphtheria, 129
Guillain-Barré, 129
myasthenia gravis, 129
Pharynx, 46–48, 132–133
Plethysmograph, 149
Plethysmography, 148–149
Pleura, 16–17
Pleural effusion, 17
Pleurodesis, 17
Pneumonia, 31, 73b–74b
Pneumothorax, 17, 71b–73b
Poliomyelitis, 128–129
Pores of Kohn, 14
Posture, 31, 70
Pressure, 52
Pulmonary afferents
C-fibre receptors (J receptors), 132
rapidly adapting (irritant) receptors (RARs), 131–132
slowly adapting pulmonary stretch receptors (PSRs), 130–131
Pulmonary blood vessels, 87–89, 88f
Pulmonary blood volume, 31
Pulmonary circulation
alveolar-arterial PO_2 gradient, 95
anatomical shunt, 94
blood flow distribution, lungs, 89–92
alveolar gas pressure, 90
cor pulmonale, 91
dead space, 90
gravity, 89–90
hypoxic pulmonary vasoconstriction (HPV), 90–91
pulmonary hypertension, 91
pulmonary vessels innervation, 91–92, 91f
regional differences in ventilation, 92, 92f
vasoconstrict, 90
vasodilate, 90
bronchial circulation, 86, 86f, 94
dead space, 93–94
function, 86–89
gross structure, 87–89
driving pressure, 88–89
mixed venous blood, 88
pulmonary blood vessels, 87–89, 88f
recruitment, 88
right ventricle, 87, 88f
massive pulmonary embolism, 96b–98b

Pulmonary circulation *(Continued)*
oxygen-carbon dioxide diagram, 93–94
perfusion, 86, 89–92
pulmonary emboli, 96b–98b
pulmonary embolus, 96b–98b
respiratory exchange ratio (R), 93
salutary tale, 95–99
shunt, 94–95
equation, 95
structure, 86–89
systemic circulation, 86
tensions, 93
thebesian veins, 94
venous admixture, 95
ventilation, 86, 89–92
Pulmonary emboli, 96b–98b
Pulmonary fibrosis, 31
Pulmonary hypertension, 19
Pulmonary vasculature, 18–19
Pulmonary ventilation
capacities, 62–63
dead space. *See* Dead space
expiratory reserve volume (ERV), 63
inspiratory reserve volume (IRV), 63
lung volumes, 62–63
minute ventilation, 62
spirometric abnormalities in disease, 63–75, 63f
spirometry, 62–63
total lung capacity (TLC), 63
vital capacity (VC), 63
Pulmonary vessels, 8b

R

Radial traction, 57–58
Rapidly adapting pulmonary receptors, 56
Rapidly adapting (irritant) receptors (RARs), 131–132
Recruitment, 88
Regional differences, 68–69, 69f
Resistance, 150
Respiration
aorta, 8b
basic science of, 3–4, 4f
bones, 8b
breathlessness, 5
centimetre, gram, second (CGS) system, 4–5
chest pain, 5
chest x- ray, clinical skill interpreting, 7b, 7f–8f
clinical skill examination, 6b
auscultation, 6b
chest inspection, 6b
cyanosis, 6b
finger clubbing, 6b
percussion, 6b
trachea, 6b
cough, 5
definition, 2
diaphragm, 8b
diffusion, 3
drugs, 5
Respiration *(Continued)*
gas transport, 3
haemoptysis, 5
heart, 8b
homeostasis, 2
lungs, 8b
need for, 2–3
pulmonary vessels, 8b
respiratory symbols, 4
sputum, 5
stridor, 5
symbols, 5t
symptoms of, 5
Système International (SI), 4
timing in circulation, 3, 3f
trachea, 8b
ventilation, 2
wheezing, 5
Respiratory centre, afferent inputs to, 130
Respiratory exchange, 66
Respiratory exchange ratio (R), 93
Respiratory muscle
disorders, 129
innervation, 127–128
Respiratory symbols, 4
Respiratory system, 59b–60b
air pollution, 23
airways, 10
histological structure of, 14–16, 15f
allergic rhinitis, 12
biologically active substances, 24
breathing, mechanics of, 20–21
ciliated epithelium, 15
conditioning air, 21
dead space, 14
diaphragm, 17–18, 17f–18f
dichotomous branching, 13–14
diffusion, 21–22
embryology, 10
empyema, 17
environment, defences against, 21
exudates, 17
folds/cords, 12
haemothorax, 17
impaction, 21–22
infective rhinitis, 12
inhaled particles, 21–23
intrathoracic airways, 13–14
laryngospasm, 12
laryngotracheal bud, 10
larynx, 12
lung, non-respiratory functions of, 24–25
blood capacity, 25
blood filtration, 24
blood fluidity, 24–25
cooling, 25
structure of, 25b
voluntary control of breathing, 25
lymphatics, 19
metabolic activity, 23–24
metabolism, 24
microcirculation, 18–19
mouth and nose, 11–12, 11f
nerves, 19–20
bronchomotor, 19–20
Respiratory system *(Continued)*
parasympathetic nerves, 19–20
sympathetic nerves, 19
visceral afferents, 19–20
parenchyma, 16–17
pleura, 16–17
pleural effusion, 17
pleurodesis, 17
pneumothorax, 17
pores of Kohn, 14
production of, 24
pulmonary hypertension, 19
pulmonary vasculature, 18–19
sedimentation, 21–22
smoking, 23
smooth muscle, 15
structure of, 26b
surfactants, 16
trachea, 13
trachealis muscle, 13
transudates, 17
turbinates, 11
vasomotor rhinitis, 12
Respiratory system, elastic properties of
compliance, 30–42
elastance, 30–42
elastic resistance, 30
intrapleural space, 30
lung compliance. *See* Lung compliance
new-born
respiratory distress syndrome in, 40b–41b
surface forces, 30
Respiratory system resistance, 46–50
airway resistance, 46–48
airway resistance sites, 46–48
assessing and measuring resistance, 52–54
interrupter technique, 52–53
pressure, 52
whole-body plethysmography, 53–54, 53f
clinical tests for changes, 54, 54f
conductance, 49–50
expiratory flow limitation, 48–49
flow-related airway collapse, 48–49
functional residual capacity (FRC), 50
inertia, 46
larynx, 46–48
nose, 46–48
Ohm's law, 46
pharynx, 46–48
tidal breathing, 49–50
tissue resistance, 46
transmural, 48–49
volume-related airway collapse, 49–50
work of breathing, 50–51
Right ventricle, 87, 88f

S

Salutary tale, 95–99
Sedimentation, 21–22

Shunt, 94–95
  equation, 95
Single-breath method, 151–152
Single-breath washout curves, 152–153
Slowly adapting pulmonary receptors, 56
Slowly adapting pulmonary stretch receptors (PSRs), 130–131
Smoking, 23
Smooth muscle, 15
Sneezing, 132
Sodium cromoglicate, 57
Somatic and visceral reflexes, 133
Spinal cord injury, 129
Spirometric abnormalities in disease, 63–75, 63f
Spirometry, 62–63, 148
Sputum, 5
States of matter
  gases, 159–160
  liquids, 159, 159f
  solids, 159
Static compliance, 30, 39–42, 150
Static lung compliance, 38–39, 38f
Steady-state method, 151
Stridor, 5
Strong acid, 112–113
Surface of liquids, 35, 35f
Surface tension, 162–163
Surfactants, 16
Swallowing, 133
Sympathetic nerves, 19, 55
Système International (SI), 4
Systemic circulation, 86

T

Tensions, 93
Thalassaemia, 109
Thebesian veins, 94
Thoracic cage, 31–32
Tidal breathing, 49–50
Timing in circulation, 3, 3f
Total blood oxygen content, 141
Total compliance, 32–33
  intrapleural pressure, 32–33, 32f
Total lung capacity (TLC), 63
Trachea, 6b, 6b, 13
Trachealis muscle, 13
Transported carbon dioxide quantities, 110–111
Transudates, 17
Trauma, 128
Turbinates, 11
Turbulent flow, 45, 45f

U

Upper airway afferents, 132–133
  coughing, 133
  laryngospasm, 133
  larynx, 132–133
  nose, 132–133
  pharynx, 132–133
  sneezing, 132
  swallowing, 133
Upper motor neurons, 127

V

Vasomotor rhinitis, 12
Venous admixture, 95
Ventilation, 2, 86, 89–92, 152–153
Ventilation regional variation, 69–75
  airway smooth muscle tone, 70
  pathological changes, 70–75
  pneumonia, 73b–74b
  pneumothorax, 71b–73b
  posture, 70
Visceral afferents, 19–20
Vital capacity (VC), 31, 63
Volatile acids, 112

W

Weak acid, 112–113
Wheezing, 5
Whole-body plethysmography, 53–54, 53f

Y

Young's Modulus, 160